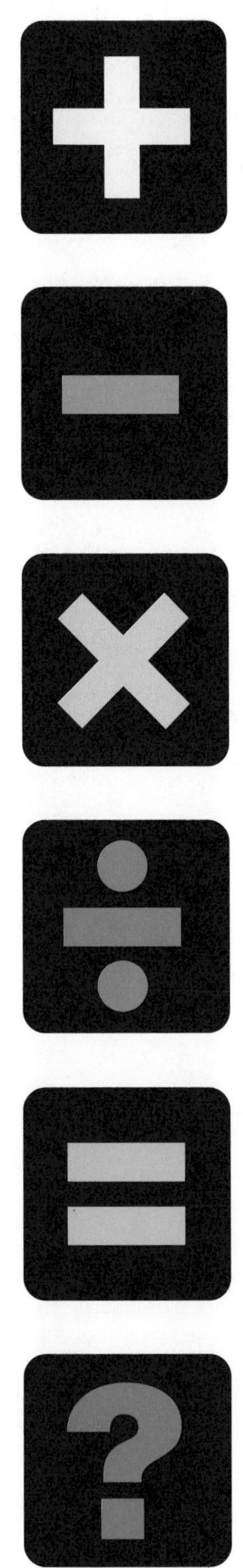

MATH FOR NURSES

A Problem Solving Approach

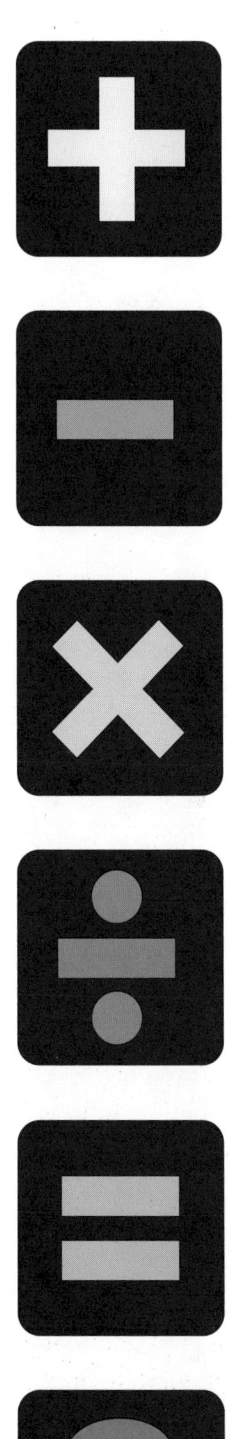

MATH FOR NURSES

SALLY IRENE LIPSEY, MA, EdD
Associate Professor of Mathematics (Retired)
Brooklyn College
Brooklyn, New York

DONNA D. IGNATAVICIUS, MS, RN, C
Instructor
MacQueen Gibbs Willis School of Nursing
Easton, Maryland
Consultant in Gerontological Nursing
Easton, Maryland

W.B. SAUNDERS COMPANY
A Division of Harcourt Brace & Company
Philadelphia London Toronto Montreal Sydney Tokyo

A Problem Solving Approach

W.B. Saunders Company
A Division of Harcourt Brace & Company
The Curtis Center
Independence Square West
Philadelphia, Pennsylvania 19106

Library of Congress Cataloging-in-Publication Data

Lipsey, Sally I. (Sally Irene)
Math for nurses: a problem solving approach/Sally I. Lipsey, Donna D. Ignatavicius.
p. cm.
Includes bibliographical references and index.
ISBN 0-7216-6481-4
1. Nursing—Mathematics. 2. Pharmaceutical arithmetic.
I. Ignatavicius, Donna D. II. Title.
RT68.L559 1994
610.73'01'51—dc20 93-19188

Math for Nurses: A Problem Solving Approach ISBN 0-7216-6481-4

Printed in the United States of America.

Last digit is the print number: 9 8 7 6 5 4 3 2 1

Dedicated
to Florence Nightingale (1820–1910)
who loved mathematics and statistics
almost as much as nursing

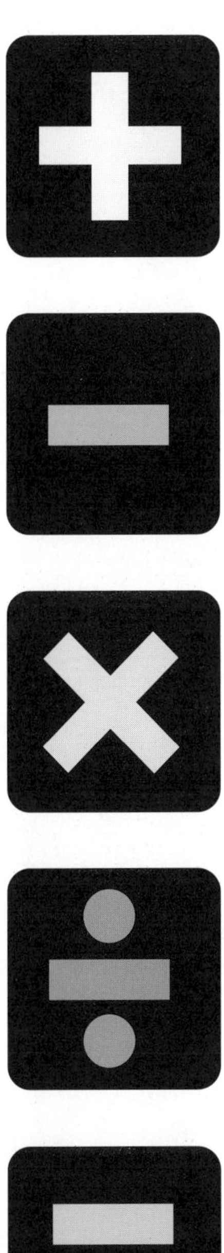

In 1840, Florence Nightingale begged her parents "to let her study mathematics instead of doing worsted work and practising quadrilles."* At first her parents refused (math was not considered a suitable subject for a young woman), but eventually they granted permission. Years later, her mathematical approach saved the British army at Scutari during the Crimean War (1854–1856) and provided the data that led to hospital reforms.†

She helped promote what was then a revolutionary idea (and a religious idea for her): "that social phenomena could be objectively measured and subjected to mathematical analysis."‡ Her work with medical statistics was so impressive that she was elected (in 1858) to membership in the Statistical Society of England.§ Her Model Hospital Statistical Form (developed with colleagues) was approved at the International Congress of Statistics in 1860.|| One of the pioneers in the graphic method of statistical presentation, she invented colorful polar-area diagrams to dramatize medical data.¶ Although other methods of persuasion had failed, Florence Nightingale's mathematical approach persuaded military authorities, Parliament, and Queen Victoria to carry out her proposed hospital reforms.

* Woodham-Smith CB: *Florence Nightingale.* New York: Atheneum, 1983:26.
† Pickering G: *Creative Malady.* New York: Oxford University Press, 1974:100.
‡ Cohen IB: Florence Nightingale. *Sci Am* 1984; 250(3):128.
§ Seymer, L: "Florence Nightingale." New York: Macmillan, 1950, p. 115.
|| Cohen, IB: *op. cit.,* p. 136.
¶ *Ibid.,* p. 129.

PREFACE

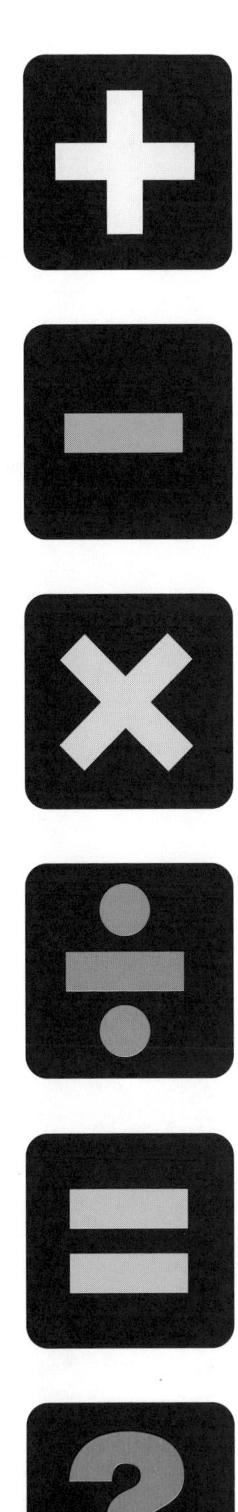

The nursing profession is undergoing profound changes. Rewards and challenges are greater than ever. Today's nurse faces many technological advances not only at the hospital but also in the home, the nursing home, the private clinic, or wherever a career may lead. She or he, equipped to handle more responsibility than ever before, will also need to be more adaptable than ever before.

In response to the needs of today's nurse, MATH FOR NURSES: A PROBLEM SOLVING APPROACH is devoted to efficient learning and timely content. Emphasis is on unifying principles for depth of understanding, mastery of skills, and flexibility with present and future (as yet unknown) applications. Shortcuts (based on principles) are presented after a strong foundation is established. Chapters and their subdivisions are arranged to ensure adequate preparation for each new concept.

Each chapter furnishes concrete examples, from simple to complex, with attention to the types of problems that are most relevant to today's nurse. Pictures of actual labels, syringes, and measuring devices accompany examples and exercises. Sometimes these pictures are enlarged to make the details visible. There are many exercises for each topic, providing a concomitant choice for a variety of students with different levels of preparation.

Students with strong preparation may move quickly through the mathematical foundation, using pre- and post-tests as guides. Others will find the step-by-step approach a means of avoiding troublesome gaps in knowledge. Pictures of actual labels, syringes, and measuring devices accompany examples and exercises. Sometimes these pictures are enlarged to make the details visible. Pedagogical devices include concrete suggestions for avoiding errors and a special, fail-safe way of using the ratio and proportion method, which parallels the nursing process. This method also serves as a basis for other popular methods (such as formulas and dimensional analysis) and for the nursing process.

Both a tool for learning and a handbook for reference, the text provides a simple but strong math foundation for the calculations to be needed. Chapters 1–3 provide the essential mathematical groundwork and some elementary applications of interest to nurses. Chapters 4 and 5 cover the prevailing systems of measurement with special emphasis on the international system.

Applications to dosage calculations appear in a great variety of settings. Dosage calculations are first formally introduced in Chapters 6 and 7 and continue in connection with individualized drug therapy in Chapter 8, intravenous therapy in Chapter 9, and documentation in Chapter 10. The material covered in Chapter 10 provides a good basis and an easy transition to a typical discussion of documentation in a text on Fundamentals of Nursing, and a quick and easy reference for the student as well as the staff nurse.

The book ends with a number of Appendices and a set of Selected References. For the many students who are nervous about or dislike math, the appendix on math anxiety includes suggestions for building self-confidence and achieving mastery. There is also an appendix on the computer, including a discussion of how different systems are used in health care, and suggestions for computer explorations. Other appendices provide lists of commonly used measurements, conversions, and abbreviations.

We are always happy to hear from readers. To ensure a response, please enclose a stamped, self-addressed envelope and send it with your comments or questions to the address listed below:

Sally I. Lipsey and/or Donna Ignatavicius
P.O. Box 207
Lake Peekskill, NY 10537

ACKNOWLEDGMENTS

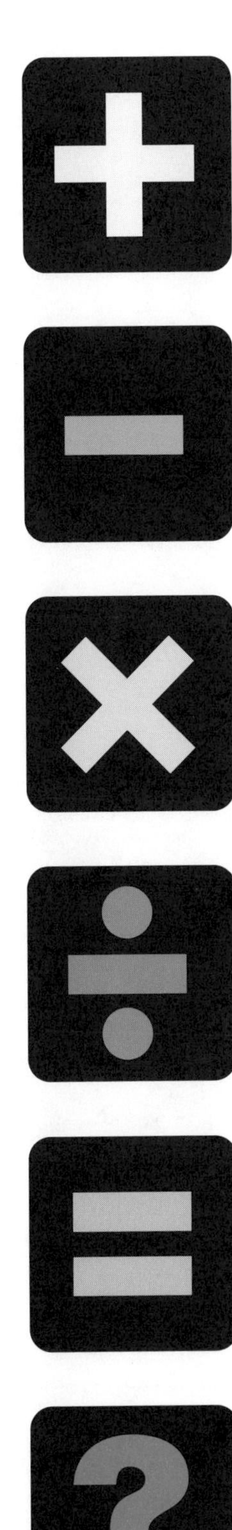

For many valuable comments and suggestions, we are grateful to our colleagues in mathematics and nursing at the following institutions: City University of New York (Bronx Community College, Brooklyn College, and Borough of Manhattan Community College); Altoona Hospital School of Nursing in Altoona, Pennsylvania; and MGW School of Nursing in Easton, Maryland. The methods that we have used are the result of years of experience with various techniques in classes of nursing students and in remedial classes in mathematics.

We thank the following reviewers for their conscientious attention to detail and their many excellent comments and suggestions: EMA, KBA, MDD, ABP, DUG, SBM, LWM, and PLV.

We appreciate the cooperation of the nurses at William Hill Manor in Easton, Maryland, and the following companies, who provided materials and granted permission to reproduce labels, syringes, and other items: Abbott Pharmaceutical Products (Abbott Laboratories), A. H. Robins (Wyeth-Ayerst Laboratories), Apex Medical, Astra Pharmaceutical Products, Becton Dickinson, Berlex Laboratories, Biocraft Laboratories, Boots Pharmaceuticals, Bristol-Myers Squibb, Burroughs Wellcome, Educational Teaching Aids, Ever Ready Thermometer, The First Years, Forest Laboratories, Glaxo, Key Pharmaceuticals (Schering-Plough), Eli Lilly, Marion Merrill Dow, Parke Davis, Sandoz, Schering, Smith Kline Beecham, Terumo Medical, and Vangard Laboratories.

To our colleagues at W.B. Saunders Company, many thanks for all their excellent help. Daniel T. Ruth, the editor of Nursing Books, introduced us and guided us all along the way; Danni Morinich, a very patient editorial assistant, smoothed the office processes greatly. Rachel Bedard, developmental editor, deserves special credit for her photographic skills. We appreciate the careful work of Linda Davoli, William Donnelly, Peter Faber, Alison Kieber, Ellen Bodner-Zanolle, Lynn Mahan, and Anne Ostroff in the production of the text.

Our families have been a great source of support and encouragement. In addition, Dr. Carol Lipsey Hersh and Dr. William Hersh were generous with scientific help. Dr. Robert Lipsey contributed his photographic talents.

CONTENTS

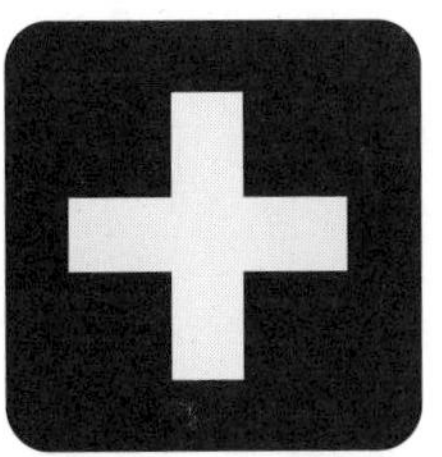

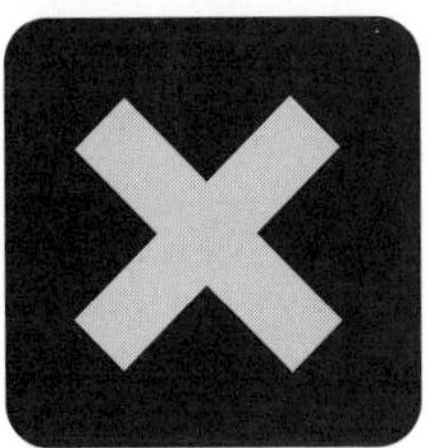

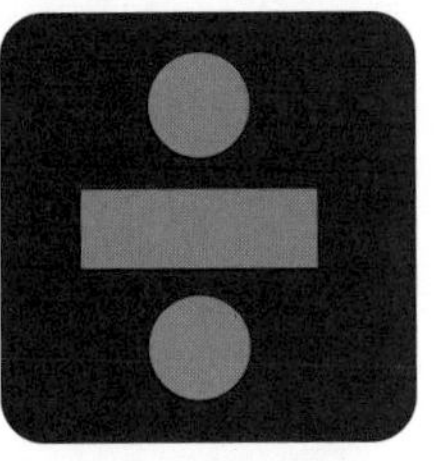

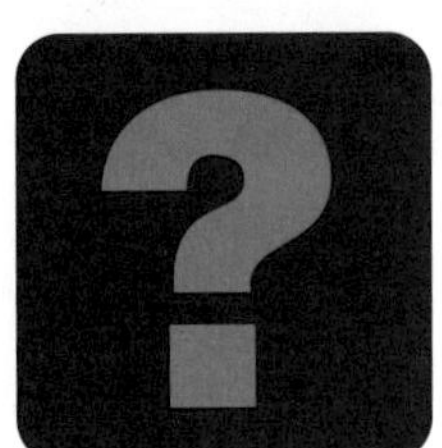

Introduction

WHY DO NURSES NEED MATH?

Nurses carry out computations in order to prepare and administer drugs according to physicians' instructions. Even in the most modern facilities, nurses must verify the computations of physicians, pharmacists, and other nurses, in order to prevent errors that all humans sometimes make. Computation is also important for the accurate, efficient collection of data, for the benefit of the client, and for the pursuit of research.

The nurse is a professional who keeps in touch with the latest information by reading journals and books and attending clinical lectures. To absorb the medical, nursing, dietetic, legal, and career information in the literature and the lectures, an understanding of mathematics is essential.

Many hospitals give prospective staff a test in dosage calculations as part of their assessment of a nurse's qualifications. Sometimes remedial assistance is provided for those who fail. Nurses are not allowed to administer medications until they pass the test.

WHAT MATH DO NURSES NEED?

To carry out their responsibilities, nurses must be comfortable with arithmetic and elementary algebra, including fractions, decimals, percents, ratio and proportion, and simple equations. They must be able to apply these concepts to dosage calculations whatever the route of administration or type of client. Nurses must use not only the most important system of measurement, SI (*Systême Internationale,* the modernized metric system), but also, on occasion, the apothecaries' system, because a few of these old units still appear; nurses must also know how to convert between the two systems and what their household equivalents are.

The process for solving math problems in nursing parallels the nursing process, a systematic approach to nursing. The nursing process includes assessment of data, analysis of the problem (a diagnosis based on a logical framework), planning and implementation of care, and evaluation of results. An analogous process is followed when computations are needed in pursuit of a nursing goal. There are four steps:

1. *T*abulate numerical information in an organized way and clarify the question.
2. *E*stimate mentally a sensible range within which the answer must lie.
3. *C*ompute carefully and clearly state the answer.
4. *C*heck results for reasonableness and accuracy.

In brief, tabulate, estimate, compute, and check (TECC). This mathematical problem solving process diminishes the chance of error and builds self-confidence.

For a quick and easy illustration of the TECC process, consider the following situation. Assume that a certain kind of nurse's uniform is on sale for $27. We need to purchase 6 uniforms. What must we pay?

Tabulate (T): 1 uniform for $27
6 uniforms for ?

How many dollars must we pay for 6 uniforms?

Estimate (E): 1 uniform costs $27, in between $20 and $30. Then 6 uniforms cost between $120 and $180.

Compute (C): $27 \times 6 = 162$

We must pay $162 for 6 uniforms.

Check (C):

1. Is the answer reasonable? Yes, because $162 is between $120 and $180.
2. Is the answer accurate? We check by reversing the order of multiplication:

$$6 \times 27 = 162 \qquad \text{(The same result as obtained before)}$$

Once the TECC process becomes habitual, it is a speedy way to maximize accuracy.

WHEN SHOULD YOU USE A CALCULATOR?

Only after the basic concepts and fundamental principles of mathematics are absolutely under your control! A calculator is a handy device to have, of course. It can perform some of our work for us and help us check whatever calculations we do. However, it certainly does not eliminate the need to understand the mathematical operations involved. The calculator carries out only the simplest operations and only after we decide what must be done and which keys to press. We must choose the numbers to use and in what order. There are no keys on the calculator to tell us, for instance, whether we should multiply or divide, which proportion or formula is appropriate in a given situation, or which of two fractions represents the larger quantity. It is important to understand the mathematical techniques thoroughly in order to know what instructions to give the calculator and to check that our results make sense.

Many instructors do not permit the use of calculators at examinations because they want to make sure that students develop enough facility with computations so that they can interpret results intelligently and are never dependent on a calculator. (Also, use of calculators is not yet permitted on standardized tests.) We should be happy that the calculator was invented, because it is a great timesaver, but we must retain our strength in depth of understanding and the ability to recognize errors.

TO THE STUDENT: SUGGESTIONS FOR STUDY

Each student has unique strengths and weaknesses. In your case, you may already know the topic of a particular chapter. To judge whether you need the review, use the Proficiency Gauge at the beginning of each chapter as a pretest, and check your answers with those given. If you have no errors, skip ahead to the next chapter.

For a quick review of a topic, or for reference, use the Summary at the end of each chapter. For further strengthening of skills, carry out the Exercises for Extra Practice that appear directly after each Summary, check your answers, and make careful corrections where necessary.

To test your understanding of a topic after you complete a chapter, take the chapter test. It will enable you to assess your skills and let you know what you have learned and what gaps in knowledge may still need to be filled in. Then you can go back to just that particular item necessary for you. In this way, you build a powerful foundation for the next part of the mathematical structure.

ONE

Review of Common Fractions

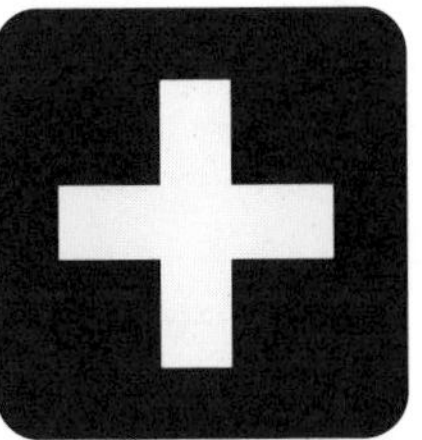

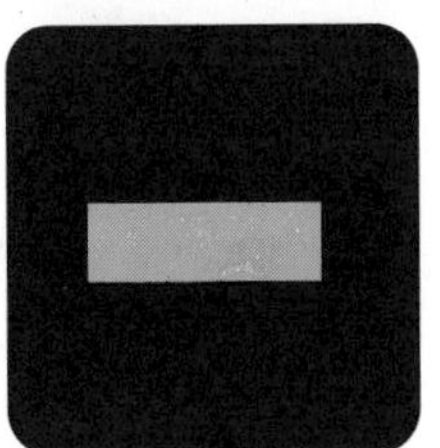

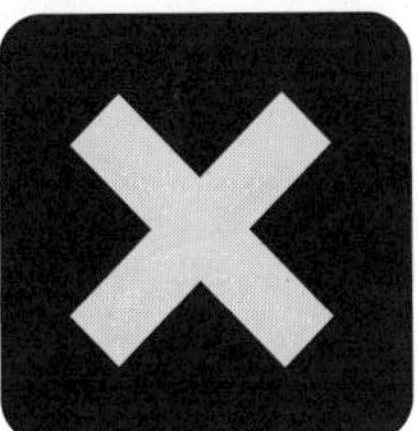

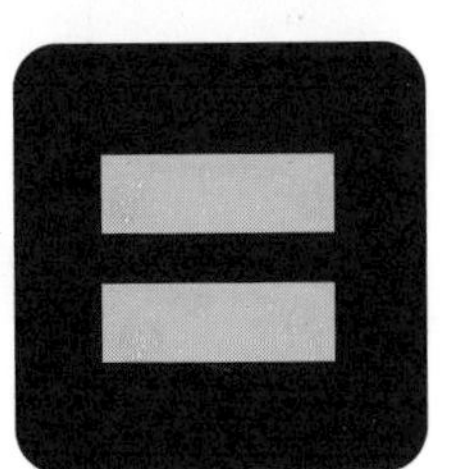

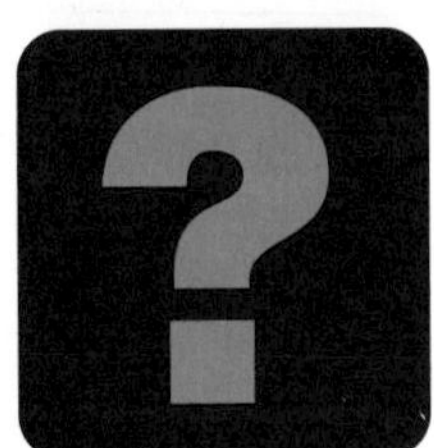

▶ OUTLINE

1-1. INTRODUCTION
1-2. MEANING OF A FRACTION
1-3. TERMS OF A FRACTION
1-4. EXPANDING AND REDUCING TERMS
1-5. MIXED NUMBERS
1-6. ADDING AND SUBTRACTING
1-7. MULTIPLYING AND DIVIDING
1-8. RELATIVE SIZE
1-9. AVOIDING ERRORS
1-10. SUMMARY

▶ OBJECTIVES

After studying this unit, you will be able to:

1. Interpret common fraction form.
2. Convert from common fractions to mixed numbers, and vice versa.
3. Expand and reduce fractions.
4. Add, subtract, multiply, and divide fractions.
5. Judge the relative size of fractions and use inequality signs.
6. Check answers for accuracy.
7. Use fractions to solve simple verbal problems.

1-1. INTRODUCTION

Why do nurses need fractions? Fractions appear in prescriptions and doctors' orders, on charts and hospital records, and in all nursing literature. Nurses must calculate with fractions in order to carry out and document patient care.

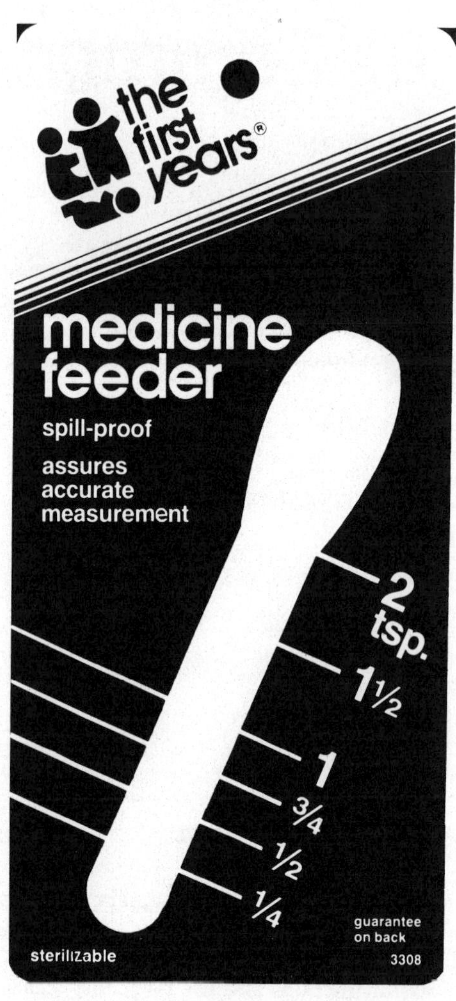

Examples

1. Sometimes it is necessary to reduce a dose of medication by $\frac{1}{4}$ because of the age of the patient or by $\frac{1}{2}$ because of the route of administration.
2. "$\frac{2}{5}$ cup tuna contains 170 calories." (From a client's diet chart)
3. "Bonus pay for evening hours = 1 1/2 × hourly rate." (From a nurse's salary schedule)
4. $X = \frac{D}{H} \times Q$ (Formula for dosage calculations)

Expertise with common fractions will help you be successful with decimal notation, percentages, ratio and proportion, and their medical applications.

Proficiency Gauge

It is possible that you understand fractions completely and can skip this chapter. Gauge your proficiency by doing the following exercises. Check your answers with those that follow the test only after you have answered all the questions.

SAMPLE EXERCISES

1. A gallon is divided into 8 pints. Each pint is what part of the gallon? 1. ____________
2. Change $\frac{23}{5}$ to a mixed number. 2. ____________
3. Express $3\frac{7}{8}$ as a fraction. 3. ____________
4. Reduce 90/108 to lowest terms. 4. ____________
5. True or false? $\frac{3}{10} < \frac{7}{8}$. 5. ____________

Exercises 6–10. Carry out the indicated operations.

6. $3\frac{7}{12} + 4\frac{2}{15}$ 6. ____________
7. $3\frac{7}{8} - 1\frac{5}{6}$ 7. ____________
8. $\frac{600}{5000} \times 25{,}000$ 8. ____________
9. $5\frac{1}{4} \times 1\frac{5}{7}$ 9. ____________
10. $1\frac{4}{5} \div 2\frac{1}{10}$ 10. ____________

ANSWERS 1. $\frac{1}{8}$ 2. $4\frac{3}{5}$ 3. $\frac{31}{8}$ 4. $\frac{5}{6}$ 5. True 6. $7\frac{43}{60}$ 7. $2\frac{1}{24}$ 8. 3000 9. 9 10. $\frac{6}{7}$

1-2. MEANING OF A FRACTION

The pharmacist may cut a scored acetazolamide (Diamox) tablet into four pieces for administration to a child. If we give a daily dose of 1 whole tablet in 4 divided doses, we understand that each dose is $\frac{1}{4}$ of the whole. Three of the doses would be $\frac{3}{4}$ of the whole.

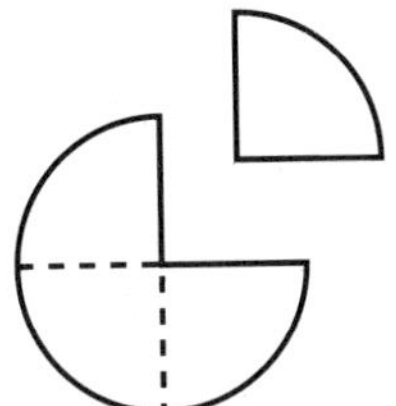

MEANING OF A FRACTION

We use fractions to compare a **part** of an object to the **whole**.

$$\frac{1}{2}, \frac{1}{3}, \frac{2}{3}, \frac{3}{4}, \ldots$$

Review of Common Fractions

Examples

1. A scored tablet may be broken into 2 equal portions. Each portion is $\frac{1}{2}$ of the tablet.

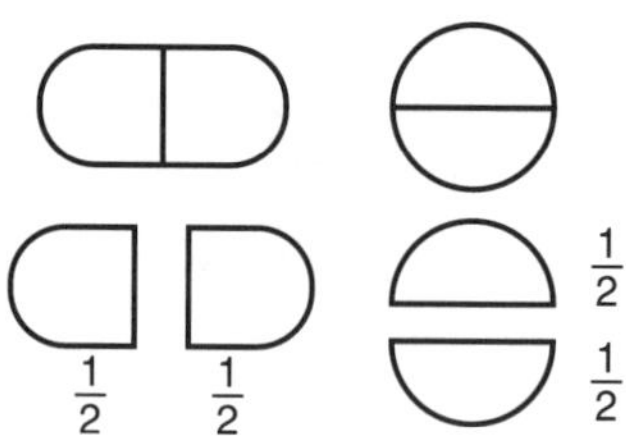

2. Suppose we cut a piece of tape into 5 equal pieces. Each piece is $\frac{1}{5}$ of the whole tape. Two pieces together are $\frac{2}{5}$ of the tape. The remainder would be $\frac{3}{5}$.

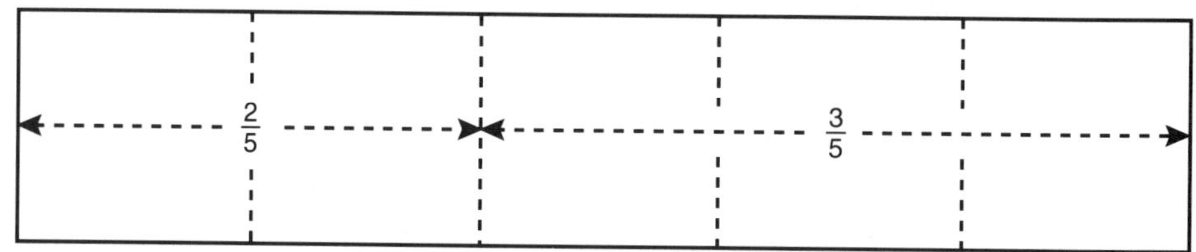

SAMPLE EXERCISES

Exercises 1–4. Suppose the pharmacist has cut a scored tablet into 4 equal pieces.

1. What fraction of the tablet is 1 piece?

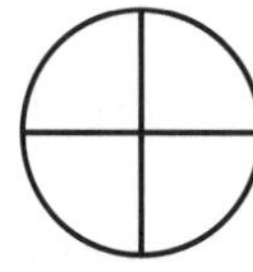

2. What fraction of the tablet do 3 of the pieces represent?
3. How many pieces does $\frac{2}{4}$ of the tablet represent?
4. A typical dose of magnesium carbonate (as an antacid) is 600 milligrams. If a patient takes only 200 milligrams, what part of the typical dose is he taking?

ANSWERS 1. 1 of the 4 pieces is $\frac{1}{4}$ of the whole tablet. 2. 3 of the 4 pieces represent $\frac{3}{4}$ of the tablet. 3. $\frac{2}{4}$ of the tablet represents 2 of the 4 pieces. 4. $\frac{200}{600}$

For medical applications, it is also helpful to think of a fraction as a symbol for division.

A FRACTION AS A DIVISION SYMBOL

A **fraction** represents **division** of two numbers.

$$\frac{10}{2} = 10 \div 2$$

Examples

1. The fraction $\frac{10}{2}$ is a shorthand way of writing $10 \div 2$. The fraction bar — is the same as the division sign without the dots. Sometimes the fraction bar is written as a slash: 10/2.
2. To simplify $\frac{10}{2}$, or 10/2, carry out the indicated division.

$$\frac{10}{2} = 10 \div 2 = 5$$

3. A supply of 10 tablets may be given in doses of 2 tablets each. The supply is enough for 5 doses because $\frac{10}{2} = 5$.

SAMPLE EXERCISES

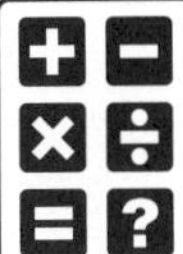

1. Write $\frac{18}{3}$ as a whole number.
2. Simplify $\frac{10}{10}$.
3. Write $7 \div 3$ as a fraction.
4. Write 5 as a fraction.

ANSWERS 1. $\frac{18}{3} = 18 \div 3 = 6$ 2. $\frac{10}{10} = 10 \div 10 = 1$

3. $7 \div 3 = \frac{7}{3}$ 4. $\frac{5}{1}$ is the simplest; among the other possibilities are $\frac{10}{2}$, and $\frac{15}{3}$.

EXERCISES

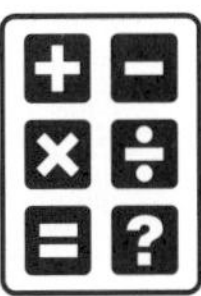

1. If the pharmacist cuts a scored tablet of trazodone hydrochloride (Desyrel) into 3 equal parts
   (a) What fraction represents 2 of the 3 parts?
   (b) What does $\frac{3}{3}$ represent?

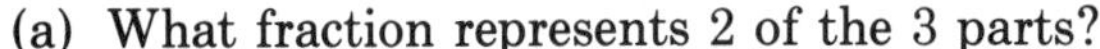

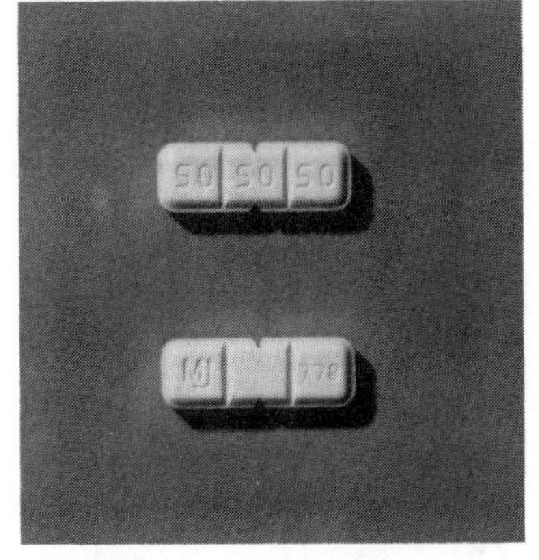

2. Assume that you have cut a tape into 8 equal pieces.
   (a) What fraction represents 5 of the 8 pieces?
   (b) What does 8/8 represent?
3. A baby drank 3 ounces of a filled 8-ounce bottle of milk. What fraction represents the part of the bottle
   (a) that was drunk?
   (b) that was not drunk?

4. A student correctly answered 117 out of 140 questions on an achievement test. What fraction represents the part of the test
   (a) that was answered correctly?
   (b) incorrectly?

5. If a typical dose of magnesium carbonate is 600 milligrams,
   (a) What fractional part of the typical dose is 100 milligrams?
   (b) What dose is represented by $\frac{359}{600}$ of the typical dose?

6. The minimum US recommended daily allowance (RDA) for vitamin C is 60 milligrams per day.
   (a) What fraction of the RDA is 40 milligrams?
   (b) How many milligrams is $\frac{27}{60}$ of the RDA?

7. A yardstick is divided into 36 inches.
   (a) Each inch is what fractional part of the yardstick?
   (b) How many inches in 25/36 yard?

8. A meterstick may be divided into 100 parts. Each part is called a centimeter.
   (a) A centimeter is what fractional part of the meterstick?
   (b) How many centimeters in $\frac{47}{100}$ of a meter?

9. A quart contains 32 ounces.
   (a) Five ounces is what part of a quart?
   (b) How many ounces is $\frac{7}{32}$ of a quart?

10. A liter contains 1000 milliliters.
    (a) What fractional part of the liter does 257 milliliters represent?
    (b) How many milliliters are in $\frac{21}{1000}$ of a liter?

Exercises 11–20. Write the fraction as a whole number.

11. $\frac{12}{3}$

12. $\frac{24}{6}$

13. $\frac{60}{10}$

14. $\frac{800}{10}$

15. 108/12

16. 154/11

17. 15/15

18. 339/339

19. $\frac{365}{1}$

20. 99/1

Exercises 21–26. Write the whole number as a fraction.

21. 10

22. 35

23. 1

24. 20

25. 1000

26. 49

ANSWERS 1. (a) $\frac{2}{3}$ (b) 1 tablet 3. (a) $\frac{3}{8}$ (b) $\frac{5}{8}$
5. (a) $\frac{100}{600}$ (b) 359 milligrams 7. (a) $\frac{1}{36}$ (b) 25 inches
9. (a) $\frac{5}{32}$ (b) 7 ounces 11. 4 13. 6 15. 9 17. 1
19. 365 21. $\frac{10}{1}$, or $\frac{20}{2}$, for instance 23. $\frac{1}{1}$ 25. $\frac{1000}{1}$

1-3. TERMS OF A FRACTION

Think of any fraction

$$\frac{1}{4}, \frac{3}{5}, \frac{10}{2}$$

as

$$\frac{N}{D}$$

The number above the fraction bar (1, 3, 10, or N) is called the **numerator;** the number *d*own below the fraction bar is called the ***d*enominator** (4, 5, 2, or D). The numerator and denominator are the **terms** of the fraction. The numerator can be any number, and the denominator can be any number except 0.

TERMS OF A FRACTION

$$\text{Every fraction} = \frac{\text{Numerator}}{\text{Denominator}} = N \div D = D\overline{)N}$$

In the division process, the numerator represents the **dividend** and the denominator represents the **divisor.** The result of the division process is the **quotient.**

Examples

1. Numerator (N): 3
   Fraction bar: —
   Denominator (D): 5
2. Numerator (N) ⟶ 3/5 ⟵ (D) Denominator
3. In the following diagram, the shaded area of the tape is $\frac{3}{5}$ of the whole tape. The denominator, 5, tells you that the tape has been cut into 5 pieces. The numerator, 3, tells you that 3 of the pieces have been shaded.

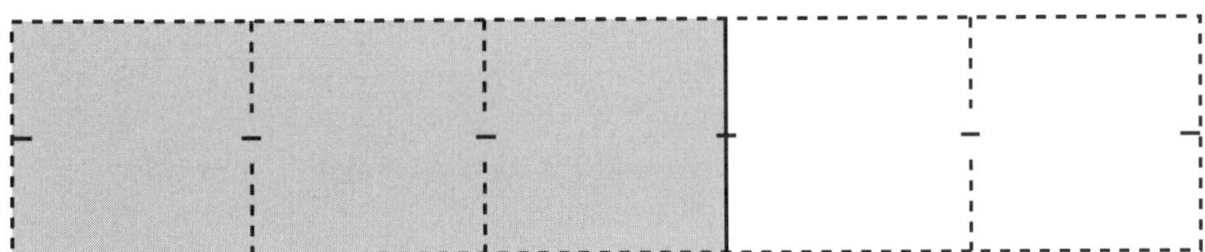

4. $\frac{3}{5} = 3 \div 5$. The **denominator,** 5, is the **divisor.**

SAMPLE EXERCISES

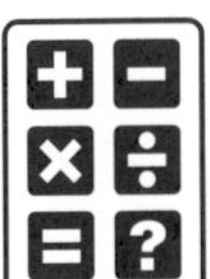

1. Name the numerator and denominator in the fraction $\frac{11}{3}$.
2. Write the fraction whose denominator is 7 and whose numerator is 2.
3. What is the denominator of a fraction that represents 50 divided by 3?
4. Which fraction has the greater numerator, $\frac{2}{9}$ or $\frac{5}{8}$?
5. If the terms of a fraction are equal, what is the value of the fraction?
6. Write the fraction that symbolizes the division $4 \div 5$.

ANSWERS 1. The numerator is the top term, 11; the denominator is the bottom term, 3. 2. Since the numerator is the top term, the fraction is $\frac{2}{7}$. 3. The fraction is $\frac{50}{3}$; the denominator is 3. 4. Looking at the top terms, we determine that $\frac{5}{8}$ has the greater numerator. 5. If the numerator is equal to the denominator, the fraction is equivalent to 1. $\frac{1}{1} = 1 \div 1 = 1$, $\frac{2}{2} = 2 \div 2 = 1$, $\frac{3}{3} = 3 \div 3 = 1$, and so on. 6. $\frac{4}{5}$

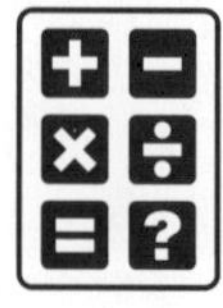

EXERCISES

Exercises 1–4. Name the numerator and denominator of the fraction.

1. $\dfrac{79}{100}$
2. $\dfrac{1000}{17}$
3. 12/1
4. $\dfrac{50}{50}$

Exercises 5–8. Write the fraction with the given terms.

	Numerator	*Denominator*
5.	44	21
6.	10	1
7.	29	5
8.	5	5

9. What is the denominator of a fraction that represents 43 divided by 22?
10. State the numerator of the fraction that represents division of 156 by 95.

Exercises 11–14. Find the fraction with the greater denominator, if there is one.

11. $\dfrac{3}{4}, \dfrac{4}{3}$
12. $\dfrac{1}{5}, \dfrac{2}{5}$
13. 2/5, 2/6
14. 4/9, 9/4
15. If the numerator of a fraction is equal to its denominator, what is the value of the fraction?

Exercises 16–20. Express the following fractions as whole numbers.

16. $\dfrac{9000}{9000}$
17. $\dfrac{40}{40}$
18. $\dfrac{2468}{2468}$
19. $\dfrac{5}{5}$
20. $\dfrac{37}{37}$

Exercises 21–28. Express each indicated quotient in fraction form.

21. $25 \div 3$
22. $7 \div 2$
23. $9 \div 10$
24. $6 \div 17$
25. $2 \div 5$
26. $5 \div 12$
27. $37 \div 100$
28. $1 \div 150$

ANSWERS 1. $N = 79, D = 100$ 3. $N = 12, D = 1$ 5. $\frac{44}{21}$ 7. $\frac{29}{5}$ 9. 22 11. $\frac{3}{4}$ 13. $\frac{2}{6}$ Exercises 15–20. 1 21. $\frac{25}{3}$ 23. $\frac{9}{10}$ 25. $\frac{2}{5}$ 27. $\frac{37}{100}$

1-4. EXPANDING AND REDUCING TERMS

When we exchange half-dollar coins for quarters, we expect to receive twice as many coins as before, because each quarter has half the value of the larger coin. In terms of fractions, $\frac{1}{2}$ dollar = $\frac{2}{4}$ dollar. We see that if we multiply both the numerator and the denominator in the fraction $\frac{1}{2}$ by 2, we find an equivalent fraction, $\frac{2}{4}$. If we divide each term of $\frac{2}{4}$ by 2, we find an equivalent fraction $\frac{1}{2}$. Both $\frac{1}{2}$ and $\frac{2}{4}$ have the same value.

EXPANDING TERMS

We may **multiply** both terms of a fraction by the **same** number (except 0) without changing the value of the fraction.

$$\frac{1}{3} = \frac{1 \times 2}{3 \times 2} = \frac{2}{6}$$

Examples

1. Eating $\frac{2}{3}$ of a pancake is the same as eating $\frac{4}{6}$ of the pancake.

$$\frac{2}{3} = \frac{2 \times 2}{3 \times 2} = \frac{4}{6}$$

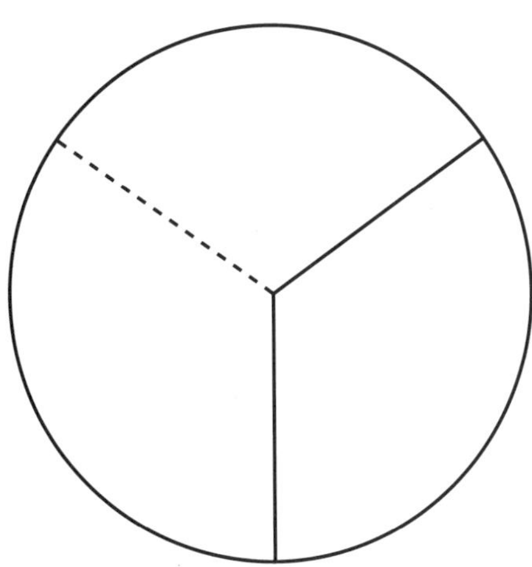

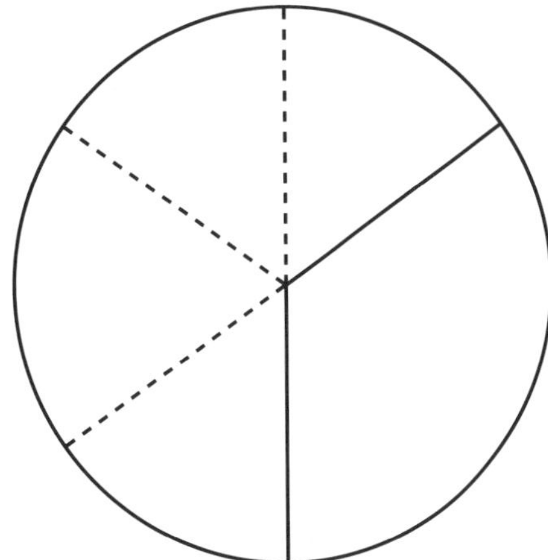

2. To expand the fraction $\frac{8}{10}$ to a fraction with a denominator of 30, we multiply both terms by 3.

$$\frac{8}{10} = \frac{8 \times 3}{10 \times 3} = \frac{24}{30}$$

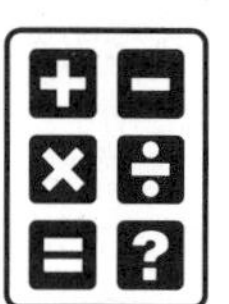

SAMPLE EXERCISES

1. Expand to higher terms as indicated:

$$\frac{3}{5} = \frac{12}{?}$$

2. Fill in the missing term: $\frac{?}{50} = \frac{7}{10}$

ANSWERS

1. Because $3 \times 4 = 12$, multiply both terms by the **same** whole number, 4.

$$\frac{3}{5} = \frac{3 \times 4}{5 \times 4} = \frac{12}{20}$$

2. Because $10 \times 5 = 50$, multiply both terms by the **same** whole number, 5.

$$\frac{7}{10} = \frac{7 \times 5}{10 \times 5} = \frac{35}{50}$$

The missing term is 35.

REDUCING TERMS

We may **divide** both terms of a fraction by the **same** whole number (except 0) without changing the value of the fraction.

$$\frac{9}{12} = \frac{9 \div 3}{12 \div 3} = \frac{3}{4}$$

Examples

1. In measurement, $\frac{6}{8}$ inch is the same length as $\frac{3}{4}$ inch:

$$\frac{6}{8} = \frac{6 \div 2}{8 \div 2} = \frac{3}{4}$$

2. To simplify $\frac{400}{8000}$, divide both terms by the common divisor, 100. Thus,

$$\frac{400}{8000} = \frac{400 \div 100}{8000 \div 100} = \frac{4}{80}$$

(A **common divisor** of both terms is a number by which both terms may be divided without a remainder.)

3. To reduce $\frac{12}{100}$ to lowest terms, divide both terms by the greatest common divisor, 4.

$$\frac{12}{100} = \frac{12 \div 4}{100 \div 4} = \frac{3}{25}$$

$\frac{3}{25}$ is in lowest terms because 3 and 25 have no common divisors.

4. To reduce $\frac{385}{1225}$ to lowest terms, we repeat the process of division as often as necessary:

Start with:	$\frac{385}{1225}$
Divide each term by 5:	$\frac{77}{245}$
Now divide each term by 7:	$\frac{11}{35}$
Stop.	11 and 35 have no further common divisors

1. Finding the missing term:

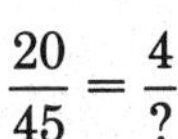

$$\frac{20}{45} = \frac{4}{?}$$

2. Reduce $\frac{60}{84}$ to lowest terms. We seek common divisors of 60 and 84. We can use 2, 3, 4, or 12 because both 60 and 84 are divisible by these numbers. The greatest of these common divisors is 12.
3. If 6 inches have been cut from an 8-inch tape, what fractional part of the tape has been cut off? (Reduce to lowest terms.)

SAMPLE EXERCISES

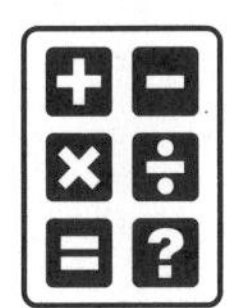

ANSWERS

1. We divide both terms by the **same** whole number, 5.

$$20 \div 5 = 4$$
$$45 \div 5 = 9$$
$$\frac{20}{45} = \frac{20 \div 5}{45 \div 5} = \frac{4}{9}$$

2. $\frac{60}{84} = \frac{60 \div 12}{84 \div 12} = \frac{5}{7}$
3. Since $6 \div 8 = \frac{6}{8} = \frac{3}{4}$, $\frac{3}{4}$ of the tape has been cut off.

EXERCISES

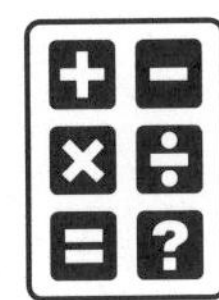

Exercises 1–8. Expand to higher terms as indicated.

1. $\frac{2}{4} = \frac{?}{8}$
2. $\frac{6}{9} = \frac{?}{27}$
3. $\frac{7}{11} = \frac{42}{?}$
4. $\frac{?}{48} = \frac{5}{12}$
5. $\frac{8}{10} = \frac{?}{30}$
6. $\frac{5}{6} = \frac{?}{24}$
7. $\frac{2}{5} = \frac{6}{?}$
8. $\frac{2}{3} = \frac{8}{?}$

Exercises 9–20. Reduce to lowest terms.

9. $\frac{56}{16} = \frac{7}{?}$
10. $\frac{38}{8} = \frac{?}{4}$
11. $\frac{360}{150} = \frac{?}{5}$
12. $\frac{18}{12} = \frac{3}{?}$
13. $\frac{6}{21}$
14. 12/15
15. $\frac{24}{84}$
16. $\frac{3}{36}$
17. $\frac{360}{1320}$
18. $\frac{90}{420}$
19. $\frac{1000}{5750}$
20. $\frac{20{,}000}{48{,}000}$

21. If 16 inches are cut from a 32-inch tape, what fractional part of the tape has been cut off? (Give your answer in lowest terms.)

22. If 18 ounces have been poured from a 30-ounce supply of syrup, what fractional part of the syrup has been poured? (Give your answer in lowest terms.)

ANSWERS 1. $\frac{4}{8}$ 3. $\frac{42}{66}$ 5. $\frac{24}{30}$ 7. $\frac{6}{15}$ 9. $\frac{7}{2}$ 11. $\frac{12}{5}$ 13. $\frac{2}{7}$ 15. $\frac{2}{7}$ 17. $\frac{3}{11}$ 19. $\frac{4}{23}$ 21. $\frac{1}{2}$

1-5. MIXED NUMBERS

To compute doses efficiently, it is often necessary to convert numbers from one form to another.

If the numerator is **greater than** the denominator, the fraction may be converted by division to a **mixed number** (the sum of a whole number and a fraction).

CHANGING A FRACTION TO A MIXED NUMBER

Divide the numerator by the denominator.

$$\frac{3}{2} = 3 \div 2 = 1\tfrac{1}{2}$$

EXAMPLES

1. $\frac{3}{2}$ tablet $= 1\frac{1}{2}$ tablets

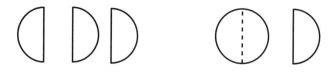

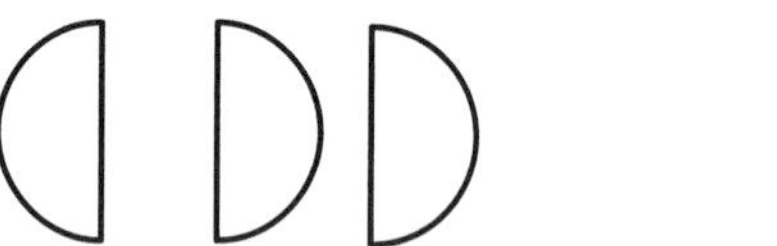

2. $\frac{39}{10} = 39 \div 10 = 3\frac{9}{10}$

3. $\frac{58}{25} = 58 \div 25 = 2\frac{8}{25}$

Details of division:

```
     2
25)58
   50
    8
```

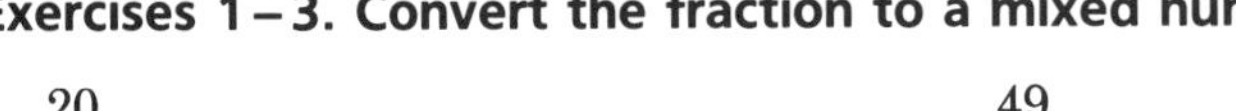

Exercises 1–3. Convert the fraction to a mixed number.

SAMPLE EXERCISES

1. $\frac{20}{3}$

2. $\frac{49}{5}$

3. $\frac{65}{12}$

ANSWERS 1. $\frac{20}{3} = 20 \div 3 = 6\frac{2}{3}$ 2. $\frac{49}{5} = 49 \div 5 = 9\frac{4}{5}$

3. $\frac{65}{12} = 65 \div 12 = 5\frac{5}{12}$

CHANGING A MIXED NUMBER TO A FRACTION

Multiply the whole number by the denominator and **add** the numerator to the product.
Keep the same denominator.

$4\frac{5}{8} = \frac{37}{8}$

EXAMPLES

1. Change $4\frac{5}{8}$ to a fraction.

Multiply:	$4 \times 8 = 32$
Add:	$32 + 5 = 37$
Keep the denominator:	$4\frac{5}{8} = \frac{37}{8}$

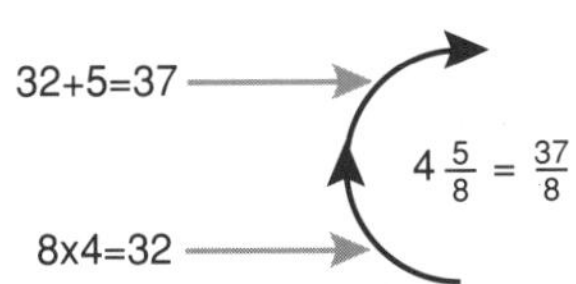

2. Change $3\frac{9}{10}$ to a fraction.

Multiply:	$10 \times 3 = 30$
Add:	$30 + 9 = 39$
Keep the denominator:	$3\frac{9}{10} = \frac{39}{10}$

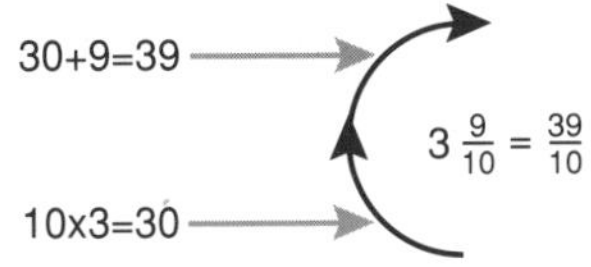

Exercises 1–2. Change the mixed number to a fraction.

SAMPLE EXERCISES

1. $2\frac{7}{12}$

2. $7\frac{39}{100}$

ANSWERS

	1.	2.
Multiply:	$2 \times 12 = 24$	$7 \times 100 = 700$
Add:	$24 + 7 = 31$	$700 + 39 = 739$
Keep denominator:	$2\frac{7}{12} = \dfrac{31}{12}$	$7\frac{39}{100} = \dfrac{739}{100}$

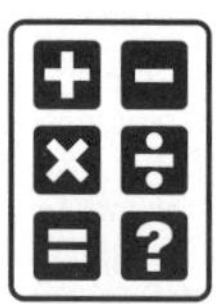

EXERCISES

Exercises 1–8. Change the fraction to a mixed number.

1. $\dfrac{13}{2}$
2. $\dfrac{15}{4}$
3. 13/5
4. 23/10
5. $\dfrac{135}{11}$
6. $\dfrac{46}{7}$
7. $\dfrac{29}{12}$
8. $\dfrac{35}{20}$

Exercises 9–16. Change the mixed number to a fraction.

9. 6 1/2
10. 2 1/5
11. $4\frac{2}{5}$
12. $11\frac{2}{3}$
13. $5\frac{1}{12}$
14. $100\frac{5}{8}$
15. $3\frac{9}{10}$
16. $5\frac{17}{100}$

Exercises 17–20. Give your answer as a fraction and as a mixed number.

17. If a total of 9 tablets are to be divided equally into 4 separate doses, how many tablets should be taken for each dose?
18. How many ounces of tuna should each of 3 patients receive if 11 ounces of tuna is to be divided evenly among them?
19. If 130 inches of tape is to be cut into 20 pieces for bandages, how long will each piece be?
20. What is the monthly salary of a worker who receives $38,000 per year?

ANSWERS 1. $6\frac{1}{2}$ 3. 2 3/5 5. $12\frac{3}{11}$ 7. $2\frac{5}{12}$ 9. 13/2 11. $\frac{22}{5}$ 13. $\dfrac{61}{12}$ 15. $\dfrac{39}{10}$ 17. $\dfrac{9}{4} = 2\ 1/4$ tablets 19. $\dfrac{130}{20} = 6\frac{1}{2}$ inches

1-6. ADDING AND SUBTRACTING

Sometimes it is important to record how much a patient drinks. If Allen P. had $\frac{1}{4}$ cup of prune juice and $\frac{3}{4}$ cup of orange juice with breakfast, how much juice did he drink? We would add $\frac{1}{4}$ to $\frac{3}{4}$. The easiest fractions to add are those with equal denominators.

ADDING AND SUBTRACTING FRACTIONS WITH EQUAL DENOMINATORS

If the denominators are **equal, add** (or subtract) the numerators, and keep the **same** denominator.

$$\frac{1}{5}+\frac{3}{5}=\frac{4}{5} \qquad \frac{4}{5}-\frac{3}{5}=\frac{1}{5}$$

Examples

1. $\frac{1}{10}+\frac{3}{10}=\frac{4}{10}$

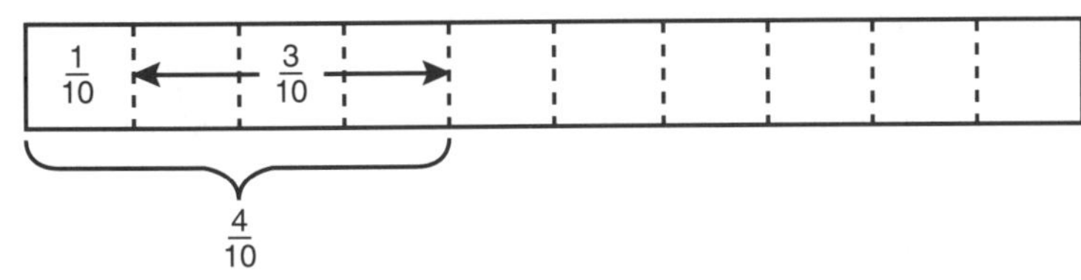

2. $\frac{7}{8}-\frac{3}{8}=\frac{4}{8}$

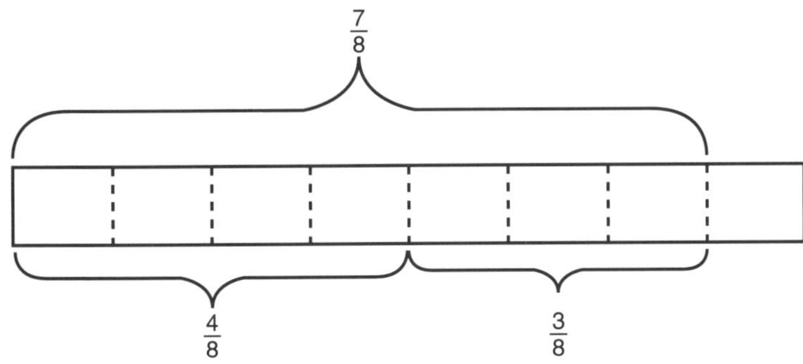

3. Find the sum of $\frac{7}{100}$ and $\frac{11}{100}$.

Method:	Note that the denominators are equal.
Add the numerators:	$7 + 11 = 18$
Keep the denominator:	100
Result:	$\frac{18}{100}$

4. Find the difference of $\frac{25}{100} - \frac{4}{100}$.

Method:	We note that the denominators are equal.
Subtract numerators:	$25 - 4 = 21$
Keep the denominator:	100
Result:	$\frac{21}{100}$

Sometimes you need to add fractions with unequal denominators. For example, Barbara K. had $\frac{2}{3}$ cup of juice before breakfast and $\frac{3}{4}$ cup after breakfast. How do we determine how much juice she drank? We need to add $\frac{2}{3}$ and $\frac{3}{4}$, fractions with unequal denominators.

ADDING AND SUBTRACTING FRACTIONS WITH UNEQUAL DENOMINATORS

If the denominators are **unequal**

1. Find the least common denominator (LCD).
2. **Expand** fractions, using the LCD.
3. **Add** (or subtract) the new numerators.
4. Keep the LCD as the **new** denominator.

$$\frac{2}{3} + \frac{3}{4} = \frac{8}{12} + \frac{9}{12} = \frac{17}{12} \text{ or } 1\tfrac{5}{12}$$

Examples

1. To find $\frac{3}{2} + \frac{1}{5}$, we want both fractions to have the same denominator. Therefore, we find the **least common denominator (LCD),** that is, the smallest number divisible by 2 and 5. Using the LCD, 10, we expand terms so that both fractions have the same denominator.

$$\begin{aligned} \frac{3}{2} &= \frac{15}{10} \\ +\frac{1}{5} &= +\frac{2}{10} \\ \frac{\text{Sum of new numerators}}{\text{LCD}} &= \frac{17}{10}, \text{ or } 1\tfrac{7}{10} \end{aligned}$$

2. Find $7\frac{1}{3} + 1\frac{1}{2}$.

Method:	Use the LCD, 6
Replace $\frac{1}{3}$ by $\frac{2}{6}$:	$7\frac{1}{3} = 7\frac{2}{6}$
Replace $\frac{1}{2}$ by $\frac{3}{6}$:	$+1\frac{1}{2} = +1\frac{3}{6}$
	$8\frac{5}{6}$

3. Find $26 - 3\frac{5}{8}$.
Replace 26 by $25\frac{8}{8}$ so that matching fractions can then be subtracted:

$$\begin{array}{r} 25\frac{8}{8} \\ -3\frac{5}{8} \\ \hline 22\frac{3}{8} \end{array}$$

4. Find $1\frac{1}{2} + 2\frac{3}{4}$

Method:	Use the LCD, 4.
Replace $\frac{1}{2}$ by $\frac{2}{4}$:	$1\frac{1}{2} = 1\frac{2}{4}$
	$+2\frac{3}{4} = +2\frac{3}{4}$
	$3\frac{5}{4}$
Replace $\frac{5}{4}$ by $1\frac{1}{4}$:	$3 + 1\frac{1}{4}$
Result:	$4\frac{1}{4}$

5. Steps in finding the LCD in cases in which it is not obvious:
   (a) Factor each denominator completely.
   (b) Write each different factor the maximum number of times it appears in any of the original denominators.
   (c) Multiply the product of the factors in (b). This product is the LCD.

   Thus, to find $\frac{7}{10} + \frac{5}{12}$,
   Find the LCD:
   (a) $10 = 2 \times 5$ and $12 = 2 \times 2 \times 3$;

(b) 2, 5, 2, 3
(c) LCD $= 2 \times 5 \times 2 \times 3 = 60$
Expand fractions, using the LCD:

$$\frac{7}{10} = \frac{42}{60} \quad \text{and} \quad \frac{5}{12} = \frac{25}{60}$$

Add the new numerators: $42 + 25 = 67$

$$\frac{7}{10} + \frac{5}{12} = \frac{67}{60} = 1\tfrac{7}{60}$$

SAMPLE EXERCISES

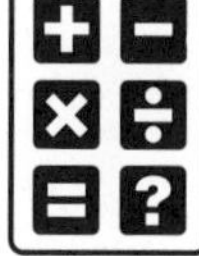

1. Find $7\frac{3}{8} + 4\frac{5}{6}$.
2. Subtract $10\frac{3}{4} - 2\frac{1}{2}$.
3. Find the difference between $3\frac{1}{6}$ and $9\frac{7}{8}$.
4. Subtract $2\frac{3}{4}$ from $5\frac{1}{2}$.
5. Subtract $1\frac{1}{2}$ from $3\frac{1}{8}$.

ANSWERS

1. Method: Use the LCD, 24.

Replace $\frac{3}{8}$ by $\frac{9}{24}$: $7\frac{3}{8} = 7\frac{9}{24}$
Replace $\frac{5}{6}$ by $\frac{20}{24}$: $+4\frac{5}{6} = +4\frac{20}{24}$
$11\frac{29}{24}$
Replace $\frac{29}{24}$ by $1\frac{5}{24}$: $11\frac{29}{24} = 11 + 1\frac{5}{24}$
Result: $12\frac{5}{24}$

2. Method: Use the LCD, 4.

$10\frac{3}{4}$
$-2\frac{2}{4}$
Result: $8\frac{1}{4}$

3. Method: Use the LCD, 24.

$9\frac{7}{8} = 9\frac{21}{24}$
$-3\frac{1}{6} = -3\frac{4}{24}$
Result: $6\frac{17}{24}$

4. Method: Use the LCD, 4.

$5\frac{1}{2} = 5\frac{2}{4} = 4\frac{6}{4}$
$-2\frac{3}{4} = -2\frac{3}{4} = -2\frac{3}{4}$
Result: $2\frac{3}{4}$

5. Method: Use the LCD, 8.

$3\frac{1}{8} = 3\frac{1}{8}$
$-1\frac{1}{2} = -1\frac{4}{8}$ But $\frac{4}{8}$ cannot be subtracted from $\frac{1}{8}$

Rewrite: $3\frac{1}{8} = 2 + 1 + \frac{1}{8} = 2 + \frac{8}{8} + \frac{1}{8} = 2\frac{9}{8}$

$3\frac{1}{8} = 2\frac{9}{8}$
$-1\frac{1}{2} = -1\frac{4}{8}$
Result: $1\frac{5}{8}$

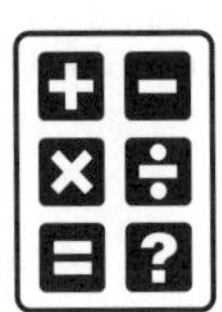

EXERCISES

Exercises 1 – 6. Add the fractions.

1. $\frac{2}{3} + \frac{3}{5}$
2. $\frac{4}{5} + \frac{5}{8}$
3. $\frac{1}{3} + \frac{1}{3} + \frac{1}{4}$
4. $\frac{3}{10} + \frac{2}{5} + \frac{5}{3}$
5. 1/3 + 5/6
6. 3/4 + 5/8 + 1/2

Exercises 7 – 12. Subtract as indicated.

7. $5\frac{3}{4} - 2\frac{1}{2}$
8. $7\frac{3}{4} - 2\frac{1}{8}$
9. $12\frac{1}{4} - 7\frac{1}{5}$
10. $11\frac{2}{3} - 2\frac{5}{12}$
11. 32 − 3 5/8
12. 18 − 5 1/4

Exercises 13 – 18. Carry out the indicated operation.

13. $2\frac{1}{4} + 3\frac{1}{8} + 1\frac{1}{2}$
14. $1\frac{3}{4} + 2\frac{5}{6}$
15. 5 3/4 − 2 1/10
16. 7 1/100 + 2 7/10
17. $18\frac{2}{3} - 2\frac{5}{12}$
18. $12\frac{9}{10} - 7\frac{1}{6}$
19. During a 12-hour period, Carl J. received intravenous therapy at first for $4\frac{1}{3}$ hours, and then later for $2\frac{1}{2}$ hours. What was the total number of hours for the therapy?
20. If, during a 24-hour period, David J. received intravenous therapy for $9\frac{3}{4}$ hours, for how many hours did he not receive IV therapy?

ANSWERS 1. $\frac{19}{15} = 1\frac{4}{15}$ 3. $\frac{11}{12}$ 5. $1\frac{1}{6}$ 7. $3\frac{1}{4}$ 9. $5\frac{1}{20}$ 11. $28\frac{3}{8}$ 13. $6\frac{7}{8}$ 15. $3\frac{13}{20}$ 17. $16\frac{1}{4}$ 19. $6\frac{5}{6}$ hours

---

1-7. MULTIPLYING AND DIVIDING

Many children receive a fractional part of a typical adult dose of medication. If little Patty R. is to receive $\frac{3}{5}$ of an adult dose of $\frac{1}{2}$ ounce, we calculate her dose by multiplying $\frac{1}{2}$ by $\frac{3}{5}$.

MULTIPLYING FRACTIONS

1. **Reduce** fractions wherever possible.
2. Multiply **numerators** and multiply **denominators**.

$$\frac{3}{5} \times \frac{1}{2} = \frac{3 \times 1}{5 \times 2} = \frac{3}{10}$$

Examples

1. $\frac{4}{15} \times \frac{7}{10}$

Multiply numerators: Multiply denominators: $\frac{4}{15} \times \frac{7}{10} = \frac{4 \times 7}{15 \times 10}$

Divide numerator and denominator by 2: $= \frac{\overset{2}{\cancel{4}} \times 7}{15 \times \underset{5}{\cancel{10}}}$

(The cancellation marks show the division.)

Result: $\frac{14}{75}$

2. Multiplication leads to a result called a **product**. The result of multiplying $\frac{4}{15}$ by $\frac{7}{10}$ is the product $\frac{14}{75}$.

3. $\frac{9}{22} \times \frac{5}{6} = \frac{\overset{3}{\cancel{9}}}{22} \times \frac{5}{\underset{2}{\cancel{6}}} = \frac{15}{44}$

4. $7 \times \frac{3}{100} = \frac{7}{1} \times \frac{3}{100}$

$= \frac{7 \times 3}{1 \times 100}$

$= \frac{21}{100}$

5. How many minutes in 4 1/2 hours?
Since 1 hour has 60 minutes, we need

4 1/2 × 60 =

$\frac{9}{\cancel{2}} \times \overset{30}{\cancel{60}} = 270$

Result: 270 minutes

6. Find 1/4 of $3\frac{1}{2}$ ounces.
Method: $1/4 \times 3\frac{1}{2} =$
$\frac{1}{4} \times \frac{7}{2} = \frac{7}{8}$
Result: $\frac{7}{8}$ ounce

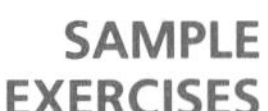

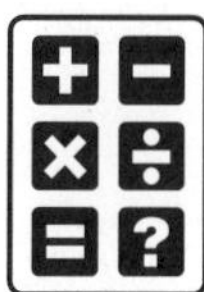

1. Find $\frac{1}{2}$ of $\frac{3}{8}$.
2. Multiply $\frac{3}{4} \times \frac{8}{15}$.
3. Find the product of $\frac{40}{500} \times 2000$

ANSWERS 1. $\frac{1}{2} \times \frac{3}{8} = \frac{1 \times 3}{2 \times 8} = \frac{3}{16}$ 2. $\frac{\overset{1}{\cancel{3}}}{\underset{1}{\cancel{4}}} \times \frac{\overset{2}{\cancel{8}}}{\underset{5}{\cancel{15}}} = \frac{2}{5}$

3. $\frac{40}{500} \times \frac{2000}{1} = \frac{40}{\cancel{500}} \times \frac{\overset{4}{\cancel{2000}}}{1} = \frac{160}{1} = 160$

If we cut 9 inches of labeling tape into $\frac{3}{4}$-inch pieces, how many labels will we have? To find the answer, we divide 9 by $\frac{3}{4}$.

DIVIDING FRACTIONS

Invert the divisor, then multiply.

$$9 \div \frac{3}{4} = 9 \times \frac{4}{3} = 12$$

Examples

1. $9 \div \frac{3}{4} = \overset{3}{\cancel{9}} \times \frac{4}{\underset{1}{\cancel{3}}} = 12$

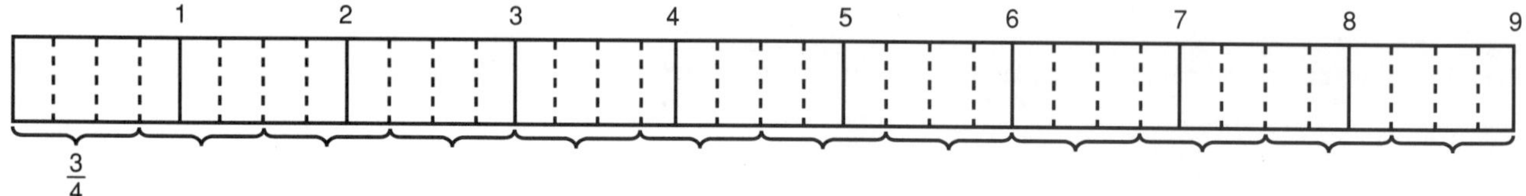

2. $\frac{3}{20} \div \frac{2}{9} = \frac{3}{20} \times \frac{9}{2} = \frac{27}{40}$

3. $\frac{15}{16} \div \frac{3}{8} = \frac{\overset{5}{\cancel{15}}}{\underset{2}{\cancel{16}}} \times \frac{\overset{1}{\cancel{8}}}{\underset{1}{\cancel{3}}} = \frac{5}{2} = 2\frac{1}{2}$

4. $\frac{21}{10} \div \frac{63}{100} = \frac{\overset{1}{\cancel{21}}}{\underset{1}{\cancel{10}}} \times \frac{10\cancel{0}}{\underset{3}{\cancel{63}}}$

$$= \frac{1}{1} \times \frac{10}{3} = \frac{10}{3} = 3\frac{1}{3}$$

5. $\frac{\frac{1}{2}}{\frac{1}{4}}* = \frac{1}{2} \div \frac{1}{4} = \frac{1}{\underset{1}{\cancel{2}}} \times \frac{\overset{2}{\cancel{4}}}{1} = 2$

We can illustrate this division by cutting a $\frac{1}{2}$-inch thread into $\frac{1}{4}$-inch pieces.

$\longleftarrow \frac{1}{2}$ inch $\longrightarrow$

$\frac{1}{4}$ inch $\frac{1}{4}$ inch

There are 2 pieces, each of $\frac{1}{4}$-inch length in a $\frac{1}{2}$-inch thread.

6. Find $5 \div \frac{1}{2}$.

$$5 \div \frac{1}{2} = 5 \times 2 = 10$$

The following diagram represents this division.

---

* $\frac{\frac{1}{2}}{\frac{1}{4}}$ is a complex fraction that indicates division of $\frac{1}{2}$ by $\frac{1}{4}$. Whenever the numerator or denominator of a fraction is itself in fractional form, the entire combination is called **a complex fraction.**

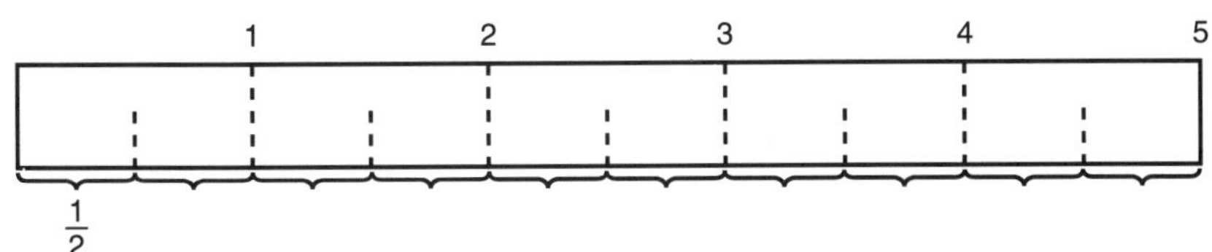

7. If an $8\frac{3}{4}$-inch cord is cut into $\frac{5}{8}$-inch pieces, how many pieces would there be?

$$8\frac{3}{4} \div \frac{5}{8} = \frac{\overset{7}{\cancel{35}}}{\underset{1}{\cancel{4}}} \times \frac{\overset{2}{\cancel{8}}}{\underset{1}{\cancel{5}}} = 14$$

Result: 14 pieces

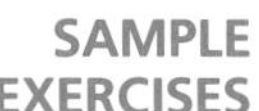

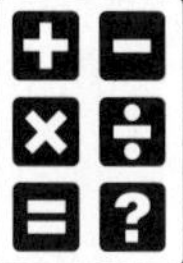

Exercises 1–3. Divide as indicated.

1. $5 \div 1/5$

2. $\frac{3}{5} \div 2$

3. $\frac{1}{300} \div \frac{1}{200}$

ANSWERS 1. $5 \div \frac{1}{5} = 5 \times 5 = 25$ 2. $\frac{3}{5} \div \frac{2}{1} = \frac{3}{5} \times \frac{1}{2} = \frac{3}{10}$

3. $\frac{1}{300} \times \frac{200}{1} = \frac{200}{300} = \frac{2}{3}$

EXERCISES

Exercises 1–12. Find the indicated value.

1. $\frac{1}{2}$ of $\frac{1}{4}$

2. $\frac{3}{5}$ of $\frac{1}{4}$

3. $\frac{9}{11} \times \frac{5}{24}$

4. $\frac{2}{3} \times \frac{7}{8}$

5. $\frac{5}{7} \times \frac{14}{15}$

6. $\frac{3}{4} \times \frac{16}{15}$

7. $\frac{50}{100} \times 5$

8. $\frac{100}{200} \times 2$

9. $\frac{2000}{250} \times 1$

10. $\frac{250{,}000}{5{,}000{,}000} \times 10$

11. $5\frac{1}{4} \times 1\frac{1}{3}$

12. $2\frac{1}{10} \times 1\frac{2}{3}$

Exercises 13–22. Divide as indicated.

13. $10 \div \frac{1}{5}$

14. $7 \div \frac{1}{9}$

15. $6 \div 2/3$

16. $8 \div 4/5$

17. $\frac{1}{16} \div \frac{1}{24}$

18. $\frac{1}{200} \div \frac{1}{10}$

19. $\frac{\frac{1}{20}}{\frac{1}{40}}$

20. $\frac{1}{10} \div \frac{3}{100}$

21. $6\frac{1}{4} \div 2\frac{1}{2}$

22. $5\frac{5}{6} \div 1\frac{2}{3}$

23. How many seconds are there in 3 1/2 minutes?

24. A ketoconazole (Nizoral) tablet contains 200 milligrams. How many milligrams are in
    (a) 2 tablets?
    (b) $\frac{1}{4}$ tablet?

25. Jean B. has 9 tablets and must take $\frac{1}{2}$ tablet each day. For how many days should her supply last?

26. James S. has 24 tablets and takes $1\frac{1}{2}$ tablets each day. How long should his supply last?

ANSWERS 1. $\frac{1}{8}$ 3. $\frac{15}{88}$ 5. $\frac{2}{3}$ 7. $2\frac{1}{2}$ 9. 8 11. 7

13. 50 15. 9 17. $\frac{3}{2} = 1\frac{1}{2}$ 19. 2 21. $\frac{25}{4} \div \frac{5}{2} = \frac{5}{2} = 2\frac{1}{2}$

23. $60 \times 3\frac{1}{2} = 210$ seconds 25. $9 \div \frac{1}{2} = 18$ days

---

1–8. RELATIVE SIZE

Drug literature may recommend that a child receive a dose "<" $\frac{3}{4}$ of the typical adult dose of a certain medication. The inequality signs, < and >, often appear in the literature instead of the words *less than,* or *greater than.*

"LESS THAN" AND "GREATER THAN" SYMBOLS

$<$ means "(is) **less than,**" as in $\frac{1}{4} < \frac{3}{4}$;

$>$ means "(is) **greater than,**" as in $\frac{3}{4} > \frac{1}{4}$.

Examples

1. The symbol $>$ is like the tip of an arrow pointing to the smaller quantity. In both "$\frac{3}{4} > \frac{1}{4}$," and "$\frac{1}{4} < \frac{3}{4}$," the tip points to $\frac{1}{4}$, the smaller quantity.
2. For some medications, a child must be $>\frac{1}{2}$ year of age, that is, older than 6 months.
3. Sometimes, a young child's dose is $<1/4$ of the adult dose of a drug. Thus, 1/4 of the adult dose would be too great for such a child.

Equal Denominators

From notes on the patient's record, we read that he drank $\frac{1}{4}$ cup of juice at breakfast and $\frac{3}{4}$ cup at lunch. By comparing $\frac{1}{4}$ with $\frac{3}{4}$, we easily can see that the patient drank more at lunch than at breakfast. It is always easy to compare fractions that have equal denominators.

EQUAL DENOMINATORS

If two fractions have **equal denominators,** the **greater fraction** has the **greater numerator.**

$$\frac{3}{4} > \frac{1}{4}$$

Examples

1. $\frac{2}{4}$ dollar $>$ $\frac{1}{4}$ dollar (2 quarters are worth more than 1). Denominators are equal and $\frac{2}{4}$ has the greater numerator.
2. One patient may receive $\frac{1}{10}$ of a typical adult dose; a second patient may receive $\frac{9}{10}$. The second patient is receiving more than the first, since $\frac{9}{10} > \frac{1}{10}$. (The denominators are equal and $\frac{9}{10}$ has the greater numerator.)

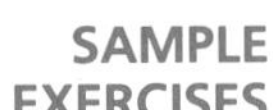

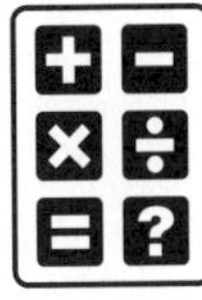

1. Insert an inequality sign between the following fractions to indicate which is larger:

$$\frac{12}{100} \quad \frac{49}{100}$$

2. Write an inequality statement comparing

$$\frac{359}{1000} \quad \text{with} \quad \frac{24}{1000}$$

ANSWERS 1. $\frac{12}{100} < \frac{49}{100}$ or $\frac{49}{100} > \frac{12}{100}$

(Denominators are equal and $\frac{49}{100}$ has the greater numerator.)

2. $\frac{359}{1000} > \frac{24}{1000}$ or $\frac{24}{1000} < \frac{359}{1000}$

(Denominators are equal and $\frac{359}{1000}$ has the greater numerator.)

Equal Numerators

One container of adhesive bandages is labeled "width, 1/4 inch," another is labeled "width, 1/2 inch." To choose the right container, we compare the fractions for size. These fractions have equal numerators.

EQUAL NUMERATORS

If two fractions have **equal numerators,** compare the denominators. The **greater fraction** has the **smaller denominator.**

$$\frac{1}{2} > \frac{1}{4}$$

Examples

1. $\frac{3}{4}$ inch > $\frac{3}{8}$ inch.
   $\frac{3}{4}$ means 3 of 4 equal parts that make a whole;
   $\frac{3}{8}$ means 3 of 8 equal parts that make a whole.
   Therefore, $\frac{3}{4} > \frac{3}{8}$.
   (Numerators are equal, and $\frac{3}{4}$ has the smaller denominator.)

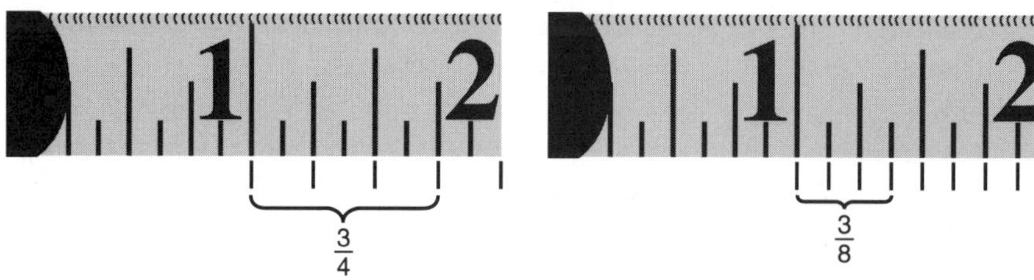

2. Imagine a brick of ice cream divided evenly into 4 portions. Similarly, imagine the same brick divided evenly into 6 portions instead. The person who received $\frac{1}{4}$ of the ice cream would have more to eat than the person who received $\frac{1}{6}$. Thus, $\frac{1}{4} > \frac{1}{6}$. (Numerators are equal and $\frac{1}{4}$ has the smaller denominator.)

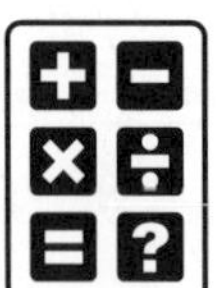

SAMPLE EXERCISES

1. Insert an inequality sign between the following fractions: $\frac{1}{100}$ $\quad$ $\frac{1}{150}$.
2. Write an inequality statement comparing $\frac{1}{4}$ dollar with $\frac{1}{2}$ dollar.

ANSWERS

1. $\frac{1}{100} > \frac{1}{150}$
   (Numerators are equal, and $\frac{1}{100}$ has the smaller denominator.)
2. $\frac{1}{4}$ dollar $<$ $\frac{1}{2}$ dollar
   (Numerators are equal, and $\frac{1}{2}$ has the smaller denominator.)

Unequal Numerators and Unequal Denominators

Where neither numerators nor denominators are equal, we compare fractions by using a least common denominator, just as we did for addition.

UNEQUAL NUMERATORS AND UNEQUAL DENOMINATORS

Expand terms so that both fractions have the **same** denominator.

$$\frac{2}{5} > \frac{3}{10}$$

Examples

1. To compare $\frac{2}{5}$ and $\frac{3}{10}$, we expand $\frac{2}{5}$ to $\frac{4}{10}$. Since $\frac{4}{10} > \frac{3}{10}$, we see that $\frac{2}{5} > \frac{3}{10}$.
2. To compare $\frac{2}{5}$ and $\frac{1}{3}$, we use the least common denominator, 15, just as we would for addition:

$$\frac{2}{5} = \frac{6}{15} \quad \text{and} \quad \frac{1}{3} = \frac{5}{15}$$

Since $\frac{6}{15} > \frac{5}{15}$, we see that $\frac{2}{5} > \frac{1}{3}$.

SAMPLE EXERCISES

1. Insert an inequality sign between the following fractions: $\frac{3}{8}$ $\quad$ $\frac{5}{12}$.
2. Which dose is greater, $\frac{11}{100}$ grain or $\frac{13}{150}$ grain?

ANSWERS 1. $\frac{3}{8} < \frac{5}{12}$ 2. $\frac{11}{100}$ grain $> \frac{13}{150}$ grain

EXERCISES

Exercises 1–4. Sometimes a patient is required to have <150 units (U) of a drug. Which of the following fit the requirement?

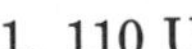

1. 110 U
2. 80 U
3. 150 U
4. 200 U

Exercises 5–8. You are asked to "notify the doctor if the patient's systolic blood pressure (SBP) > 100." In which of the following cases would you notify the doctor?

5. SBP = 110
6. SBP = 80
7. SBP > 110
8. SBP < 95

Exercises 9–30. Write an inequality statement comparing the given quantities.

9. 1/4 cup, 3/4 cup
10. 1/2 cup, 1/3 cup
11. $\frac{3}{4}, \frac{3}{10}$
12. $\frac{2}{5}, \frac{3}{5}$
13. $\frac{2}{9}, \frac{5}{9}$
14. $\frac{3}{7}, \frac{3}{4}$

15. $\frac{1}{5}, \frac{1}{6}$

16. $\frac{5}{7}, \frac{3}{7}$

17. $\frac{1}{10}, \frac{1}{20}$

18. $\frac{5}{100}, \frac{5}{1000}$

19. $\frac{1}{150}, \frac{1}{200}$

20. $\frac{1}{500}, \frac{1}{250}$

21. $\frac{3}{4}$ cup, $\frac{2}{3}$ cup

22. $\frac{3}{5}, \frac{5}{9}$

23. $\frac{3}{5}, \frac{2}{3}$

24. $\frac{4}{5}, \frac{5}{8}$

25. $\frac{2}{5}, \frac{7}{10}$

26. $\frac{3}{10}, \frac{7}{20}$

27. $\frac{3}{4}, \frac{7}{10}$

28. $\frac{3}{4}, \frac{5}{6}$

29. $\frac{5}{6}, \frac{7}{8}$

30. $\frac{7}{150}, \frac{11}{200}$

ANSWERS 1. yes 3. no 5. yes 7. yes 9. 1/4 cup < 3/4 cup 11. $\frac{3}{4} > \frac{3}{10}$ 13. $\frac{2}{9} < \frac{5}{9}$ 15. $\frac{1}{5} > \frac{1}{6}$ 17. $\frac{1}{10} > \frac{1}{20}$ 19. $\frac{1}{150} > \frac{1}{200}$ 21. $\frac{3}{4}$ cup > $\frac{2}{3}$ cup 23. $\frac{3}{5} < \frac{2}{3}$ 25. $\frac{2}{5} < \frac{7}{10}$ 27. $\frac{3}{4} > \frac{7}{10}$ 29. $\frac{5}{6} < \frac{7}{8}$

1-9. AVOIDING ERRORS

Errors are natural. All health professionals—doctors, pharmacists, technicians, as well as nurses—make errors at times. In fact, over many years, studies have shown that one in every five doses of medication is likely to be wrong. But as Michael Cohen observes, "an informed and aware nurse . . . can be the final defense in preventing a medication error from reaching the patient."* Preventive recommendations include, over and over again, the words **check** and **recheck.** The habit of checking, an essential part of the problem solving process, becomes ingrained by practice and builds self-confidence.

A common method of checking is simply repeating a calculation. Although this method has some merit, its defect is that we can be repeating the error. The secret of a good check is to change some aspect of the calculation.

A good way to check addition and multiplication is to switch the order of the numbers.

* Cohen M.R. *200 Medication Errors and How to Avoid Them.* Springhouse, PA: Springhouse Corporation, 1991:iii.

CHECKING ADDITION AND MULTIPLICATION

Reverse the order of the numbers.

$$\frac{1}{2} \times \frac{2}{3} = \frac{1}{3}$$

Check: $$\frac{2}{3} \times \frac{1}{2} = \frac{1}{3}$$

Examples

1. Compute: $25 + 34 = 59$.
   Check: $34 + 25 = 59$ also.
2. The computation may be done vertically.

Add down

$$\begin{array}{r} 25 \\ +\,34 \\ \hline 59 \end{array}$$

59 ↑ Check by adding up

3. Compute: $\frac{1}{3} + \frac{3}{4} = 1\frac{1}{12}$

   Check: $\frac{3}{4} + \frac{1}{3} = 1\frac{1}{12}$

SAMPLE EXERCISES

1. Add and check: $\frac{1}{2} + \frac{3}{8} + \frac{1}{4}$.

2. Find the sum of $2\frac{5}{10}$ and $4\frac{7}{10}$, and check.

Exercises 3–4. Find the indicated product and check.

3. $\frac{2}{3}$ of $2\frac{1}{4}$

4. $5\frac{1}{4} \times \frac{2}{7}$

ANSWERS

1. Method: $\frac{1}{2} + \frac{3}{8} + \frac{1}{4} = \frac{4 + 3 + 2}{8} = \frac{9}{8} = 1\frac{1}{8}$

   Check: $\frac{1}{4} + \frac{3}{8} + \frac{1}{2} = \frac{2 + 3 + 4}{8} = \frac{9}{8} = 1\frac{1}{8}$ also.

2. *Computation* *Check*

$7\frac{2}{10} = 7\frac{1}{5}$ also.

Add down

$$\begin{array}{r} 2\frac{5}{10} \\ +\,4\frac{7}{10} \\ \hline 6\frac{12}{10} \\ 7\frac{2}{10} = 7\frac{1}{5} \end{array}$$

Add up

3. Method: $\frac{2}{3} \times 2\frac{1}{4} = \frac{2}{3} \times \frac{9}{4} = \frac{3}{2}$

   Check: $2\frac{1}{4} \times \frac{2}{3} = \frac{9}{4} \times \frac{2}{3} = \frac{3}{2}$ also.

4. Method: $5\frac{1}{4} \times \frac{2}{7} = \frac{21}{4} \times \frac{2}{7} = \frac{3}{2} = 1\frac{1}{2}$

   Check: $\frac{2}{7} \times 5\frac{1}{4} = \frac{2}{7} \times \frac{21}{4} = 1\frac{1}{2}$ also.

To check subtraction and division in the recommended way, we use a different method; we backtrack.

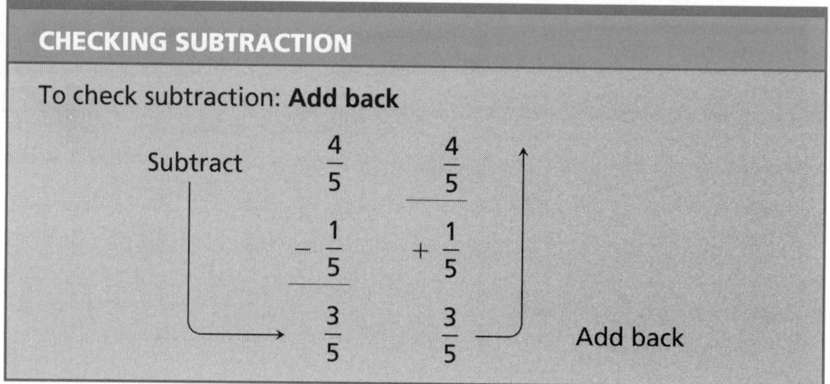

Examples

1. Compute $\frac{2}{3} - \frac{1}{4} = \frac{5}{12}$

   Check: Add back. Take the answer, $\frac{5}{12}$. Add the number that we subtracted, $\frac{1}{4}$. The sum should be the number we started with, $\frac{2}{3}$.

$$\frac{5}{12} + \frac{1}{4} = \frac{2}{3}$$

2. Subtract

$$\begin{array}{r} \frac{2}{3} \\ -\frac{1}{4} \\ \hline \frac{5}{12} \end{array} \qquad \begin{array}{r} \frac{2}{3} \\ \hline +\frac{1}{4} \\ \frac{5}{12} \end{array}$$

Add back

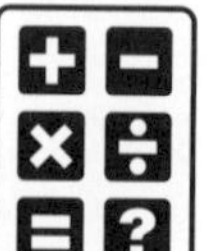

SAMPLE EXERCISES

1. Subtract and check: $\frac{3}{8} - \frac{1}{4}$.
2. Subtract $3\frac{1}{5}$ from $7\frac{3}{5}$, and check.

ANSWERS

1. Compute: $\frac{3}{8} - \frac{1}{4} = \frac{3-2}{8} = \frac{1}{8}$

   Check: $\frac{1}{8} + \frac{1}{4} = \frac{1+2}{8} = \frac{3}{8}$

2.

	Computation	*Check*	
Subtract →	$7\frac{3}{5}$	$7\frac{3}{5}$	Add back ↑
	$-\ 3\frac{1}{5}$	$+\ 3\frac{1}{5}$	
	$4\frac{2}{5}$	$4\frac{2}{5}$	

We use the same backtracking to check division that we use for subtraction.

CHECKING DIVISION

To check division: **multiply back**

$$\frac{3}{4} \div \frac{1}{4} = 3$$

$$\text{Check:} \quad 3 \times \frac{1}{4} = \frac{3}{4}$$

Examples

1. Compute $8 \div 2 = 4$.
Check: Multiply back. Take the quotient, 4, and multiply by the divisor, 2. The result should be the number we started with, 8.

$$4 \times 2 = 8$$

2. Compute $\frac{1}{4} \div \frac{5}{8} = \frac{2}{5}$.
Check: Multiplying back, take the quotient, $\frac{2}{5}$, and multiply by the divisor, $\frac{5}{8}$. The result should be the number we started with, $\frac{1}{4}$.

$$\frac{2}{5} \times \frac{5}{8} = \frac{1}{4}$$

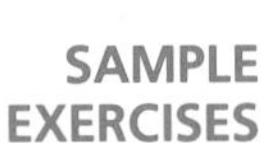

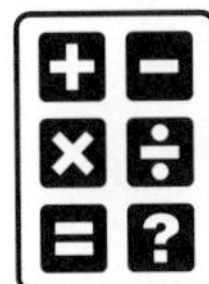

1. Divide $5\frac{1}{3}$ by $\frac{4}{9}$, and check.
2. Simplify

$$\frac{\frac{1}{100}}{\frac{1}{10}}$$

and check.
3. Change $\frac{13}{4}$ to a mixed number and check.

ANSWERS

1. *Computation*

$5\frac{1}{3} \div \frac{4}{9}$

$\frac{16}{3} \times \frac{9}{4}$

12

Check

Does $12 \times \frac{4}{9} = 5\frac{1}{3}$?

$12 \times \frac{4}{9}$

$\frac{16}{3} = 5\frac{1}{3}$

2. Method: $\dfrac{\frac{1}{100}}{\frac{1}{10}} = \dfrac{1}{100} \div \dfrac{1}{10}$

$\dfrac{1}{100} \div \dfrac{1}{10} = \dfrac{1}{100} \times \dfrac{10}{1} = \dfrac{1}{10}$

Check: Does $\dfrac{1}{100} \div \dfrac{1}{10} = \dfrac{1}{10}$?

Yes, because $\dfrac{1}{10} \times \dfrac{1}{10} = \dfrac{1}{100}$.

3. Method: $\dfrac{13}{4} = 13 \div 4 = 3\frac{1}{4}$

Check: Does $\dfrac{13}{4} = 3\frac{1}{4}$?

Yes, because $3\frac{1}{4} \times 4 = \frac{13}{4} \times 4 = 13$.

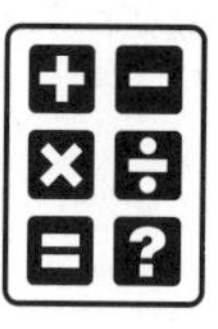

EXERCISES

Exercises 1–16. Compute as indicated, and check.

1. $\dfrac{3}{4} + \dfrac{4}{5}$
2. $\dfrac{5}{6} + \dfrac{1}{4}$
3. $\dfrac{3}{10} + \dfrac{9}{100}$
4. $8\frac{2}{3} + 5\frac{5}{6}$
5. $3\frac{27}{100} + 4\frac{3}{1000}$
6. $3\frac{5}{6} + 1\frac{2}{3} + 7\frac{3}{4}$
7. $\dfrac{5}{6} - \dfrac{2}{3}$
8. $32\frac{99}{100} - 11\frac{3}{10}$
9. $4\frac{3}{10} - 1\frac{1}{100}$
10. $8 - 3\frac{4}{5}$
11. $\dfrac{3}{8} \times \dfrac{7}{10}$
12. $\dfrac{3}{7} \times 14$
13. $\dfrac{6}{25} \times \dfrac{5}{9}$
14. $2\frac{1}{5} \times 2\frac{3}{11}$
15. $\dfrac{\frac{1}{3}}{\frac{4}{9}}$
16. $5\frac{5}{6} \div 10$

Exercises 17–18. Change to a mixed number and check.

17. $\dfrac{17}{6}$
18. $\dfrac{23}{3}$

Exercises 19–20. Change to a fraction and check.

19. $8\frac{2}{5}$
20. $3\frac{7}{10}$

21. Ronda K. receives a total daily dose of $4\frac{1}{2}$ caffeine tablets. If the total daily dose is divided into 3 equal doses, what is the amount of each dose?

22. A certain antimalarial tablet contains 25 milligrams of drug. If a child takes $\frac{3}{4}$ of the tablet, how many milligrams of drug are taken?

ANSWERS 1. $\dfrac{3}{4} + \dfrac{4}{5} = 1\frac{11}{20} = \dfrac{4}{5} + \dfrac{3}{4}$ 3. $\dfrac{39}{100}$ 5. $7\frac{273}{1000}$ 7. $\dfrac{5}{6} - \dfrac{2}{3} =$

$\frac{1}{6}$; $\frac{1}{6} + \frac{2}{3} = \frac{5}{6}$ 9. $3\frac{29}{100}$ 11. $\frac{3}{8} \times \frac{7}{10} = \frac{21}{80} = \frac{7}{10} \times \frac{3}{8}$ 13. $\frac{2}{15}$

15. $\frac{3}{4}$ 17. $2\frac{5}{6}$ 19. $\frac{42}{5}$ 21. $\frac{3}{2}$ tablet, or 1 1/2 tablet

1-10. SUMMARY

1. MEANING OF FRACTIONS
   (a) To compare a **part** to the **whole**

   ← ½ inch →

   ←—— 1 inch ——→

   (b) To indicate **division:** $\frac{6}{3} = 6 \div 3$.

2. TERMS OF A FRACTION

   $\dfrac{\textbf{Numerator}}{\textbf{Denominator}}$ or **Numerator / Denominator** $= N \div D$ or $D\overline{)N}$

Numerator:	3
Fraction bar:	–
Denominator:	5

   Numerator ⟶ 3/5 ⟵ Denominator

3. EXPANDING AND REDUCING TERMS

   We may **multiply** or **divide** the numerator and denominator by the **same whole number** (except 0) without changing the value of the fraction.

   Examples: $\frac{2}{3} = \frac{10}{15}$ since $\frac{2}{3} = \frac{2 \times 5}{3 \times 5}$

   $\frac{20}{12} = \frac{5}{3}$ since $\frac{20}{12} = \frac{20 \div 4}{12 \div 4}$

4. REDUCING TO LOWEST TERMS

   Divide both terms by the same whole number. Repeat until no further common divisors exist. (To use a shortcut, divide both terms by the greatest common divisor.)
   Example: To reduce $\frac{30}{36}$, divide both terms by 2. Thus, $\frac{30}{36} = \frac{15}{18}$. Now divide both terms by 3. Thus, $\frac{15}{18} = \frac{5}{6}$.
   (Shortcut: Divide both terms of $\frac{30}{36}$ by 6.)

5. CHANGING TO ANOTHER FORM
   (a) To change a fraction **to** a mixed number, **divide.**

   $$\frac{3}{2} = 3 \div 2 = 1\tfrac{1}{2}$$

   (b) To change **from** a mixed number to a fraction, **multiply** the whole number by the denominator and **add** the numerator to the product. Keep the **same denominator.**

   $$4\tfrac{5}{8} = \frac{32 + 5}{8} = \frac{37}{8}$$

6. ADDING AND SUBTRACTING

(a) If the **denominators** are **equal,** add (or subtract) the **numerators,** and keep the same denominator.

$$\frac{1}{5}+\frac{3}{5}=\frac{4}{5}; \qquad \frac{4}{5}-\frac{3}{5}=\frac{1}{5}$$

(b) If the **denominators** are **not equal,** use the least common denominator (LCD) to expand terms. Add (or subtract) the new numerators and keep the **LCD as the denominator** of the result.

$$\frac{3}{8}+\frac{1}{6}=\frac{9}{24}+\frac{4}{24}=\frac{13}{24}$$

7. MULTIPLYING

Reduce fractions wherever possible. **Multiply numerators** and **multiply denominators.**

$$\frac{4}{5}\times\frac{1}{6}=\frac{\overset{2}{\cancel{4}}}{5}\times\frac{1}{\underset{3}{\cancel{6}}}$$

$$=\frac{2\times 1}{5\times 3}$$

$$=\frac{2}{15}$$

8. DIVIDING

Invert the divisor (second term) and multiply.

$$9\div\frac{3}{4}=\overset{3}{\cancel{9}}\times\frac{4}{\underset{1}{\cancel{3}}}$$

$$=12$$

9. INEQUALITY SIGNS

$>$ means "(is) greater than"; $<$ means "(is) less than"; (the tip points to the smaller quantity).

Examples: (a) $\frac{2}{3}>\frac{1}{3}$ and $\frac{1}{3}<\frac{2}{3}$

(b) Systolic blood pressure >150 may be dangerous for some patients.

10. RELATIVE SIZE

In a pair of fractions with

(a) **Equal denominators,** the larger fraction has the larger **numerator**

$$\frac{3}{4}>\frac{1}{4}$$

(b) **Equal numerators,** the **smaller** fraction has the **larger denominator**

$$\frac{1}{4}<\frac{1}{2}$$

(c) **Unequal numerators** and **unequal denominators,** expand terms, so that both fractions have the **same denominator**

$$\frac{3}{4}>\frac{7}{10} \quad \text{because} \quad \frac{15}{20}>\frac{14}{20}$$

11. CHECKING

(a) Addition and multiplication: Reverse order.

$$\frac{1}{2} \times \frac{2}{3} = \frac{1}{3}; \quad \frac{2}{3} \times \frac{1}{2} = \frac{1}{3}$$

(b) Subtraction and division: Backtrack (use the inverse operation).

$$\frac{4}{5} - \frac{1}{5} = \frac{3}{5} \quad \text{and} \quad \frac{3}{5} + \frac{1}{5} = \frac{4}{5};$$

$$\frac{4}{5} \div \frac{1}{5} = 4 \quad \text{and} \quad \frac{1}{5} \times 4 = \frac{4}{5}$$

EXERCISES FOR EXTRA PRACTICE

Exercises 1–4. Express the fraction as a whole number.

1. $\frac{25}{25}$
2. $\frac{64}{4}$
3. 48/12
4. 490/10

Exercises 5–8. Reduce the fraction to lowest terms.

5. $\frac{12}{150}$
6. $\frac{50}{75}$
7. $\frac{280}{440}$
8. $\frac{20}{180}$

Exercises 9–12. Change the fraction to a mixed number and check.

9. 6/5
10. $\frac{83}{20}$
11. $\frac{37}{12}$
12. $\frac{89}{40}$

Exercises 13–26. Compute as indicated and check.

13. $7\frac{1}{6} + 3\frac{5}{8}$
14. $12\frac{1}{10} + 6\frac{7}{1000}$
15. $10\frac{7}{8} - 4\frac{1}{4}$
16. $12 - 2\frac{7}{10}$
17. $\frac{2}{3} \times \frac{9}{10}$
18. $\frac{9}{16} \times \frac{10}{21}$
19. $\frac{5}{10} \times 1000$
20. $\frac{250}{450} \times 500$
21. $1\frac{1}{2} \times \frac{4}{9}$
22. $2\frac{2}{3} \times 1\frac{5}{16}$
23. $9 \div \frac{3}{5}$
24. $\frac{5}{6} \div \frac{5}{9}$
25. $\frac{\frac{1}{100}}{\frac{1}{200}}$
26. $\frac{\frac{1}{100}}{\frac{1}{10}}$

Exercises 27–30. Insert the appropriate inequality sign between the fractions.

27. $\frac{6}{14} \quad \frac{6}{10}$
28. $\frac{8}{300} \quad \frac{8}{200}$

29. $\frac{5}{7}$ $\frac{4}{7}$ 30. $\frac{23}{150}$ $\frac{38}{150}$

31. If pyridostigmine bromide (Regonol) is given orally, the dose may be 180 milligrams. If the same medication is given by injection, the dose is $\frac{1}{30}$ of the oral dose. How many milligrams are given in the injection?

32. Each serving of fish weighs $3\frac{1}{2}$ ounces. What is the weight of $2\frac{2}{3}$ servings?

33. Find the number of minutes in $5\frac{3}{4}$ hours.

34. Find the number of minutes in $10\frac{1}{3}$ hours.

Exercises 35–36. Express the result as a fraction and as a mixed number.

35. How many hours are in 1385 minutes?

36. How many days are in 180 hours?

ANSWERS 1. 1 3. 4 5. $\frac{2}{25}$ 7. $\frac{7}{11}$ 9. 1 1/5 11. $3\frac{1}{12}$

13. $10\frac{19}{24}$ 15. $6\frac{5}{8}$ 17. $\frac{3}{5}$ 19. 500 21. $\frac{2}{3}$ 23. 15 25. 2

27. $\frac{6}{14} < \frac{6}{10}$ 29. $\frac{5}{7} > \frac{4}{7}$ 31. 6 milligrams 33. 345 minutes

35. $23\frac{1}{12}$ hours

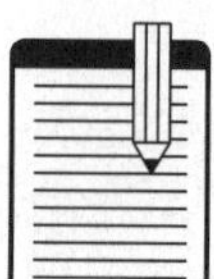

CHAPTER TEST

1. Change $\frac{99}{4}$ to a mixed number. ________

2. Change $5\frac{2}{3}$ to a fraction. ________

3. Simplify $\frac{400}{20} \times 10$. ________

4. Reduce $\frac{48}{54}$ to lowest terms. ________

5. Insert an inequality sign between the following fractions: $\frac{1}{9}$ $\frac{1}{10}$. ________

Questions 6–9. Compute as indicated.

6. $8\frac{1}{6} + 9\frac{1}{2}$ ________

7. $35 - 11\frac{2}{3}$ ________

8. $4\frac{1}{2} \times 9\frac{1}{3}$ ________

9. $5\frac{5}{6} \div 10$ ________

10. To relieve angina, a patient took 4 nitroglycerin tablets in one day. The amount of drug in each tablet was 1/400 grain. What was the total amount of nitroglycerin taken? ________

ANSWERS 1. $24\frac{3}{4}$ 2. $\frac{17}{3}$ 3. 200 4. $\frac{8}{9}$

5. $\frac{1}{9} > \frac{1}{10}$ or $\frac{1}{10} < \frac{1}{9}$ 6. $17\frac{2}{3}$ 7. $23\frac{1}{3}$ 8. 42 9. $\frac{7}{12}$

10. 1/100 grain

TWO

Decimal Fractions

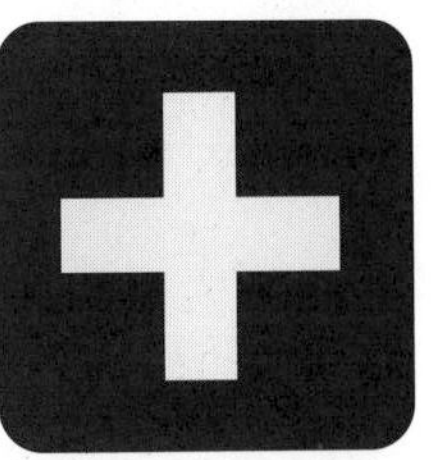

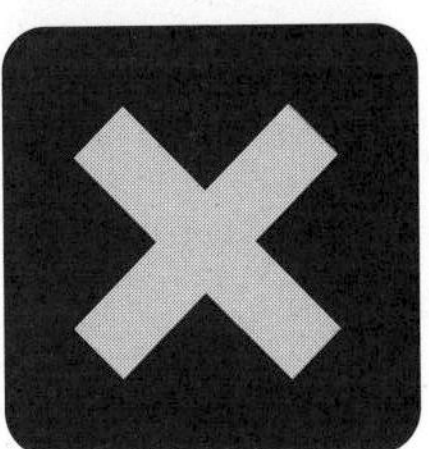

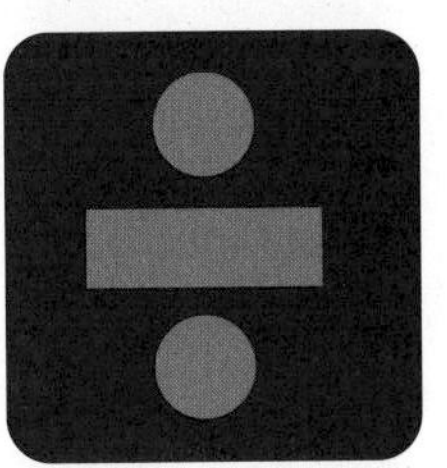

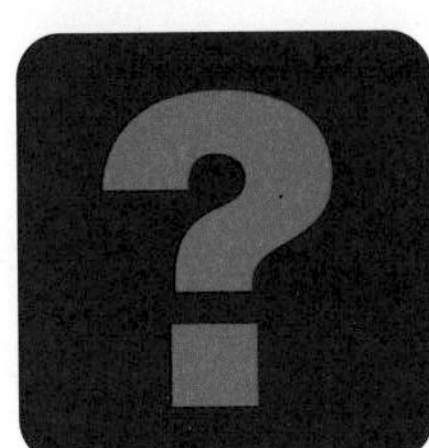

▶ OUTLINE

2-1. INTRODUCTION
2-2. MEANING OF DECIMAL FRACTIONS
2-3. RELATIVE SIZE OF MIXED DECIMALS
2-4. ADDING AND SUBTRACTING MIXED DECIMALS
2-5. MULTIPLYING MIXED DECIMALS
2-6. DIVIDING MIXED DECIMALS
2-7. SHORTCUTS FOR MULTIPLYING AND DIVIDING BY 10s
2-8. ROUNDING
2-9. AVOIDING ERRORS: ESTIMATION
2-10. SUMMARY

▶ OBJECTIVES

After studying this unit, you will be able to:

1. Interpret decimal form.
2. Convert from decimal form to fraction form, and vice versa.
3. Add, subtract, multiply, and divide decimals.
4. Judge the relative size of decimals.
5. Round numbers.
6. Estimate results.
7. Use decimals to solve simple verbal problems.

2-1. INTRODUCTION

Decimal fractions are a shorthand way of writing common fractions. Statements using decimal fractions are simpler, and computations are faster. (As with all shortcuts, special care must be taken to prevent errors.)

Examples

1. "Draw the solution +0.5 cc of air into the syringe." (Instructions for an intramuscular injection)
2. "Dilute with 0.9% normal saline." (Instructions for intravenous therapy)
3. "0.25 mg/kg" (Doctor's order for daily dosage of a medication)

Proficiency Gauge

It is possible that you understand the concepts explained in this chapter and can skip it. Gauge your proficiency by working out the following exercises. Uncover the answers that follow the test only after you have answered all the questions.

1. Write $\frac{3}{8}$ in decimal form. 1. ____________
2. Write 0.003 as a common fraction. 2. ____________
3. Arrange in order of size, smallest first: 1.101, 0.01, 0.0001, 0.10, 1.001. 3. ____________
4. Round 159.127 to hundredths. 4. ____________

Exercises 5–9. Compute as indicated.

5. $2.1 + 3.002 + 0.21$ 5. ____________
6. $21.35 - 2.001$ 6. ____________
7. $\frac{24.35}{100}$ 7. ____________
8. 3.125×8.2 8. ____________
9. $8.0136 \div 1.06$ 9. ____________
10. A baby is drinking about 4.25 ounces of liquid 6 times a day. About how much liquid is the baby drinking each day? 10. ____________

ANSWERS 1. 0.375 2. $\frac{3}{1000}$ 3. 0.0001, 0.01, 0.10, 1.001, 1.101 4. 159.13 5. 5.312 6. 19.349 7. 0.2435 8. 25.625 9. 7.56 10. 25.5 ounces

---

2-2. MEANING OF DECIMAL FRACTIONS

By a temperature reading of 102.1°F, we mean 102 degrees **and** $\frac{1}{10}$ of a degree. The decimal fraction is a shortcut for writing the common fraction $\frac{1}{10}$.

A **decimal fraction** denotes a common fraction whose **denominator** is 10, or 100, 1000, and so on.

$$0.4 = \frac{4}{10}, \quad 0.76 = \frac{76}{100}, \quad 0.234 = \frac{234}{1000}$$

Examples

1. Instead of $\frac{1}{10}$, or $\frac{2}{10}$, $\frac{3}{10}$, $\frac{4}{10}$, $\frac{5}{10}$, and so on, we may write

   0.1, 0.2, 0.3, 0.4, 0.5, . . .

   The decimal point replaces the fraction bar (or slash) and the denominator. The "0" to the left of the decimal point indicates a value <1.*
2. The decimal fractions 0.23, 0.145, and 0.098 are shortcuts for the common fractions $\frac{23}{100}$, $\frac{145}{1000}$, and $\frac{98}{1000}$. Here again, we see how the decimal point replaces the fraction bar and the denominator.
3. All common fractions can be expressed exactly or approximately as fractions with denominators 10 or 100, 1000, and so forth. For instance, $\frac{3}{4} = 0.75$ exactly, and $\frac{1}{3} = 0.33$ approximately.

While the decimal point replaces the fraction bar and the denominator, it is the number of decimal places that tells us whether the denominator is 10 or 100, 1000, and so on.

DECIMAL PLACES

The **number of decimal places** in a decimal fraction is equal to the number of digits **to the right** of the decimal point, which is also equal to the number of **zeros** in the denominator of the corresponding common fraction.

$$0.76 = \frac{76}{100}$$

2 decimal places — 2 zeros in the denominator

Examples

1. Each of the decimal fractions 0.1, 0.2, 0.3, . . . 0.9 has **one** decimal place because there is **one** digit to the **right** of the decimal

* It is important to write the zero before the decimal point. In "200 Medication Errors and How to Avoid Them" (Springhouse, PA: Springhouse Corp., 1991, p. 24), Michael Cohen relates the case of a patient who was overdosed because ".5" (which should have been written as "0.5") was read as "5."

point. The corresponding fractions, $\frac{1}{10}$, $\frac{2}{10}$, $\frac{3}{10}$, and so on, have **one** zero in the denominator.

2. In decimal form, $\frac{1}{100} = 0.01$; we use two decimal places because there are two zeros in the denominator.
3. There are three decimal places in $0.492 = \frac{492}{1000}$.
4. To read a decimal fraction, we simply pronounce the common fraction that it represents.

$$0.1 = \frac{1}{10} = \text{one tenth}$$

$$0.123 = \frac{123}{1000} = \text{one hundred twenty-three thousandths}$$

$$1.23 = 1\tfrac{23}{100} = \text{one and twenty-three hundredths}$$

5. We may also count off decimal places to tell which denominator is intended.

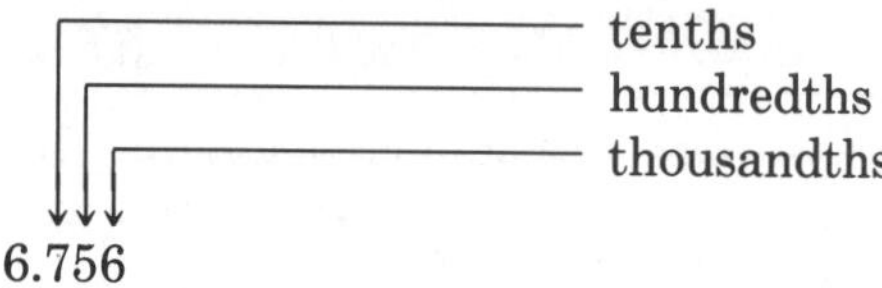

6.756

7 in the first decimal place, represents $\frac{7}{10}$
5 in the second decimal place, represents $\frac{5}{100}$
6 in the third decimal place, represents $\frac{6}{1000}$

$$\text{Thus, } 6.756 = 6 + \frac{7}{10} + \frac{5}{100} + \frac{6}{1000} = 6\tfrac{756}{1000}.$$

6. On the label of the unit dose digoxin tablet, we see the dosage strength, "0.125 mg," which means $\frac{125}{1000}$ milligram.

60 mL NDC 0081-0264-27

LANOXIN®
(DIGOXIN)
ELIXIR PEDIATRIC
Each mL contains
50 μg (0.05 mg)
PLEASANTLY FLAVORED

Alcohol 10%, Methylparaben 0.1% (added as a preservative)
For indications, dosage, precautions, etc., see accompanying package insert.
Store at 15° to 25°C (59° to 77°F) and protect from light.
CAUTION: Federal law prohibits dispensing without prescription.

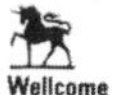

BURROUGHS WELLCOME CO.
RESEARCH TRIANGLE PARK, NC 27709
Made in U.S.A. 542399

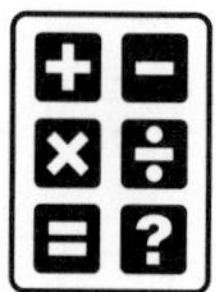

SAMPLE EXERCISES

Exercises 1–5. Complete the following table.

	Common Fraction	*Corresponding Decimal*	*Words*
1.			three tenths
2.	$\frac{27}{100}$		
3.		0.03	
4.		0.495	
5.	$\frac{3}{1000}$		

ANSWERS

1. $\frac{3}{10}$	0.3	three tenths
2. $\frac{27}{100}$	0.27	twenty-seven hundredths
3. $\frac{3}{100}$	0.03	three hundredths
4. $\frac{495}{1000}$	0.495	four hundred ninety-five thousandths
5. $\frac{3}{1000}$	0.003	three thousandths

It is often convenient to expand or reduce the number of decimal places in a decimal fraction, just as we expand or reduce the terms of a common fraction. (See Section 1–4.)

EXPANDING DECIMAL PLACES

We may **add** or **drop** zeros to the **right** of the **last** digit in a decimal fraction **without** changing the value of the fraction.

$$0.76 = 0.7600$$

because

$$\frac{76}{100} = \frac{7600}{10{,}000}$$

Examples

1. We may write 0.7 as 0.700, a three-place decimal, since

$$\frac{7}{10} = \frac{700}{1000}$$

2. When we add zeros in a decimal fraction, we must be careful **not** to insert them directly to the right of the decimal point, between the decimal point and other digits. Such an insertion **decreases** the value of the fraction.

$$0.7 > 0.\overset{\downarrow}{0}7$$

because

$$\frac{7}{10} > \frac{7}{100}$$

3. We may write 0.70000 as a one-place decimal, 0.7, because

$$\frac{70{,}000}{100{,}000} = \frac{7}{10}$$

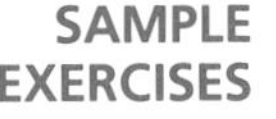

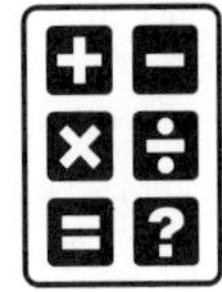

Exercises 1–2. Make the indicated change without changing the value of the decimal fraction.

1. Change 0.012 to a four-place decimal.
2. Change 0.2300 to a two-place decimal.

ANSWERS 1. 0.0120 2. 0.23

EXERCISES

Exercises 1–10. Change to decimal form.

1. $\frac{76}{100}$
2. $\frac{7}{10}$
3. $\frac{63}{1000}$
4. $\frac{731}{10,000}$
5. $\frac{3}{100}$
6. $\frac{9}{1000}$
7. $\frac{77}{10,000}$
8. $\frac{852}{100,000}$
9. $\frac{40}{100}$
10. $\frac{30,000}{100,000}$

Exercises 11–18. Fill in the table.

	Common Fraction	*Corresponding Decimal*	*Words*
11.	$\frac{84}{100}$		
12.	$\frac{7}{10,000}$		
13.		0.365	
14.		0.89	
15.			two hundred forty-six thousandths
16.			eighty-eight hundredths
17.		0.301	
18.		0.0004	

19. Change 93.002 to a five-place decimal.
20. Change 22.95 to a three-place decimal.
21. Change 4.090 to a two-place decimal.
22. Change 34.96000 to a three-place decimal.

ANSWERS 1. 0.76 3. 0.063 5. 0.03 7. 0.0077 9. 0.40

11.	$\frac{84}{100}$	0.84	eighty-four hundredths
13.	$\frac{365}{1000}$	0.365	three hundred sixty-five thousandths
15.	$\frac{246}{1000}$	0.246	two hundred forty-six thousandths

17. $\frac{301}{1000}$ 0.301 three hundred one thousandths

19. 93.00200 21. 4.09

2-3. RELATIVE SIZE OF MIXED DECIMALS

The recommended maximum daily dose of acetohexamide is 1.5 grams. The amount 1.5 is an example of a mixed decimal, the sum of a decimal fraction and a whole number. A mixed decimal is just like a mixed number with a common fraction.

A **mixed decimal** is the sum of a **whole** number and a **decimal fraction.**

$$4.76 = 4 + 0.76$$

Examples

	Mixed Number	*Mixed Decimal*	*Words*
1.	$1\frac{9}{10}$	1.9	one **and** nine tenths
2.	$23\frac{7}{100}$	23.07	twenty-three **and** seven hundredths

SAMPLE EXERCISES

Exercises 1–3. Complete the table.

	Mixed Number	*Mixed Decimal*	*Words*
1.	$49\frac{29}{100}$		
2.		3.102	
3.			five hundred and thirty-seven thousandths

ANSWERS 1. 49.29 = forty-nine and twenty-nine hundredths
2. $3\frac{102}{1000}$ = three and one hundred two thousandths 3. $500\frac{37}{1000}$ = 500.037

Relative Size

The recommended maximum dose of alprazolam is 0.5 milligrams. A particular patient may need a smaller amount. It is easy to compare amounts if they have the same number of decimal places.

COMPARING MIXED DECIMALS

To compare mixed decimals: **align decimal points** and decimal places; then **add zeros** so that all quantities have the same number of decimal places.

0.250
0.500 (Largest amount)
0.099

Examples

1. We compare 0.25, 0.5, and 0.099 by changing them all to three-place decimals and aligning them:

   0.250
   0.500
   0.099

   Now it is easy to see that 500 thousandths > 250 thousandths > 99 thousandths. This process is the same as comparing common fractions that have the same denominator.
2. To compare 0.2 with 0.007, we change 0.2 to a three-place decimal and align the numbers:

   0.200
   0.007

   It becomes clear that 200 thousandths > 7 thousandths.
3. We can compare the mixed numbers 2.1 and 1.999 by writing:

   2.100
   1.999

   In this case the whole numbers take precedence. We see clearly that the top amount is greater because it is more than 2 and the bottom number is less than 2.

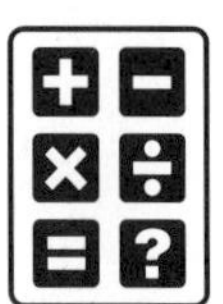

SAMPLE EXERCISES

Exercises 1–2. Insert an inequality sign (< or >) between the amounts.

1. 0.7 0.45
2. 0.999 3.2

ANSWERS 1. 0.7 > 0.45 2. 0.999 < 3.2

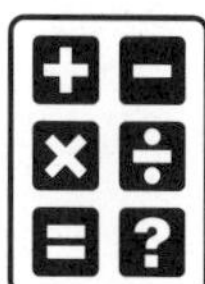

EXERCISES

Exercises 1–12. Complete the table.

	Mixed Number	*Mixed Decimal*	*Words*
1.		2.5	
2.		4.9	

3. $2\frac{3}{10}$		
4. $5\frac{61}{100}$		
5.	72.6	
6.	18.92	
7.		thirty-two and seventeen hundredths
8.		nine hundred twenty-five and sixteen thousandths
9. $34\frac{7}{1000}$		
10. $285\frac{31}{1000}$		
11.	62.04	
12.	23.08	

Exercises 13–16. Label the statement true or false.

13. 1.7 grams = 1.70 grams
14. 1.2 grams = 1.02 grams
15. 8.5 ounces = 8.500 ounces
16. 3.0 liters = 3 liters

Exercises 17–20. Sometimes a patient is required to have <0.6 milligram of a drug. Do the following given amounts fit the requirement?

17. 0.19 milligram
18. 5 milligrams
19. 1.1 milligrams
20. 0.07 milligram

Exercises 21–24. The recommended oral dose of triprolidine hydrochloride (Actifed) for a child older than 6 is 1.25 milligrams. Compare the following given amounts with the recommended dose.

21. 1.025 milligrams
22. 1.250 milligrams
23. 2.00 milligrams
24. 0.99 milligram

Exercises 25–32. Use "<" or ">" to compare the given quantities.

25. 0.5 inch 0.06 inch
26. 1.3 inches 1.009 inches
27. 0.442 1.442
28. 9.01 0.910
29. 4.3 4.25
30. 5.67 5.0679
31. 125.2 121.9
32. 37.001 370.01

Exercises 33–36. For certain patients, a dose of butorphanol tartrate should be $>$ 0.5 milligram, but $<$ 2 milligrams. Are the following given doses within the required limits?

33. 0.25 milligram
34. 2.5 milligrams
35. 0.75 milligram
36. 2.0 milligrams

ANSWERS

1. $2\frac{5}{10}$	2.5	two and five tenths
3. $2\frac{3}{10}$	2.3	two and three tenths
5. $72\frac{6}{10}$	72.6	seventy-two and six tenths
7. $32\frac{17}{100}$	32.17	thirty-two and seventeen hundredths
9. $34\frac{7}{1000}$	34.007	thirty-four and seven thousandths
11. $62\frac{4}{100}$	62.04	sixty-two and four hundredths

13. true 15. true 17. yes 19. no 21. Less than, 1.025 milligrams < 1.25 milligrams 23. More than, 2.00 milligrams > 1.25 milligrams 25. 0.5 inch > 0.06 inch 27. 0.442 < 1.442 29. 4.3 > 4.25 31. 125.2 > 121.9 33. no, too little 35. yes

2-4. ADDING AND SUBTRACTING MIXED DECIMALS

Suppose that a patient is receiving succinylcholine chloride by intravenous therapy: 2 milligrams during the first minute, 2.47 milligrams during the second minute, and 2.5 milligrams during the third minute. It is easy to find the total amount by aligning the decimal points and adding.

Adding

ADDING

Align decimal points and decimal places; then **add zeros** to equalize the number of decimal places. Place the decimal point in the answer. Add without regard to the decimal point. Check by reversing the order.

$$2 + 2.47 + 2.5 = \begin{array}{r} 2.00 \\ 2.47 \\ +\ 2.50 \\ \hline 6.97 \end{array}$$

Examples

1. To find the sum of 2 milligrams, 2.47 milligrams, and 2.5 milligrams, set up the addition by aligning the decimal point and adding zeros to equalize decimal places:

$$\text{Add} \downarrow \begin{array}{r} 2.00 \\ 2.47 \\ \underline{2.50} \\ 6.97 \end{array} \quad \begin{array}{c} 6.97 \\ \uparrow \end{array} \text{ Check}$$

2. A baby gained 1.4 pounds during her first month, 0.8 pounds during the second, and 1 pound during the third. We can find the total number of pounds gained by adding 1.4, 0.8, and 1.

$$\text{Add} \downarrow \begin{array}{r} 1.4 \\ 0.8 \\ \underline{1.0} \\ 3.2 \end{array} \quad \begin{array}{c} 3.2 \\ \uparrow \end{array} \text{ Check}$$

3. To find the sum of 10.052, 7.8, and 3.12, align decimal points and decimal places, adding zeros where necessary:

```
                        20.972
Add  |  10.052            ↑
     |   7.800            |
     |   3.120            |   Check
     ↓  20.972
```

SAMPLE EXERCISES

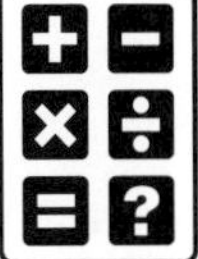

Exercises 1–2. Compute as indicated.

1. 0.2 + 0.05 + 0.111
2. 7.3 + 2.4 + 0.06

ANSWERS 1. 0.361 2. 9.76

Subtracting

SUBTRACTING

Align decimal points and decimal places; then **add zeros** to equalize the number of decimal places. Place the decimal point in the answer. Subtract without regard to the decimal point. Check by adding back.

```
10.3 − 0.009 =   10.300
               −  0.009
                 10.291
```

Examples

```
1. Subtract    10.300    10.300
   |         −  0.009      ↑   Add back
   ↓           10.291      |   to check

2. Subtract    0.20       0.20
   |         − 0.05        ↑   Add back
   ↓           0.15        |   to check
```

SAMPLE EXERCISES

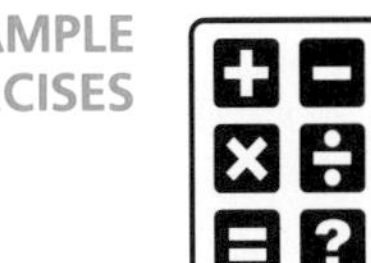

Exercises 1–2. Compute as indicated.

1. 0.542 − 0.31
2. 76.25 − 23.154

ANSWERS 1. 0.232 2. 53.096

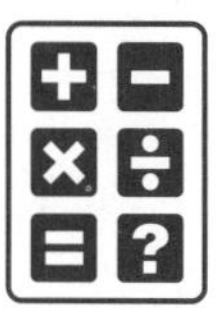

EXERCISES

Exercises 1–6. Find the sum of the mixed decimals and check.

1. 8.25 + 2.34
2. 9.134 + 7.215
3. 49.2 + 37.11
4. 83.5 + 6.53
5. 226.64 + 18.035
6. 58.002 + 12.24

Exercises 7–12. Find the difference between the mixed decimals and check.

7. 9.16 − 3.25
8. 12.215 − 8.316
9. 58.3 − 46.02
10. 92.6 − 7.44
11. 317.57 − 27.126
12. 67.103 − 21.33

Exercises 13–18. Compute as indicated.

13. \$25.32 + \$63.41
14. \$72.50 − \$34.41
15. 1.23 inches + 7.5 inches
16. 6.75 inches + 4.2 inches
17. 0.025 gram + 1.25 grams
18. 35.4 grams + 12.005 grams
19. A stethoscope costs \$20.38 and a blood pressure measurement apparatus (sphygmomanometer) costs \$31.12. What was the total cost of both items?
20. An infant measured 19.75 inches at birth. One month later, he was 22.5 inches. How much had he grown?

ANSWERS 1. 10.59 3. 86.31 5. 244.675 7. 5.91 9. 12.28 11. 290.444 13. \$88.73 15. 8.73 inches 17. 1.275 grams 19. \$51.50

2–5. MULTIPLYING MIXED DECIMALS

Multiplying

If a patient takes 3.5 tablets every day, each containing 0.025 gram of hydrochlorothiazide, it is easy to find the total daily amount by multiplying 0.025 by 3.5.

MULTIPLYING MIXED DECIMALS

Ignore decimal points and multiply; then count the **total number of decimal places** in the quantities multiplied; then place the decimal point in the product. The product has the **same** number of decimal places as the total number of decimal places in the original quantities.

0.02 5	3 decimal places	3.5	
× 3.5	+ 1 decimal place	× 0.02 5	
12 5		17 5	
75		70	
0.0 87 5	4 decimal places	0.0 87 5	Check by reversing order

Examples

1.

$$\begin{array}{rl} 0.4 & \text{1 decimal place} \\ \underline{\times 0.2} & + \text{1 decimal place} \\ 0.08 & \text{2 decimal places} \end{array}$$

In common fraction form, this multiplication would be

$$\frac{4}{10} \times \frac{2}{10} = \frac{8}{100}$$

2.

$$\begin{array}{rl} 0.04 & \text{2 decimal places} \\ \underline{\times 0.002} & + \text{3 decimal places} \\ 0.00008 & \text{5 decimal places} \end{array}$$

In common fraction form, this multiplication would be

$$\frac{4}{100} \times \frac{2}{1000} = \frac{8}{100{,}000}$$

3. A tablet of clemastine fumarate may contain 1.34 milligrams. If a patient takes 3 tablets every day, we can compute the total daily dose by multiplying 1.34 by 3.

$$\begin{array}{rl} 1.34 & \text{2 decimal places} \\ \underline{\times \ 3} & + \text{0 decimal places} \\ 4.02 & \text{2 decimal places} \end{array}$$

4.

Finding a Product	Checking the Product	
3.25	1.45	Check by reversing the order
× 1.45	× 3.25	
16 25	7 25	
1 30 0	29 0	
3 25	4 35	
4.71 25	4.71 25	

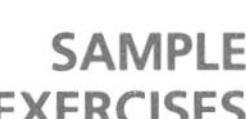

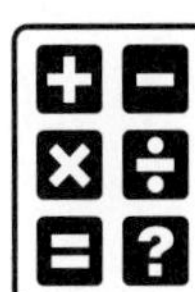

1. Insert the decimal point in the product:

$$\begin{array}{r} 0.23 \\ \underline{\times 4.51} \\ 1\ 0\ 3\ 7\ 3 \end{array}$$

Exercises 2–4. Multiply as indicated and check.

2. 0.03 × 15

3. 0.8 × 0.005

4. 87.92 × 10

ANSWERS 1. 1.0373 2. 0.45 3. 0.0040 = 0.004 4. 879.2

EXERCISES

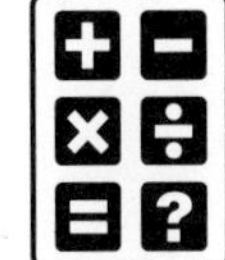

Exercises 1–8. Insert the decimal point in the product.

1.

$$\begin{array}{r} 1.21 \\ \underline{\times 2.056} \\ 2\ 4\ 8\ 7\ 7\ 6 \end{array}$$

2.

$$\begin{array}{r} 1.4896 \\ \underline{\times 0.2} \\ 2\ 9\ 7\ 9\ 2 \end{array}$$

3. $\begin{array}{r} 8.11 \\ \times\ 3.22 \\ \hline 2\ 6\ 1\ 1\ 4\ 2 \end{array}$

4. $\begin{array}{r} 2.0034 \\ \times\ 1.33 \\ \hline 2\ 6\ 6\ 4\ 5\ 2\ 2 \end{array}$

5. $2.53 \times 15 = 3\ 7\ 9\ 5$

6. $42.3 \times 0.2 = 8\ 4\ 6$

7. $0.61 \times 0.72 = 4\ 3\ 9\ 2$

8. $0.31 \times 0.03 = 9\ 3$

Exercises 9–16. Find the product and check.

9. 0.625×4
10. 0.025×6
11. 1.38×0.5
12. 25.32×2.3
13. 4.5×60
14. 23.01×82.5
15. 36.5×7.5
16. 6.05×0.15
17. A child is receiving 0.5 milligram of dexchlorpheniramine maleate 6 times a day. What is the total amount of drug each day?
18. A recommended minimum dose of methantheline bromide for a child younger than 1 year is 12.5 milligrams 4 times a day. What is the recommended minimum total dose per day?
19. At $0.64 per pound, what is the cost of 2.5 pounds of bicarbonate of soda?
20. To comfort a baby, 0.12 ounce of sugar may be added to every ounce of sterile water that the baby drinks. How much sugar would be added to 14.75 ounces of sterile water?

ANSWERS 1. 2.48776 3. 26.1142 5. 37.95 7. 0.4392 9. 2.5 11. 0.69 13. 270 15. 273.75 17. 3 milligrams 19. $1.60

2-6. DIVIDING MIXED DECIMALS

Suppose that we need to give 22.5 milligrams of chlorazepate dipotassium and that tablets containing 3.75 milligrams are on hand. We can find the number of tablets needed by dividing 22.5 by 3.75. Once the decimal points are arranged, it is easy to divide.

> Move **both** decimal points an **equal** number of places to the **right** so that the divisor becomes a **whole number.** Mark the decimal point in the quotient **immediately.** Then divide without regard to the decimal point.
>
> $3.75\overline{)22.50} = 375.\overline{)2250.}$

Examples

1. $3.75\overline{)22.50} = 375.\overline{)2250.}$ with quotient $6.$

Moving the decimal point two places to the right is the same as multiplying both terms of a fraction by 100.

$$\frac{22.5^*}{3.75} = \frac{22.5 \times 100}{3.75 \times 100} = \frac{2250}{375}$$

2. We may use long division to simplify $\frac{42.721}{0.35}$. Set up the division and mark the decimal point:

$$0.35\,\overline{)\,42.721} = 35.\,\overline{)\,4272.1}$$

Carry out the division without regard to the decimal point. For accuracy, keep neat columns.

$$\begin{array}{r} 122.06 \\ 35\overline{)\,4272.10} \\ \underline{35} \\ 77 \\ \underline{70} \\ 72 \\ \underline{70} \\ 210 \\ \underline{210} \end{array}$$

3. To check division, multiply back. (Multiply the quotient by the divisor.) Is the above quotient correct? Does $\frac{42.721}{0.35} = 122.06$? Yes, because $122.06 \times 0.35 = 42.721$.
4. To change $\frac{5}{8}$ to decimal form, divide 5 by 8

$$8\overline{)\,5.000}$$

Does $\frac{5}{8} = 0.625$? Yes, because $0.625 \times 8 = 5$.

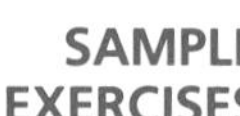

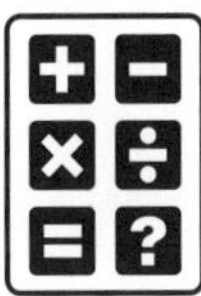

Exercises 1–3. To make the divisor a whole number, how must each decimal point be moved (if at all) in the indicated division?

1. $2.3\overline{)\,24.6882}$
2. $0.56\overline{)\,2016}$
3. $4\overline{)\,5.22228}$

Exercises 4–6. Divide and check.

4. $5\overline{)\,74.05}$
5. $9.8\overline{)\,0.49}$
6. $8\overline{)\,1}$
7. If 1.2 milliliters of penicillin G procaine contain 600,000 units of penicillin, how many units of penicillin are in 1 milliliter? (*Hint:* Divide 600,000 by 1.2.)

ANSWERS 1. 1 place to the right 2. 2 places to the right 3. not at all 4. 14.81 5. 0.05 6. 0.125 7. 500,000

* $\frac{22.5}{3.75}$ is a complex fraction that indicates division of 22.5 by 3.75. Whenever the numerator and/or denominator of a fraction is in decimal form, the fraction is called **complex.**

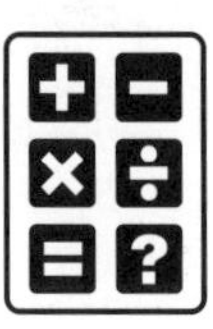

EXERCISES

Exercises 1–8. To make the divisor a whole number, how must each decimal point be moved (if at all) in the indicated division?

1. $7.81\overline{)30.0685}$
2. $12.43\overline{)18.645}$
3. $0.3\overline{)0.435}$
4. $250\overline{)1187.5}$
5. $0.025\overline{)24}$
6. $0.003\overline{)0.27}$
7. $375\overline{)1312.5}$
8. $500\overline{)225}$

Exercises 9–12. Change the common fraction to decimal form.

9. $\frac{15}{16}$
10. $\frac{7}{64}$
11. $\frac{375}{500}$
12. $\frac{13125}{75}$

Exercises 13–16. Divide as indicated and check.

13. $2.5\overline{)593.5}$
14. $0.04\overline{)0.32}$
15. $72 \div 0.018$
16. $8.4 \div 0.105$
17. A patient needs 0.5 milligram of a drug that comes in 0.25-milligram tablets. How many tablets are needed? (*Hint:* Divide 0.5 by 0.25.)
18. Suppose that a day's supply of 6.4 milliliters of medication is to be given in 4 equal doses. How many milliliters would you give per dose?
19. A patient takes 1.25 grams of levodopa each day. If 0.25-gram tablets are on hand, how many tablets are used per day?
20. If 2.5-milligram tablets of fluphenazine hydrochloride are available, how many tablets would be needed for a dose of 10 milligrams?

ANSWERS 1. 2 places to right 3. 1 place to right 5. 3 places to right 7. not at all 9. 0.9375 11. 0.75 13. 237.4 15. 4000 17. 2 tablets 19. 5 tablets

---

2-7. SHORTCUTS FOR MULTIPLICATION AND DIVISION BY 10s

Multiplying

In the decimal system, there is a simple shortcut for multiplying by a power of 10. By a power of 10, we mean 10 or 100, 1000, and so on. It is just a matter of moving the decimal point 1, 2, 3, or more places to the right, according to the number of zeros in the power of 10.

MULTIPLYING BY POWERS OF 10

To **multiply** by 10, 100, 1000, and so on, move the decimal point to the **right** 1, 2, 3, or more decimal places (as many places as there are zeros).

$0.1234 \times 10 = 1.234$ $\quad$ $0.1234 \times 100 = 12.34$

$0.1234 \times 1000 = 123.4$

Examples

Shortcut Decimal Form	*Common Fraction Form*
1. $0.1234 \times 10 = 1.234$	$\frac{1234}{10{,}000} \times 10 = \frac{1234}{1000}$
2. $0.1234 \times 100 = 12.34$	$\frac{1234}{10{,}000} \times 100 = \frac{1234}{100}$
3. $0.1234 \times 1000 = 123.4$	$\frac{1234}{10{,}000} \times 1000 = \frac{1234}{10}$
4. $0.1234 \times 10{,}000 = 1234$	$\frac{1234}{10{,}000} \times 10{,}000 = 1234$

5. \$2548.32 × 10 = \$25,483.20. Whenever we multiply by a power of 10, the product is more than the original number. If it is our money that is being multiplied, we become **richer.** This helps us to remember to move the decimal point to the **right.**

SAMPLE EXERCISES

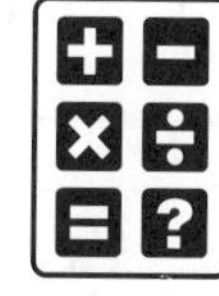

Exercises 1–4. Use the shortcut to find the indicated product.

1. $0.915 \times 10 = ?$
2. $1.805 \times 100 = ?$
3. $23.001 \times 1000 = ?$
4. $45.2 \times 1000 = ?$

ANSWERS 1. 9.15 2. 180.5 3. 23,001 4. 45,200

Dividing

There is a similar shortcut for dividing by a power of 10. In division, we move the decimal point 1, 2, 3, or more places to the left, according to the number of zeros in the power of 10.

DIVIDING BY POWERS OF 10

To **divide** by 10, 100, 1000, and so on, move the decimal point to the **left** 1, 2, 3, or more decimal places (as many places as there are zeros).

$123.4 \div 10 = 12.34$ $\quad$ $123.4 \div 100 = 1.234$

$123.4 \div 1000 = 0.1234$

Examples

Shortcut Decimal Form	*Common Fraction Form*
1. 1 2 3.4 ÷ 10 = 12.34	$\frac{1234}{10} \div 10 = \frac{1234}{10} \times \frac{1}{10} = \frac{1234}{100}$
2. 1 2 3.4 ÷ 100 = 1.234	$\frac{1234}{10} \div 100 = \frac{1234}{10} \times \frac{1}{100} = \frac{1234}{1000}$
3. 1 2 3.4 ÷ 1000 = 0.1234	$\frac{1234}{10} \div 1000 = \frac{1234}{10} \times \frac{1}{1000} = \frac{1234}{10{,}000}$

4. Every time we divide a number by a power of 10, the quotient is less than the original number. This reminds us to move the decimal point to the left.

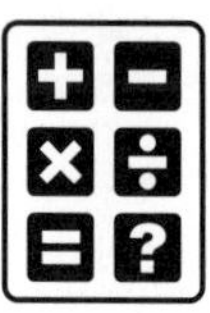

SAMPLE EXERCISES

Exercises 1–4. Use the shortcut to find the indicated quotient.

1. 20.9 ÷ 10 = ?
2. 180.5 ÷ 100 = ?
3. 0.1 ÷ 100 = ?
4. 45.2 ÷ 1000 = ?
5. A child is to receive a dose of 35 milligrams of chlorpromazine hydrochloride. If each tablet contains 10 milligrams, how many tablets should be given?

ANSWERS 1. 2.09 2. 1.805 3. 0.001 4. 0.0452 5. 3.5 tablets

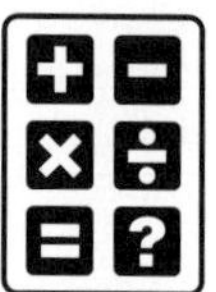

EXERCISES

Exercises 1–6. Complete the table.

Operation	*How to Move Decimal Point*	*Result Compared with Original Number*
1. Multiply by 10	1 place to right	More
2. Divide by 10	1 place to left	Less
3. Divide by 100		
4. Multiply by 100		
5. Multiply by 1000		
6. Divide by 1000		

Exercises 7–11. Use the shortcut to multiply each quantity by 10, 100, and 1000.

7. 69.237
8. 0.73296
9. 183.28
10. 6.3856
11. 0.0286

Exercises 12–16. Use the shortcut to divide each quantity by 10, 100, and 1000.

12. 59,123
13. 0.36296
14. 3648.3
15. 5.2846
16. 0.03

Exercises 17–24. Use the shortcut to compute as indicated.

17. 0.00034 × 100
18. 3.1416 × 1000
19. 70.04 ÷ 10
20. 0.00065 ÷ 100
21. 0.03 × 10,000
22. 0.0374 × 100,000
23. 10.012 × 10
24. 14.214 ÷ 1000

Exercises 25–26. In the following cases, the given quantity is the number of milligrams in a pemoline tablet. Find the total number of milligrams contained in 10 such tablets.

25. 18.75
26. 37.5

Exercises 27–28. One cup of milk contains 100 calories. How many calories are in the following number of cups?

27. 2.5
28. 3.25
29. The hospital paid a total amount of $7643.50 in bonuses equally to 10 nurses. How much did each nurse receive?
30. The dietitian weighed out equal portions of salad for 100 patients. The total amount of salad available for the whole group weighed 352.5 ounces. How many ounces did each patient receive?

ANSWERS

3. Divide by 100	2 places to left	Less
5. Multiply by 1000	3 places to right	More

7. 692.37, 6923.7, 69,237 9. 1832.8, 18,328, 183,280 11. 0.286, 2.86, 28.6 13. 0.036296, 0.0036296, 0.00036296 15. 0.52846, 0.052846, 0.0052846 17. 0.034 19. 7.004 21. 300 23. 100.12 25. 187.5 milligrams 27. 250 calories 29. $764.35

2-8. ROUNDING

Louise P. has accepted a position at $30,000 a year. It is easy to compute her weekly earnings: divide $30,000 by 52. The result is $576.92308, but we drop the digits after the second decimal place because the appropriate monetary expression is $576.92. The technical procedure for dropping digits after a specified decimal place is called **rounding.** By rounding, we are **approximating** a result instead of giving a more exact value. The approximation is as close as possible to the original number and often more useful.

RULES FOR ROUNDING TO A SPECIFIED DECIMAL PLACE

Underline the decimal places to be dropped. Look at the first digit to be dropped. Is it **less than 5?** If yes, simply **drop all underlined digits.** If no, first **add 1** to preceding digit, and then **drop** all underlined digits.

27.6485	= 27.6	rounded to tenths,
	= 27.65	rounded to hundredths, and
	= 27.649	rounded to thousandths

If a result is to be rounded to a specified decimal place, we need to compute only to one place **more** than the specified decimal place.

Examples

1. To round 27.6485 to tenths ("to the nearest tenth" or "to the first decimal place")
   Underline the decimal places to be dropped: 27.6$\underline{485}$
   Look at the first digit to be dropped: ↑
   Is 4 < 5? Yes.
   Drop all underlined digits.
   Result: 27.6
2. To round 27.6485 to hundredths ("to the nearest hundredth," or "to the second decimal place")
   Underline the decimal places to be dropped: 27.64$\underline{85}$
   Look at the first digit to be dropped: ↑
   Is 8 < 5? No.
   Add 1 to preceding digit and then drop all underlined digits.
   Result: 27.65
3. Round 4.2871 to 2 decimal places.
   Underline the decimal places to be dropped: 4.28$\underline{71}$
   Look at the first digit to be dropped: ↑
   Is 7 < 5? No.
   Add 1 to the preceding digit, and drop the last digits.
   Result: 4.29
4. Round 4.2871 to 3 places (thousandths).
   Underline the decimal places to be dropped: 4.287$\underline{1}$
   Look at the first digit to be dropped: ↑
   Is 1 < 5? Yes.
   Keep the preceding digit and drop the last digit.
   Result: 4.287
5. Round 2.75001 to the nearest tenth.
   Underline the decimal places to be dropped: 2.7$\underline{5001}$
   The first digit to be dropped is 5. ↑
   Is 5 < 5? No.
   Add 1 to the preceding digit and drop the last digits.
   Result: 2.8

6. Suppose that the numbers 8.13 and 8.17 are to be rounded to tenths (first decimal place). Both numbers lie between 8.1 and 8.2 (8.10 and 8.20). By following the rules, we round 8.13 **down** to 8.1 but we round 8.17 **up** to 8.2. This makes sense because 8.13 is nearer to 8.10 than to 8.20 but 8.17 is nearer to 8.20 than to 8.10.

SAMPLE EXERCISES

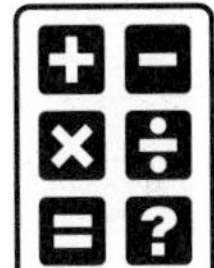

Exercises 1–3. Round as specified and fill in the table.

Problem	*Result*	*Reasoning*
1. Round 1.73 to the nearest tenth		Is $3 < 5$?
2. Round 4.28746 to the nearest hundredth		Is $7 < 5$?
3. Round 294.385001 to the nearest hundredth		Is $5 < 5$?

4. Change $\frac{2}{3}$ to a decimal fraction, rounding the result to 2 decimal places. (It is only necessary to compute to 3 decimal places.)
5. Divide 12.25 by 17 and round the result to the nearest tenth.

ANSWERS

1. Round 1.73 to the nearest tenth	1.7	Is $3 < 5$?	Yes
2. Round 4.28746 to the nearest hundredth	4.29	Is $7 < 5$?	No
3. Round 294.385001 to the nearest hundredth	294.39	Is $5 < 5$?	No

4. 0.67 5. 0.7

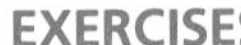

EXERCISES

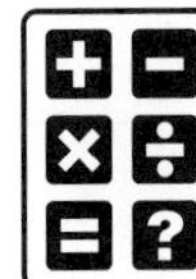

Exercises 1–8. Round the number to the nearest tenth.

1. 4.76
2. 4.651002
3. 4.65
4. 8.13
5. 8.17
6. 9.28
7. 35.21
8. 76.154

Exercises 9–14. Round the number to hundredths.

9. 4.215
10. 374.256
11. 2.467
12. 8.3752
13. 89.323
14. 6.825

Exercises 15–22. Round the numbers in the following table.

Number to be Rounded	*To 2 Places*	*To 3 Places*
15. 6.2871		
16. 544.287		
17. 4.28746		
18. 35.2149		
19. 76.1545		
20. 29.2575		

Exercises 21–26. Change each expression to decimal form, rounded to: (a) 1 decimal place, (b) 2 decimal places, (c) 3 decimal places.

21. $\frac{12}{35}$

22. $\frac{1}{15}$

23. $\frac{37.5}{11}$

24. $\frac{125.75}{3.5}$

25. $\frac{0.625}{17} \times 1.8$

26. $\frac{4.5}{17} \times 2.1$

ANSWERS 1. 4.8 3. 4.7 5. 8.2 7. 35.2 9. 4.22
11. 2.47 13. 89.32

15. 6.2871	6.29	6.287
17. 4.28746	4.29	4.287
19. 76.1545	76.15	76.155

21. 0.3, 0.34, 0.343 23. 3.4, 3.41, 3.409 25. 0.1, 0.07, 0.066

2-9. AVOIDING ERRORS: ESTIMATION

If we are purchasing items that cost \$8.10, \$2.30, and \$3.90, we get a quick idea if we have enough cash by mentally adding \$8, \$2, and \$4, noting that our total bill will be a little more than \$14. If the salesclerk gives us a bill for \$24.30, we sense an error and do not pay. Before any computation, it is important to make a quick and easy estimate of the result. With such an estimate in mind, we can spot gross errors immediately, even before we check. Estimations are our own approximations, ones that make mental computations easy.

ESTIMATING RESULTS

Choose easy approximations for mental computation

$$8.1 + 2.3 + 3.9 \approx 8 + 2 + 4 = 14 \text{ *}$$

14 is an estimate of 14.3

Examples

1. Before computing $8.1 + 2.3 + 3.9$
   Estimate: $8 \quad + 2 \quad + 4 \quad = 14$
   (Each quantity is replaced by the nearest whole number.)
2. Before computing $1.62 - 0.27$
   Estimate: $1.6 \quad - 0.3 \quad = 1.3$
3. An easy estimate of $5\frac{1}{4} \times 7\frac{1}{2}$ can be done by dropping the fractions: $5 \times 7 = 35$
4. You can quickly detect an error in a dosage computation. You see $4.5 \times 90 = 4050$. Your mental estimate of 360 (so much smaller than 4050) immediately alerts you to redo the multiplication.

---

* The symbol $\approx$ means "is approximately equal to."

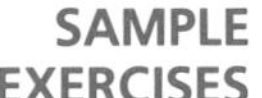

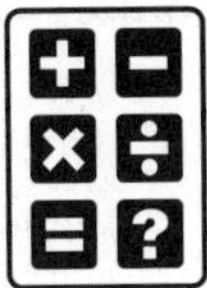

Exercises 1–6. Estimate mentally the result of the indicated computation.

1. $7.9 + 1.8 + 9.1$
2. $128.2 - 32.5$
3. 794×63
4. 7.2×6.3
5. $59.9 \div 3.1$
6. $2\frac{1}{3} + 9\frac{3}{4}$

Exercises 7–8. Explain why the following results are obviously wrong.

7. $20 \times 4.2 = 8.40$
8. $71.25 \div 10 = 712.5$

ANSWERS 1. $8 + 2 + 9 = 19$ 2. $130 - 30 = 100$ 3. $800 \times 60 = 48{,}000$ 4. $7 \times 6 = 42$ 5. $60 \div 3 = 20$ 6. $2 + 10 = 12$ 7. $20 \times 4 = 80$, so 8.4 is too small 8. $70 \div 10 = 7$, much smaller than 712.5

Estimating before computing and checking after computing are essential for saving time and money, and most important of all, for saving **lives.** A computation is incomplete without an **estimate and a check.**

COMPLETE COMPUTATION PROCEDURE
Estimate first, then **compute,** then **check.**

Examples

1. Before computing $8.1 + 2.3 + 3.9$

   Estimate: 14

   Compute: ↓ 8.1 + 2.3 + 3.9 = 14.3 ↑ *Check:* 14.3 (Add up)

   (Result is reasonably close to the estimate.)

2. Find $1.62 - 0.27$.

   Estimate: 1.3

   Compute: ↓ 1.62 − 0.27 = 1.35 ↑ *Check:* 1.62 (Add back)

   (Result is reasonably close to the estimate.)

3. Find $5\frac{1}{4} \times 7\frac{1}{2}$.

   Estimate: 35

   Compute: $39\frac{3}{8}$

   Check: $7\frac{1}{2} \times 5\frac{1}{4} = 39\frac{3}{8}$

   (Result is reasonably near estimate.)

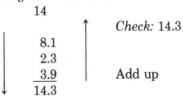

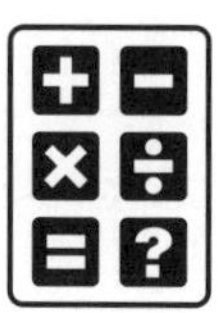

EXERCISES

Exercises 1–8. Estimate the result of the computation.

1. $3.8 + 2.1$
2. $18.3 - 11.8$
3. 7×8.5
4. $80.5 \div 2.3$
5. 52.98×278.22
6. $829 \div 10.3$
7. $1\frac{2}{3} + 5\frac{1}{8}$
8. $5\frac{1}{150} \times 2\frac{1}{200}$

Exercises 9–18. Estimate, compute, and check.

9. $2.9 + 6.8 + 1.7$
10. $2.3 + 4.9 + 1.8 + 3.3$
11. $23.4 + 49.8$
12. 3.9×8
13. $163.2 \div 4.8$
14. $277.2 - 42.3$
15. $49.3 + 7.4 + 134.8$
16. $2\frac{1}{3} + 5\frac{3}{4}$
17. $15\frac{1}{8} - 4\frac{3}{5}$
18. $1\frac{2}{3} \div 1\frac{7}{8}$

Exercises 19–24. Explain why the following results, drawn from actual student quizzes, are obviously wrong and should have been caught by the students before they handed in their papers.

19. $60 \times 8.5 = 380$
20. $37.4 \times 23 = 112.2$
21. $9.6 \div 10 = 96$
22. $1000 \div 450 = 22$
23. $19.3 \times 2 = 386$
24. $0.8 \times 250 \div 1.7 = 1176.4$

ANSWERS 1. 6 3. 63 5. 15,000 7. 7 9. 12, 11.4, 11.4 11. 70, 73.2, 73.2 13. 30, 34, 34 15. 190, 191.5, 191.5 17. 10, $10\frac{21}{40}$, $10\frac{21}{40}$ 19. $60 \times 8 = 480 > 380$ 21. $10 \div 10 = 1 < 96$ 23. $20 \times 2 = 40 < 386$

2-10. SUMMARY

1. A decimal fraction denotes a common fraction whose denominator is a power of 10 (that is, 10, 100, or 1000, etc.). The number of decimal places in a decimal fraction is equal to the number of zeros in the denominator of the corresponding common fraction.

2 zeros in 100	$\frac{76}{100} = 0.76$	2 decimal places
3 zeros in 1000	$\frac{17}{1000} = 0.017$	3 decimal places

2. Adding or dropping zeros to the right of the rightmost digit in a decimal fraction does not change the value of the fraction.

$$5.17 = 5.170 = 5.1700 = 5.17000 = 5.170000$$

3. To add, subtract, or compare mixed decimals, align decimal points and decimal places; then add zeros so that all quantities have the same number of decimal places.

To add 4.01272, 0.3, 10.101, and 0.0099:

$$\begin{array}{r} 4.01272 \\ 0.30000 \\ 10.10100 \\ \underline{0.00990} \\ 14.42362 \end{array}$$

Ranked in decreasing order, the numbers are: 10.10100 > 4.01272 > 0.30000 > 0.00990.

4. The product of mixed decimals has the same number of decimal places as the sum of the decimal places in the original numbers.

2.137	3 decimal places
× 4.11	2 decimal places
8.78307	5 decimal places

5. To divide mixed decimals, move both decimal points an equal number of places to the right so that the divisor becomes a whole number. Mark the decimal point in the quotient immediately, and then divide without regard to the decimal point.

$$3.75\overline{)23.25} = 375.\overline{)2325.}$$

$$\begin{array}{r} 6.2 \\ 375\overline{)2325.0} \\ \underline{2250} \\ 750 \\ \underline{750} \\ 0 \end{array}$$

6. Shortcuts for multiplication and division by powers of 10.

Operation	How to Move Decimal Point	Example
Multiply by 10	Right, 1 place	65.123 × 10 = 651.23
Divide by 10	Left, 1 place	65.123 ÷ 10 = 6.5123
Multiply by 100	Right, 2 places	65.123 × 100 = 6512.3
Divide by 100	Left, 2 places	65.123 ÷ 100 = 0.65123
Multiply by 1000	Right, 3 places	65.123 × 1000 = 65,123
Divide by 1000	Left, 3 places	65.123 ÷ 1000 = 0.065123
Multiply by, or divide by any power of 10	Right or left as many places as zeros in the power of 10	

7. To round to a specified decimal place, compute to 1 place **more** than the decimal place specified. Look at the first digit to be dropped. If it is less than 5, keep the preceding digit; otherwise, add 1 to the preceding digit. Then drop all digits to the right.

Rounded to tenths:	$27.6\underline{485} = 27.6$
Rounded to hundredths:	$27.64\underline{85} = 27.65$
Rounded to thousandths:	$27.648\underline{5} = 27.649$

8. To prevent errors in computations, first estimate, then compute, then check.

   To estimate, use approximations that make mental computation easy. Check addition or multiplication by changing the order of the numbers; check subtraction or division by adding or multiplying back.

   Find 1.62 − 0.27.

   Estimate: 1.3

   Compute: *Check:* 1.62

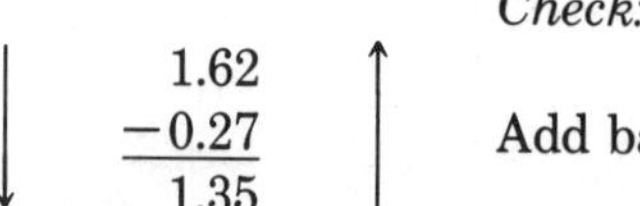

   (Result is reasonably close to the estimate.)

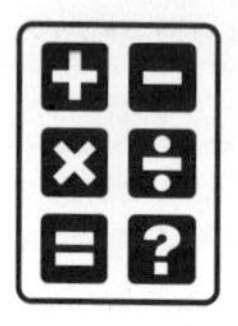

EXERCISES FOR EXTRA PRACTICE

Exercises 1–4. Change the decimal fraction to a common fraction in lowest terms.

1. 2.7
2. 3.24
3. 41.02
4. 1.2003

Exercises 5–12. Change the common fraction to decimal form.

5. $\frac{3}{10}$
6. $\frac{77}{100}$
7. $\frac{87}{1000}$
8. $\frac{3}{1000}$
9. $\frac{7}{8}$
10. $\frac{5}{16}$
11. $\frac{32}{125}$
12. $\frac{25}{32}$

Exercises 13–16. Insert "<" or ">" between the numbers.

13. 0.23 0.2003
14. 0.007 0.06
15. 0.1734 0.01744
16. 0.101095 0.10111

Exercises 17–24. Compute as indicated.

17. $0.1 + 2.005 + 0.3201$
18. $5.004 - 4.2$
19. $600 - 350.25$
20. 749.32×1000
21. 7.056×23
22. 1.035×7.2
23. $\frac{9.02}{1000}$
24. $\frac{73.1}{1.7}$

Exercises 25–28. Complete the table by rounding as indicated.

Number to be Rounded	*To 1 place*	*To 2 places*
25. 45.6529		
26. 2.0576		
27. 56.83556		
28. 549.873		

Exercises 29–30. Compute as indicated and give the result correct to the nearest tenth.

29. $96.75 \div 18.3$

30. $\frac{0.48}{1.7} \times 250$

Exercises 31–34. Some children with edema should have <1.6 milligrams of acetazolamide each day. Do the following amounts fit the requirement?

31. 1.28 milligrams

32. 1.06 milligrams

33. 15 milligrams

34. 1.60 milligrams

35. If each ounce of a certain cough syrup contains 0.045 gram of a drug, how much drug would be contained in 6.25 ounces? (Round to the nearest hundredth.)

36. If 0.001 gram of alteplase is being administered each minute, how much alteplase will have been administered in 35 minutes?

37. If a cup of cooked kale contains 2.8 grams of fiber, how much fiber is in 1/3 cup? (Round to the first decimal place.)

38. If 4.2 grams of fiber are in a cup of quick-cooking dry oats, how many cups are needed for 5.25 grams?

ANSWERS 1. $2\frac{7}{10}$ 3. $41\frac{1}{50}$ 5. 0.3 7. 0.087 9. 0.875
11. 0.256 13. 0.23 > 0.2003 15. 0.1734 > 0.01744 17. 2.4251
19. 249.75 21. 162.288 23. 0.00902

25. 45.6529 45.7 45.65
27. 56.83556 56.8 56.84
29. 5.3 31. yes 33. no 35. 0.28 gram 37. 0.9 gram

CHAPTER TEST

1. Write 263.067 in fraction form. ______
2. Arrange in order of size (smallest first): 0.199, 0.0901, 1.01 ______
3. Express $\frac{9}{16}$ in decimal form, and round to the nearest hundredth. ______

Problems 4–9. Compute as indicated.

4. $100.001 + 0.1001 + 0.0101 + 1.01$ ______
5. $23.57 - 8.364$ ______
6. 1.89×1000 ______
7. $\frac{64.8}{1000}$ ______
8. 73.2×0.023 ______
9. $\frac{0.0616}{0.4}$ ______

10. A patient needs 0.375 milligram of a drug. If 0.25-milligram tablets are on hand, how many tablets are needed? ________

ANSWERS 1. $263\frac{67}{1000}$ 2. 0.0901, 0.199, 1.01 3. 0.56 4. 101.1212 5. 15.206 6. 1890 7. 0.0648 8. 1.6836 9. 0.154 10. 1.5 tablets

THREE

Ratio, Proportion, and Percent

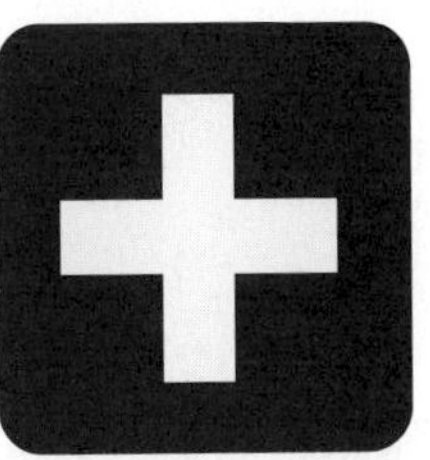
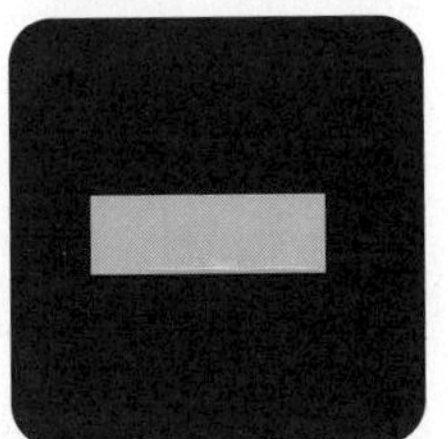
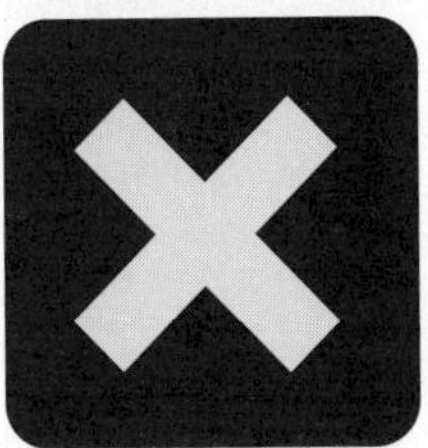

▶ OUTLINE

▶ OBJECTIVES

After studying this unit, you will be able to:

1. Express a comparison of two quantities in ratio form.
2. Simplify ratios.
3. Define "proportion."
4. Write and solve proportions.
5. Apply the concepts of ratio and proportion to the solution of rate problems.
6. Change any number from percent form to fraction or mixed number form or vice versa.
7. Find a percent of a given quantity.

3-1. INTRODUCTION

How do nurses use ratio, proportion, and percent? We use a ratio (the indicated division of two quantities) to make comparisons and a proportion to state that two ratios are equal. Percent is a special kind of ratio. Because so much information is presented in ratio (or percent) language, it helps to be fluent in that language. But most important, nurses need to be skillful with ratios in order to **prepare or check doses** and to **administer medications.**

Examples

1. "Epinephrine, 1:100,000" (ratio printed on a label)

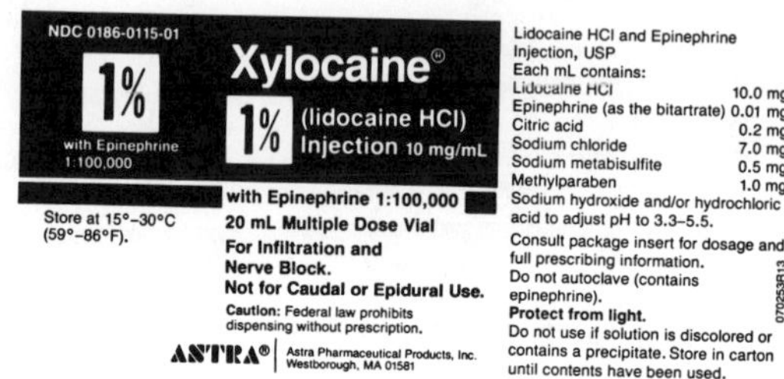

2. "100 milligrams/kilogram of body weight daily" (oral dosage of ampicillin ordered for a child)
3. Dextrose solution 20% is used for renal failure, but dextrose solution 50% is used to maintain blood volume.
4. If the patient is very young or very old, the dose must conform to restrictions that may be given by the ratio of the patient's age, weight, or body surface area to that of the average adult.

Proficiency Gauge

It is possible that you understand ratios and percents and can skip Chapter 3. Gauge your proficiency by working out the following exercises. Check your answers with those that follow the test only after you have answered all the questions.

If any rounding is required, round to two decimal places.

1. Find, in lowest terms, the ratio of the value of 1 dime to the value of 3 quarters. 1. ______
2. Simplify the ratio $\frac{1}{5}:3$. 2. ______
3. Solve the proportion $3:x = 1:40$. 3. ______
4. Solve the proportion $\frac{x}{100} = \frac{50}{2500}$. 4. ______
5. Change 2/3 to percent form. 5. ______
6. Change 0.102 to percent form. 6. ______
7. Change 0.1% to decimal form. 7. ______
8. A faucet is leaking at a rate of 50 drops/minute. How many drops will have leaked out in an hour? 8. ______

9. A patient received medication at a rate of 25 milligrams/hour. After 72 minutes, how much medication had he received? 9. ______

10. A bank gives 5.25% interest at the end of each year. If your balance at the beginning of the year was $2800, how much interest should you receive at the end of the year? 10. ______

ANSWERS 1. $\frac{2}{15}$, or 0.13 2. $\frac{1}{15}$, or 0.07 3. 120 4. 2 5. 66.67% 6. 10.2% 7. 0.001 8. 3000 drops 9. 30 milligrams 10. $147

3-2. RATIOS IN FRACTION AND COLON FORM

Sometimes, as in critical care areas, the patient-to-nurse ratio is $\frac{8}{4}$ (or "8 to 4"). This means that there are 8 patients to every 4 nurses, or twice as many patients as nurses.

> A **ratio** of two quantities is a comparison by **division** and appears in **fraction** or **colon** form.
>
> 8/4 = 8:4 = 8 ÷ 4

Examples

1. In one long-term care unit, there are 64 patients and 8 nurses. Thus, the ratio of patients to nurses is

$$\frac{\text{Number of patients}}{\text{Number of nurses}} = \frac{64}{8}, \text{ or “64 to 8.”}$$

Just as a fraction indicates the division of two numbers, a ratio indicates the division of two quantities.

2. In colon form, the ratio 64:8 means 64 ÷ 8. The colon : is an old-fashioned, shorthand way of writing the division sign. Fraction form is used much more often.

3. If we know that the patient-to-nurse ratio is $\frac{64}{8}$, then we also know the nurse-to-patient ratio:

$$\frac{\text{Number of nurses}}{\text{Number of patients}} = \frac{8}{64}$$

4. It is often convenient to reduce or expand terms.

Reducing the ratio $\frac{8}{64}$

In fraction form: $\frac{8}{64} = \frac{4}{32} = \frac{2}{16} = \frac{1}{8}$

In colon form: $8:64 = 4:32 = 2:16 = 1:8$

Instead of saying "There are 8 nurses for every 64 patients," we may say "There is 1 nurse for every 8 patients."

Expanding the ratio $\frac{8}{64}$

In fraction form: $\frac{8}{64} = \frac{16}{128} = \frac{32}{256}$

In colon form: 8:64 = 16:128 = 32:256

To say "There are 32 nurses for every 256 patients" is another way of saying "There are 8 nurses for every 64 patients."

5. We may eliminate decimal points by expanding terms, applying the shortcut for multiplying by 10's. By moving the decimal point the **same number** of places to the right in **both** terms, we do not change the value of the ratio.

$$\frac{1.1}{2.34} = \frac{1.10}{2.34} \quad \text{Each term is multiplied by 100}$$

$$= \frac{110}{234}$$

6. To simplify a ratio with fractional terms, we carry out the indicated division. The ratio

$$\frac{\frac{1}{2}}{\frac{1}{3}} = \frac{1}{2} \div \frac{1}{3}$$

$$= \frac{1}{2} \times \frac{3}{1} = \frac{3}{2}$$

7. If a term of a ratio is unknown, we use x to represent the unknown quantity until we find the information. Thus, $\frac{x}{5}$, or x:5 ("x to 5") represents the ratio of an unknown quantity to 5.

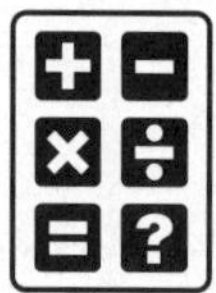

SAMPLE EXERCISES

1. Where the patient-to-nurse ratio is $\frac{8}{1}$, how many patients are there for every nurse?
2. Assume that the ratio of patients to nurses is "15 to 2." Write this ratio in fraction and colon forms.
3. Change 90:12 to fraction form and reduce the ratio to lowest terms.
4. Change $\frac{12.79}{5.3}$ to an equivalent ratio without decimals.
5. Simplify

$$\frac{3\frac{1}{2}}{5}.$$

ANSWERS 1. 8 patients 2. $\frac{15}{2} = 15:2$ 3. $\frac{90}{12} = \frac{15}{2}$ 4. $\frac{1279}{530}$

5. $\frac{7}{2} \div \frac{5}{1} = \frac{7}{2} \times \frac{1}{5} = \frac{7}{10}$

EXERCISES

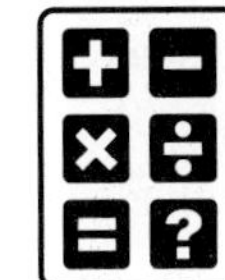

Exercises 1–6. Write the given ratio and the required ratio in fraction and colon form.

1. (a) In hospital H, the ratio of patients to nurses is 40 to 7.
   (b) In the same hospital, what is the ratio of nurses to patients?
2. (a) The ratio of doctors to US inhabitants is 23 per 10,000.
   (b) What is the ratio of US inhabitants to doctors?
3. (a) More women than men have osteoporosis; the ratio is about 5 to 1.
   (b) Fewer men than women have osteoporosis; what is the approximate ratio?
4. (a) In an infant's drink, the ratio of sugar to sterile water is about $\frac{1}{3}$ to 24.
   (b) In the same drink, what is the ratio of water to sugar?
5. (a) In pork sausage, the fat-to-protein ratio is about 16.3 to 8.4.
   (b) What is the protein-to-fat ratio?
6. (a) A waist-to-hip circumference ratio greater than 0.8 may be unhealthy.
   (b) A hip-to-waist circumference ratio less than what fraction may be unhealthy?

Exercises 7–10. Reduce the ratio to lowest terms.

7. $\frac{12}{20}$
8. $\frac{50}{10{,}000}$
9. 25:30
10. 18:33

Exercises 11–18. In a certain hospital, there are 50 attending physicians, 400 nurses, 3200 patients, and an unknown number (x) of volunteers. Write the specified ratio, reduced to lowest terms.

11. Number of nurses to number of patients
12. Number of patients to number of physicians
13. Number of nurses to number of physicians
14. Number of physicians to number of nurses
15. Number of physicians to number of patients
16. Number of patients to number of nurses
17. Number of patients to number of volunteers
18. Number of volunteers to number of nurses

Exercises 19–24. Simplify the ratio.

19. $\frac{1}{2}:\frac{1}{4}$
20. 1/3:3/4
21. $\frac{1/100}{9/1000}$
22. $\frac{\frac{7}{8}}{\frac{11}{16}}$
23. $8\frac{1}{3}:5$
24. $4\frac{1}{2}:\frac{1}{8}$
25. Which ratio is greater, $\frac{5}{6}:\frac{8}{9}$ or 30:32?
26. Which ratio is greater, (a) $\frac{0.1}{1000}$, or (b) $\frac{0.01}{10{,}000}$?

ANSWERS 1. (a) $\frac{40}{7} = 40:7$ (for every 40 patients, there are 7 nurses) (b) $\frac{7}{40} = 7:40$ 3. (a) $\frac{5}{1} = 5:1$; (b) $\frac{1}{5} = 1:5$ 5. (a) $\frac{16.3}{8.4} = 16.3:8.4$; (b) $\frac{8.4}{16.3} = 8.4:16.3$ 7. $\frac{3}{5}$ 9. $\frac{5}{6}$ 11. $\frac{400}{3200} = \frac{1}{8}$ 13. $\frac{400}{50} = \frac{8}{1}$ 15. $\frac{50}{3200} = \frac{1}{64}$ 17. $\frac{3200}{x}$ 19. $\frac{1}{2}:\frac{1}{4} = \frac{1}{2} \times \frac{4}{1} = \frac{2}{1}$ 21. $\frac{1}{100}:\frac{9}{1000} = \frac{1}{100} \times \frac{1000}{9} = \frac{10}{9}$ 23. $\frac{25}{3}:\frac{5}{1} = \frac{25}{3} \times \frac{1}{5} = \frac{5}{3}$ 25. neither; both ratios $= \frac{15}{16}$

3-3. TYPES OF RATIOS

In every ratio, we must take great care with units of measurement. Misunderstandings about units can be dangerous. We may omit units when they are identical in numerator and denominator, but must **never** omit them when they are **not** identical. A ratio with no units is called a **pure ratio.**

PURE RATIOS

In a **pure ratio** (a ratio of numbers without units), **both terms** of the original ratio must have **identical units.**

$$\frac{5 \text{ inches}}{12 \text{ inches}} = \frac{5}{12}$$

The pure ratio is a relationship between measurements that holds true no matter what common unit is used.

Examples

1. Since 12 inches = 1 foot,

$$\frac{5 \text{ inches}}{1 \text{ foot}} = \frac{5 \cancel{\text{inches}}}{12 \cancel{\text{inches}}} = \frac{5}{12}$$

(Identical units may be omitted, or "canceled.")

2. 5 inches to 1 foot is **not** 5:1, because the units (inch and foot) are not identical. It is clear that the quantity 5 inches is not 5 times greater than 1 foot!
3. The ratio of 3 pints of vanilla ice cream to 1 quart of chocolate ice cream is **not** $\frac{3}{1}$, because the units (pint and quart) are different. We do not have 3 times as much vanilla ice cream as chocolate!
4. Because there are 2 pints in every quart,

$$\frac{3 \text{ pints}}{1 \text{ quart}} = \frac{3 \cancel{\text{pints}}}{2 \cancel{\text{pints}}} = \frac{3}{2}$$

5. Because 8 ounces = 1 cup, we can change

$$\frac{16 \text{ ounces}}{1 \text{ cup}} \quad \text{to} \quad \frac{2 \cancel{\text{cups}}}{1 \cancel{\text{cup}}} \quad \text{or} \quad 2:1$$

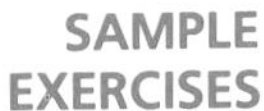

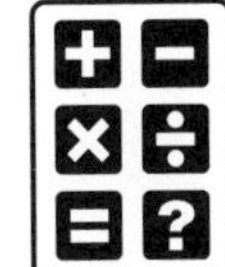

Exercises 1–6. Express the given comparison as a pure ratio, a ratio in which the units are not specified.

1. \$5 to \$2
2. 5 cents to 2 cents
3. \$5 to 2 cents
4. 5 cents to \$2
5. 5 inches to 2 feet
6. 5 feet to 2 inches

ANSWERS 1. $\frac{5}{2}$ 2. $\frac{5}{2}$ 3. $\frac{500}{2} = \frac{250}{1}$ 4. $\frac{5}{200} = \frac{1}{40}$

5. $\frac{5 \cancel{\text{inches}}}{24 \cancel{\text{inches}}} = \frac{5}{24}$ 6. $\frac{60 \cancel{\text{inches}}}{2 \cancel{\text{inches}}} = \frac{60}{2} = \frac{30}{1}$

If 72 beats/minute ("72 beats per minute") is a normal pulse rate, how many beats do you expect to count in 30 seconds? This question illustrates the importance of the type of ratio called a rate.

RATES

A **rate** is a ratio comparing two **different** types of measurements whose units must be shown.

72 beats / minute

Examples

1. Normal pulse rate is 72 beats/minute. To find the number of beats in 30 seconds, we may replace 1 minute by 60 seconds and reduce the terms.

$$\frac{72 \text{ beats}}{1 \text{ minute}} = \frac{72 \text{ beats}}{60 \text{ seconds}} = \frac{\overset{36}{\cancel{72}} \text{ beats}}{\underset{30}{\cancel{60}} \text{ seconds}} = \frac{36 \text{ beats}}{30 \text{ seconds}}$$

We should expect to count 36 beats every 30 seconds.

2. A salary rate is \$600/week ("\$600 per week"). To find the yearly salary, we may expand the terms of the ratio.

$$\frac{\$600}{1 \text{ week}} = \frac{\$600 \times 52}{1 \text{ week} \times 52} = \frac{\$31{,}200}{52 \text{ weeks}} = \frac{\$31{,}200}{1 \text{ year}}$$

3. There are about 6 grams of fiber in every 4 ounces of cooked black-eyed peas. The ratio of fiber content to weight of peas is

$$\frac{6 \text{ grams}}{4 \text{ ounces}} = \frac{\overset{3}{\cancel{6}} \text{ grams}}{\underset{2}{\cancel{4}} \text{ ounces}} = \frac{3 \text{ grams}}{2 \text{ ounces}}, \quad \text{or} \quad \frac{3}{2} \text{ grams/ounce}$$

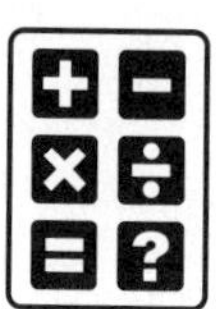

SAMPLE EXERCISES

1. We find that a dripping faucet has filled an 8-ounce glass in 4 hours. At what rate per hour has the faucet been dripping?
2. The milk container states: "2000 units vitamin A added per quart." Per ounce, how many units of vitamin A are added? (*Reminder:* 32 ounces = 1 quart.)
3. At a constant rate of 55 miles per hour, how many miles does an auto travel in 4.25 hours?
4. What is Ms. K.'s weight gain per month if she gained 12.8 pounds in 2 1/2 months?

ANSWERS 1. $\frac{\text{8 ounces}}{\text{4 hour}} = \frac{\text{2 ounces}}{\text{1 hour}} = \text{2 ounces/hour}$

2. $\frac{\text{2000 units}}{\text{1 quart}} = \frac{\text{2000 units}}{\text{32 ounces}} = \text{62.5 units/ounce}$

3. $\frac{\text{55 miles}}{\text{1 hour}} = \frac{55 \times \text{4.25 miles}}{1 \times \text{4.25 hours}} = \frac{\text{233.75 miles}}{\text{4.25 hours}}$. The auto travels 233.75 miles in 4.25 hours. 4. 5.1 pounds per month because $12.8 : \frac{5}{2} = 12.8 \times \frac{2}{5} = \frac{25.6}{5} = \frac{5.1}{1}$

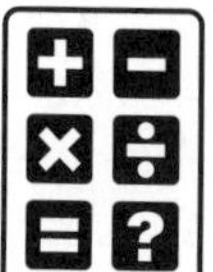

EXERCISES

Exercises 1–8. Express the given comparison as a pure ratio (a ratio in which the units are not specified).

1. $1 to $3
2. 1 cent to 3 cents
3. 5 ounces to 1 pound
4. 6 pints to 1 quart
5. 2 cents to $5
6. 1 nickel to $1
7. 3 inches to 2 feet
8. 3 quarters to $3

Exercises 9–14. Express the rate in lowest terms. (Units must be stated.)

9. The ratio of 50 grams to 10 ounces
10. The ratio of 400 miles to 4 hours
11. The ratio of 60 drops to 60 seconds
12. The ratio of 30 drops to 2 milliliters
13. The ratio of $150 to 6 uniforms
14. The ratio of 35 pens to $7

Exercises 15–16. It is important to notify the physician if the patient's rate of respiration is <12/minute. For the following given rate of respiration, would you notify the physician?

15. 20 respirations in 2 minutes
16. 42 respirations in 3 minutes

17. You may need to help a patient increase fluid intake during waking hours to 2000 milliliters in every 12 hours. What rate is this per hour? (Round to the nearest tenth.)

18. There are 4 grams of fiber in 6 ounces of dry oat bran. How much fiber is there per ounce of the bran? (Round to the nearest tenth.)

Exercises 19–22. If a patient gains the indicated amount of weight in 1 month, what is the approximate rate of weight gain per week? (Use 1 month = $4\frac{1}{3}$ weeks and round to the nearest tenth.)

19. 8 pounds

20. 10.5 pounds

21. $3\frac{1}{2}$ pounds

22. 2 pounds

ANSWERS 1. $\frac{1}{3}$ 3. $\frac{5}{16}$ 5. $\frac{2}{500} = \frac{1}{250}$ 7. $\frac{3}{24} = \frac{1}{8}$
9. 5 grams/ounce 11. 1 drop/second 13. $25/uniform 15. yes
17. 166.7 milliliters/hour 19. 1.8 pounds/week 21. 0.8 pound/week

3-4. PROPORTIONS

When we say that a human figure is "in proportion," we mean that the parts of the body are related in a similar way whether the person is small or big. For instance, the ratio of the length of the head to the length of the torso is about the same whether the person is short or tall (compare parts A and B of Fig. 3–1.) The mathematical statement that two ratios are equal is called a **proportion.** The use of proportions is an easy and dependable technique for solving many types of problems.

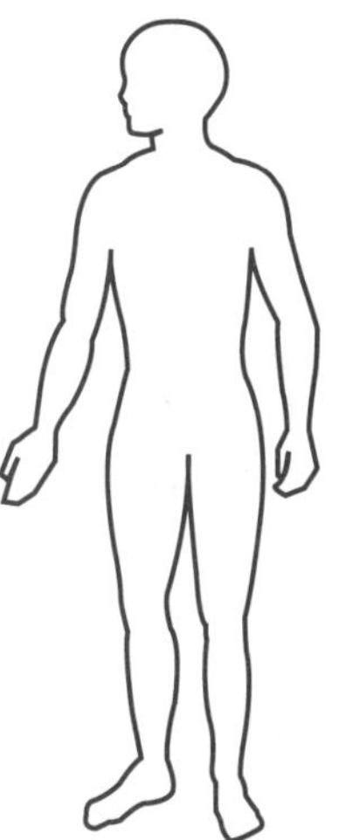

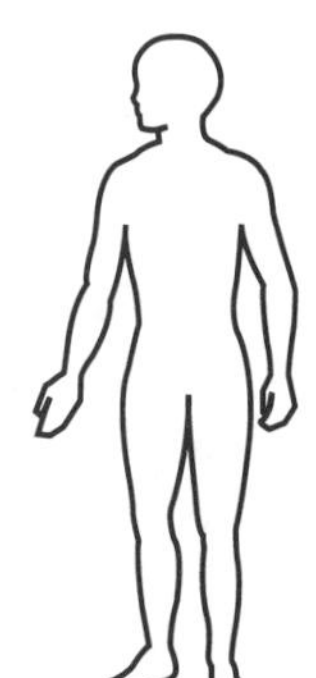

A B

Figure 3–1. Proportionate human figures.

PROPORTIONS

A **proportion** is an **equality** of **two ratios.**

$$\frac{10}{30} = \frac{1}{3} \quad \text{or} \quad 10:30 = 1:3$$

"10 is to 30 as 1 is to 3."

Examples

1. The ratio of length of head to length of torso is $\frac{9 \text{ inches}}{27 \text{ inches}}$ for Sally, but $\frac{10 \text{ inches}}{30 \text{ inches}}$ for Bob. The measurements are in proportion: $\frac{9}{27} = \frac{10}{30}$.

2. $\frac{3}{4} = \frac{6}{8}$
   or $3:4 = 6:8$
   or "3 is to 4 as 6 is to 8."

3. $\frac{0.5}{9} = \frac{1}{18}$
   or $0.5:9 = 1:18$
   or "0.5 is to 9 as 1 is to 18"

4. $\frac{x}{6} = \frac{15}{9}$
   or $x:6 = 15:9$
   or "x is to 6 as 15 is to 9."

5. $\frac{5}{1.2} = \frac{x}{2.4}$
   or $5:1.2 = x:2.4$
   or "5 is to 1.2 as x is to 2.4"

6. See Figure 3–2.

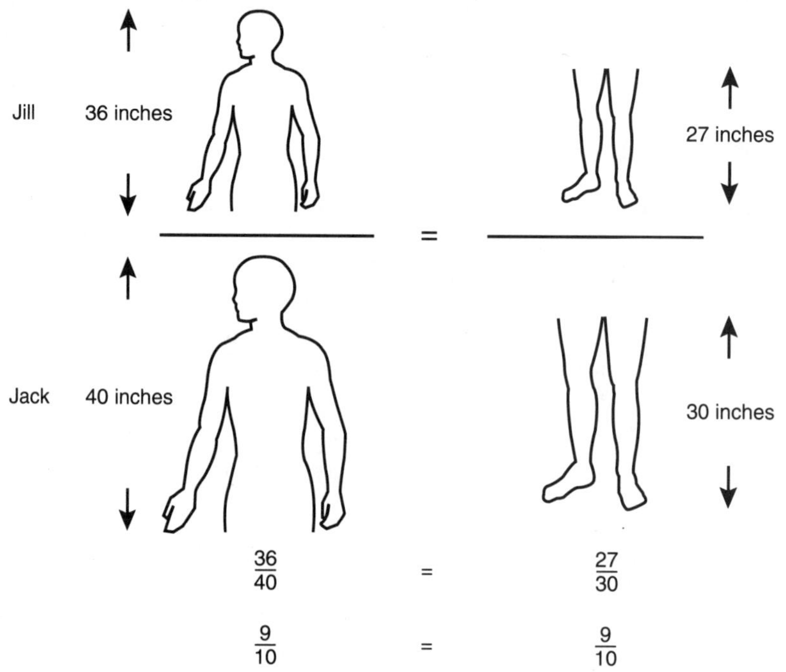

Figure 3–2. Body parts "in proportion."

SAMPLE EXERCISES

Exercises 1–5. Is the given equality a proportion?

1. $3 + 2 = 4 + 1$
2. $3 \times 2 = 6 \times 1$
3. $9:10 = 18:20$
4. $\frac{3}{2} = \frac{6}{4}$
5. $\frac{x}{7} = \frac{3}{21}$
6. $\frac{2}{3} + 1 = \frac{5}{3}$
7. Write a proportion involving the ratio $\frac{5}{12}$.

ANSWERS 1. no, not a statement that two ratios are equal. 2. no, not a statement that two ratios are equal. 3. yes 4. yes 5. yes 6. no, not a statement that two ratios are equal.
7. $\frac{5}{12} = \frac{10}{24}$ or $\frac{5}{12} = \frac{15}{36}$, etc.

From every proportion, we can derive another useful equality by cross multiplication. To obtain cross products, multiply the numerator of each ratio by the denominator of the other ratio.

CROSS MULTIPLICATION

In every proportion, the **cross products** are **equal**.

$\frac{1}{3} = \frac{10}{30}$ $\quad 10 \times 3 \quad 1 \times 30$

$1:3 = 10:30 \quad 1 \times 30 = 3 \times 10$

Examples

Proportion	*Cross Products*
1. $\frac{3}{4} = \frac{6}{8}$	Does $6 \times 4 = 3 \times 8$? Yes, $24 = 24$
2. $0.5:9 = 1:18$	Does $0.5 \times 18 = 9 \times 1$? Yes, $9 = 9$
3. $\frac{\frac{1}{2}}{\frac{3}{4}} = \frac{12}{18}$	Does $12 \times \frac{3}{4} = \frac{1}{2} \times 18$? Yes, $9 = 9$
4. But $\frac{2}{3} \neq$* $\frac{3}{4}$	Does $3 \times 3 = 2 \times 4$? No! 8 is **not** 9

5. If one of the terms of the proportion is x (representing an unknown quantity), then the cross product must contain x.

Proportion: $\frac{9}{5} = \frac{4}{x}$

Cross products: $4 \times 5 = 9 \times x$
$20 = 9x$ ($9x$ represents both $9 \times x$ and $x \times 9$)
also $9x = 20$ (Either order is correct)

Exercises 1–6. Find the cross products of the proportion.

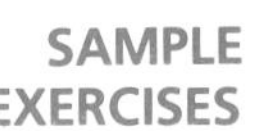

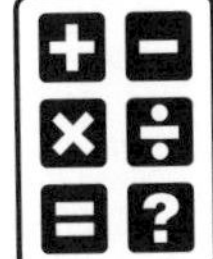

1. $\frac{7}{1} = \frac{21}{3}$

2. $\frac{3}{0.8} = \frac{12}{3.2}$

* The symbol $\neq$ means "is not equal to."

3. $1/2:1/3 = 3:2$

4. $\frac{8}{2} = 4$

5. $\frac{x}{2} = \frac{10}{4}$

6. $1:x = 3:9$

ANSWERS 1. $21 \times 1 = 7 \times 3 = 21$ 2. $12 \times 0.8 = 3 \times 3.2 = 9.6$
3. $1/2 \times 2 = 1/3 \times 3 = 1$ 4. $4 \times 2 = 8 \times 1 = 8$ 5. $20 = 4x$
6. $3x = 9$

Equality of cross products gives us a general method for solving a proportion (finding the value of x).

SOLVING A PROPORTION

To solve a proportion, cross multiply and **divide** by the **multiplier** (coefficient) of x.

$$\frac{9}{5} = \frac{4}{x}$$

$$9x = 20$$

$$x = \frac{20}{9}$$

Examples

1. To solve the proportion $\frac{9}{5} = \frac{4}{x}$ find the value of x.

   Cross multiply: $9x = 20$
   This tells us the value of $9x$.

   Divide both sides of the equality by the multiplier (coefficient) of x: $\frac{9x}{9} = \frac{20}{9}$

   $x = \frac{20}{9}$

   Simplify (round to the nearest tenth): $x = 2.2$

2. Find x in $\frac{7}{15} = \frac{2}{x}$

   Cross multiply: $7x = 30$

   Divide by the multiplier of x: $x = \frac{30}{7}$

   Simplify (round to tenths): $x = 4.3$

3. Find x in $\frac{7}{x} = \frac{8}{25}$

   Cross multiply: $8x = 175$

   Divide by the multiplier of x: $x = \frac{175}{8}$

   Simplify: $x = 21.9$

4. To check a solution to a proportion, replace x by the solution. Refer to Examples 2 and 3 above.

Check:	Does $\frac{7}{15} = \frac{2}{4.3}$?	Does $\frac{7}{21.9} = \frac{8}{25}$?
Yes:	$0.5 = 0.5$	$0.3 = 0.3$

SAMPLE EXERCISES

Exercises 1–4. Solve the proportion (find the value of x) and check.

1. $\frac{x}{2} = \frac{10}{4}$
2. $\frac{1}{x} = \frac{3}{9}$
3. $\frac{5}{2}:3 = 15:x$
4. $\frac{2}{0.5} = \frac{x}{100}$

ANSWERS 1. $x = 5$ 2. $x = 3$ 3. $x = 18$ 4. $x = 400$

EXERCISES

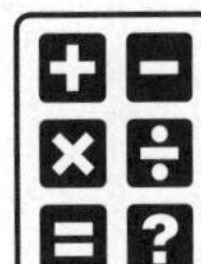

Exercises 1–10. Is the given equality a proportion?

1. $2:3 = 4:6$
2. $\frac{3}{4} + \frac{1}{2} = \frac{5}{4}$
3. $\frac{7}{2} - 1 = \frac{5}{2}$
4. $1.5:200 = 6:800$
5. $\frac{2.1}{15} = \frac{0.7}{5}$
6. $\frac{6}{1.8} = \frac{60}{18}$
7. $\frac{5}{x} = \frac{15}{60}$
8. $x = 0.9 - 0.1$
9. $x = \frac{3}{5} \times \frac{1}{4}$
10. $\frac{1}{3} = \frac{x}{30}$

Exercises 11–24. Find the cross products of the proportion.

11. $\frac{3}{8} = \frac{12}{32}$
12. $\frac{10}{34} = \frac{5}{17}$
13. $5:2 = 30:12$
14. $2:7 = 3:10.5$
15. $\frac{2.1}{15} = \frac{0.7}{5}$
16. $\frac{6}{1.8} = \frac{60}{18}$
17. $12:16 = 1:\frac{4}{3}$
18. $\frac{12.5}{100} = \frac{15}{120}$
19. $\frac{6.25}{1.5} = \frac{12.5}{3}$
20. $\frac{1}{50}:1 = \frac{1}{25}:2$
21. $\frac{x}{6} = \frac{15}{9}$
22. $\frac{x}{3} = \frac{160}{24}$
23. $\frac{2}{3} = \frac{x}{15}$
24. $\frac{7}{x} = \frac{21}{15}$

Exercises 25–40. Solve the proportion and check.

25. $\frac{x}{7} = \frac{5}{1}$

26. $\frac{x}{6} = \frac{2}{3}$

27. $\frac{3}{x} = \frac{12}{80}$

28. $\frac{7}{x} = \frac{21}{15}$

29. $\frac{3}{4} = \frac{x}{6}$

30. $\frac{1}{10} = \frac{x}{1000}$

31. $\frac{1000}{x} = \frac{25}{1}$

32. $\frac{x}{1} = \frac{3}{1.5}$

33. $\frac{x}{2.6} = \frac{3}{1}$

34. $\frac{1}{x} = \frac{2.2}{10}$

35. $\frac{x}{250} = \frac{7.5}{5}$

36. $\frac{x}{2.5} = \frac{0.4}{1}$

37. $\frac{x}{0.9} = \frac{6}{1}$

38. $\frac{x}{30} = \frac{4.2}{5}$

39. $\frac{4}{7}:200 = 1:x$

40. $\frac{1}{2}:\frac{1}{3} = x:8$

ANSWERS 1. yes 3. no 5. yes 7. yes 9. no 11. 96 13. 60 15. 10.5 17. 16 19. 18.75 21. $9x = 90$ 23. $3x = 30$ 25. $x = 35$ 27. $x = 20$ 29. $x = 4.5$ 31. $x = 40$ 33. $x = 7.8$ 35. $x = 375$ 37. $x = 5.4$ 39. $x = 350$

3-5. USING PROPORTIONS TO SOLVE RATE PROBLEMS

At $59 for every 4 hours worked, how long does it take to earn $2500? To answer this question, we can write and solve our own proportion.

SOLVING RATE PROBLEMS

1. Set up a **table.**
2. Write a **proportion.**
3. **Solve** the proportion.
4. State the result with **units.**

The rationale for setting up a table is to clarify the data and the question, and to ensure understanding of the case presented. With practice, the whole procedure becomes automatic and efficient and decreases the chance of error.

Examples

1. At $59 for every 4 hours worked, how long does it take to earn $2500?

   Set up a table to clarify the data and the question.

	Hours	Earnings ($)
(A)	*x*	2500
(B)	4	59

Write a proportion. Use line (A) for numerators; line (B) for denominators. Omit units identical in numerator and denominator. (Because the rate of pay is constant, the ratio of hours worked must equal the ratio of **corresponding** earnings.)

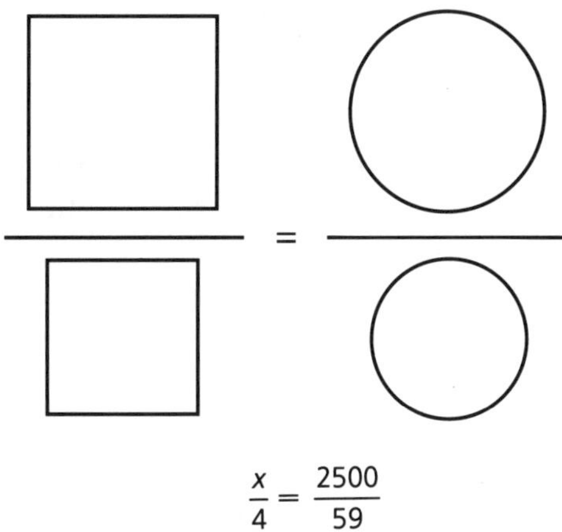

$$\frac{x}{4} = \frac{2500}{59}$$

Cross multiply: $59 \times x = 4 \times 2500$

$59x = 10{,}000$

Divide by the coefficient of x: $x = \frac{10{,}000}{59} = 169.5$

State the result with units: 169.5 hours

2. To find out how long it takes to cover 300 miles when traveling at 55 mph ("miles per hour"), we may use x to represent the unknown number of hours.

Table:

	Number of Hours	Number of Miles
(A)	*x*	300
(B)	1	55

Proportion: $\frac{x}{1} = \frac{300}{55}$

(Ratio of hours elapsed = ratio of **corresponding** miles covered)

Cross multiply: $55 \times x = 300 \times 1$

$55x = 300$

Divide: $x = \frac{300}{55} = 5.5$

Result:
(always state units): 5.5 hours

3. Tablets of ascorbic acid are labeled 100 milligrams per tablet. To find how many tablets to give for a dose of 250 milligrams we use x to represent the number of tablets.

Table:

	Number of Tablets	Dose (Milligrams)
(A)	x	250
(B)	1	100

Proportion: $\frac{x}{1} = \frac{250}{100}$

(Ratio of number of tablets = ratio of **corresponding** doses)

Cross multiply: $100 \times x = 250 \times 1$

$100x = 250$

Divide: $x = \frac{250}{100}$

Result: 2.5 tablets

4. To find the number of teaspoons/ounce in 4 tablespoons/cup the procedure is the same, except that we must first change to **identical units.**

Reminder: 3 teaspoons = 1 tablespoon;
8 ounces = 1 cup

Table:

	Teaspoons	Ounces
(A)	x teaspoons	1 ounce
(B)	4 tablespoons	1 cup

Revised table with identical units:

Teaspoons	Ounces
x teaspoons	1 ounce
12 teaspoons	8 ounces

Proportion: $\frac{x}{12} = \frac{1}{8}$

(Ratio of amounts in teaspoons = ratio of **corresponding** amounts in ounces)

Cross multiply: $8x = 12$

Divide: $x = \frac{12}{8}$

Result: 1.5 teaspoons/ounce

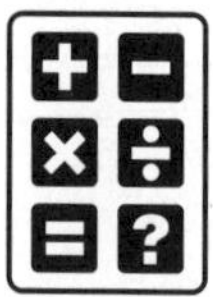

SAMPLE EXERCISES

Where necessary, round to the nearest tenth.

Exercises 1–2. Given that in 4 ounces of protein, there are 448 calories, find:

1. How many calories there are in 6.5 ounces of protein.
2. How much protein we need for 325 calories.
3. A medication available for injection is labeled 150 milligrams/ounce. If a patient needs 675 milligrams, how many ounces should you give?

ANSWERS

1. *Table:*

	Calories	Ounces of Protein
(A)	x	6.5
(B)	448	4

Proportion: $\frac{x}{448} = \frac{6.5}{4}$

Cross multiply: $4x = 448 \times 6.5$

Divide by 4: $x = 728$

Result: 728 calories in 6.5 ounces of protein

2. *Table:*

Ounces of Protein	Calories
x	325
4	448

Proportion: $\frac{x}{4} = \frac{325}{448}$

Cross multiply: $448x = 4 \times 325$

Divide by 448: $x = 2.9$

Result: 2.9 ounces of protein needed for 325 calories

3. 4.5 ounces

EXERCISES

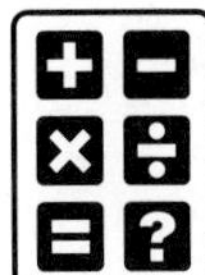

Exercises 1–2. If 72 beats/minute is a normal pulse rate, how many beats do you expect to count in the given amount of time?

1. 15 seconds
2. 2 minutes

Exercises 3–6. Assuming earnings of $700/week, find the earnings for the following periods.

3. 4 weeks
4. 26 weeks
5. 1 year
6. 1.5 years

Exercises 7–10. At a speed of 55 miles per hour, how far can you go in the following amounts of time?

7. 2 hours
8. 3.5 hours
9. 30 minutes
10. 45 minutes

Exercises 11–16. At a speed of 60 miles per hour, how long does it take to cover the following distances? (Round to the nearest tenth, where necessary.)

11. 120 miles
12. 200 miles
13. 321 miles
14. 575 miles
15. 30 miles
16. 50 miles

Exercises 17–20. Tablets of ascorbic acid are labeled 100 milligrams/tablet. Find the number of tablets needed for the following specified doses.

17. 200 milligrams
18. 150 milligrams
19. 350 milligrams
20. 250 milligrams

Exercises 21–26. Suppose that an intravenous pump rate is 60 drops/minute. How many drops flow in the following amounts of time?

21. 2 minutes
22. 1.5 minutes
23. 30 seconds
24. 10 seconds
25. 1 hour
26. $\frac{1}{2}$ hour

Exercises 27–30. If an IV pump delivers medication to a patient at a constant rate of 25 milligrams/hour, how many milligrams does the pump deliver in the following specified times?

27. 6 hours
28. 8.5 hours

29. 30 minutes

30. $\frac{1}{4}$ hour

Exercises 31–34. Using the same rate as in Exercises 27–30, determine how much time it takes to deliver the given amounts of drug.

31. 175 milligrams

32. 62.5 milligrams

33. 110 milligrams

34. 35 milligrams

ANSWERS 1. 18 beats 3. $2800 5. $36,400 7. 110 miles 9. 27.5 miles 11. 2 hours 13. 5.4 hours 15. 0.5 hour 17. 2 tablets 19. 3.5 tablets 21. 120 drops 23. 30 drops 25. 3600 drops 27. 150 milligrams 29. 12.5 milligrams 31. 7 hours 33. 4.4 hours

---

3-6. PERCENT AS A SPECIAL RATIO

In many cases, the approximate extent of a burn injury in adults may be calculated by the **rule of nines,** which divides the total body surface into areas of 1%, 9%, 18%, and 36% (Fig. 3–3). The total body surface area is represented by 100%.

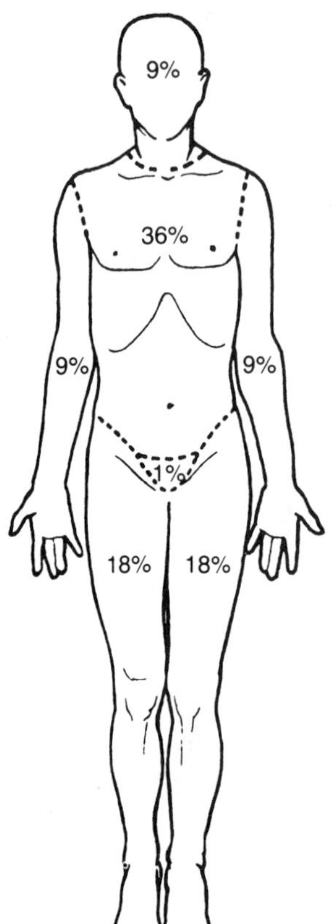

Figure 3–3. Estimation of extent of injury by the rule-of-nines method. (From Ignatavicius DD and Bayne MV. *Medical-Surgical Nursing.* Philadelphia, W.B. Saunders, 1992, p. 376.)

The word *percent* comes from Latin *per centum,* meaning "per hundred." Some alternative expressions are "out of a hundred" and "in a hundred." Since percents are symbols for ratios with a denominator of 100, the percent sign % means "divided by 100." We delete the % sign when we show the division.

PERCENTS

Percent means a ratio whose **denominator is 100.** To change from percent to another form, **divide** by 100 and **delete** %.

$9\% = \frac{9}{100}$ Fraction form

$9\% = 0.09$ Decimal form

Examples

1. In the figure below, the large square is divided into 100 parts. Each small square represents $\frac{1}{100}$ of the large square, or 1%.

100 squares represent 100%

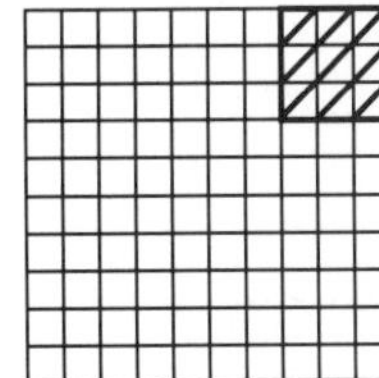

9 squares represent 9%

2. $1\% = \frac{1}{100} = 0.01$
3. $9\% = \frac{9}{100} = 0.09$
4. $0.5\% = \frac{0.5}{100} = 0.005$
5. $\frac{1}{2}\% = \frac{\frac{1}{2}}{100} = \frac{1}{200}$
6. Information about medications is often given in terms of percent. For instance, if a cream contains 0.02 gram of mupirocin in 100 grams of ointment, the cream is designated as mupirocin ointment, 0.02%.

SAMPLE EXERCISES

Exercises 1–3. Change the expression to fraction form.

1. 80%
2. 25%
3. $\frac{3}{4}\%$

Exercises 4–10. Change the expression to decimal form.

4. 80%
5. 25%
6. $\frac{3}{4}\%$
7. 18%
8. 36%
9. 0.02%
10. 300%

ANSWERS 1. $\frac{80}{100} = \frac{4}{5}$ 2. $\frac{25}{100} = \frac{1}{4}$ 3. $\frac{\frac{3}{4}}{100} = \frac{3}{4} \times \frac{1}{100} = \frac{3}{400}$

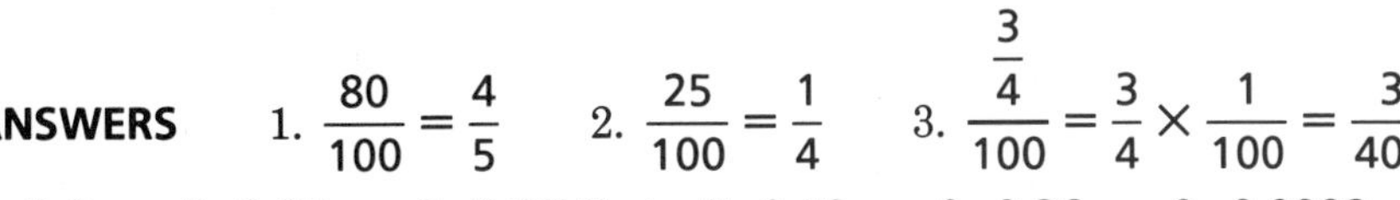

4. 0.8 5. 0.25 6. 0.0075 7. 0.18 8. 0.36 9. 0.0002
10. 3

(Whenever you see %, note that the % symbol bears a resemblance to a tipped-over division sign [÷]. This should remind you that % means "divided by 100.")

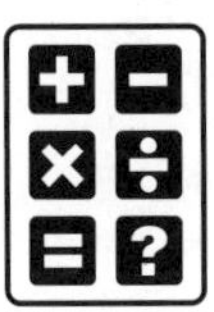

EXERCISES

Exercises 1–14. Complete the following table of commonly used percents.

	Decimal Form	*Fraction Form*	*Whole Number*
1. 0%			
2. 5%			
3. 10%			
4. 12.5%			
5. 20%			
6. $33\frac{1}{3}$%			
7. 37.5%			
8. 40%			
9. 62.5%			
10. $66\frac{2}{3}$%			
11. 75%			
12. 87.5%			
13. 90%			
14. 100%			

Exercises 15–20. Complete the following table. Simplify all fractions.

	Decimal Form	*Fraction Form or Mixed Number*	*Whole Number*
15. 2%			
16. 123%			
17. $2\frac{1}{2}$%			
18. 425%			
19. 200%			
20. 0.9%			

Exercises 21–24. Change the percent expression to decimal and fraction forms.

21. About 25% of nursing students decide upon their career early in life.

22. About 55% of all women work away from home.

23. Of all women who want to work, 7.2% are unemployed.

24. 9.25% of all working women have children under 3 years of age.

ANSWERS

	Decimal Form	*Fraction Form*	*Whole Number*
1. 0%	0		0
3. 10%	0.1	$\frac{1}{10}$	
5. 20%	0.2	$\frac{1}{5}$	
7. 37.5%	0.375	$\frac{3}{8}$	
9. 62.5%	0.625	$\frac{5}{8}$	
11. 75%	0.75	$\frac{3}{4}$	

13. 90%	0.9	$\frac{9}{10}$	
15. 2%	0.02	$\frac{2}{100} = \frac{1}{50}$	
17. 2 1/2%	0.025	$\frac{1}{40}$	
19. 200%	2		2

21. $00.25 = \frac{1}{4}$ 23. $0.072 = \frac{9}{125}$

3-7. FINDING A PERCENT OF A QUANTITY

Before administering medication to a patient, the nurse checks that the dose is not more than 10% above, or less than 10% below, the standard dose recommended by the *Physicians' Desk Reference* or another authoritative reference source. To check that a dose is within the recommended range, we first compute 10% of the dose.

PERCENTS OF QUANTITIES

To find a percent of a quantity, multiply the **percent** by the **quantity.** (Change percent form to fraction or decimal form.)

$$\begin{aligned} 10\% \text{ of } 325 \text{ milligrams} &= 0.1 \times 325 \text{ milligrams} \\ &= 32.5 \text{ milligrams} \end{aligned}$$

Examples

1. 10% of $325 = 0.1 \times 325$
   $= 32.5$
2. 10% more than a dose of 325 milligrams = 325 milligrams + 32.5 milligrams = 357.5 milligrams.
3. 10% less than a dose of 325 milligrams = 325 milligrams − 32.5 milligrams = 292.5 milligrams.
4. Suppose that in 1 year, the price of a medication is expected to decrease by 20%. If the medication costs $10 at the beginning of the year, we can find the expected cost at the end of the year.
   Amount of decrease: 20% of $10 = 0.2 × $10 = $2
   New price: $10 − $2 = $8

SAMPLE EXERCISES

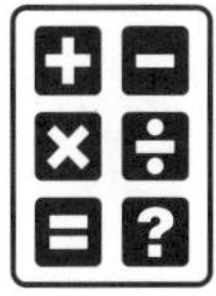

Exercises 1–3. Find the indicated amount, correct to the nearest tenth.

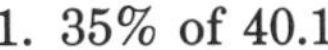

1. 35% of 40.1
2. 0.9% of 20 ounces
3. $\frac{1}{4}$% of 160 milliliters
4. Determine the amount that is 10% greater than 28.5 milligrams.

ANSWERS 1. 14.0 2. 0.2 ounce 3. 0.4 milliliter 4. 31.4 milligrams

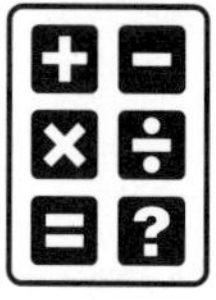

EXERCISES

Where appropriate, round to the nearest tenth.

Exercises 1–10. Find the indicated amount.

1. 10% of 125
2. 22% of 60.4
3. 25% of 80 milligrams
4. 250% of 30 units
5. 45% of 2.4 liters
6. 7.5% of 500 milliliters
7. 0.1% of 64 ounces
8. 0.9% of 32 ounces
9. $\frac{1}{2}$% of 200 milliliters
10. $\frac{1}{3}$% of 600 milliliters

Exercise 11–20. Determine the amount that is 10% greater than the indicated dose.

11. 350 milligrams
12. 40 milligrams
13. 36 milligrams
14. 1740 milligrams
15. 25 milligrams
16. 2.5 milligrams
17. 11.4 milligrams
18. 20,000 units
19. 1.5 grams
20. 0.12 milligram

Exercises 21–30. Determine the amount that is 10% less than the indicated doses in Exercises 11–20.

31. A solution containing 48 milliliters of water lost 20% of its water content because of evaporation. How many milliliters of water are left?
32. Doctor's orders for a new medication require starting the patient with 100 milliliters on the first day and then increasing by 5% per day on each of the 3 following days. Write out the dose (correct to 1 decimal place) to be given each day.

ANSWERS 1. 12.5 3. 20 milligrams 5. 1.1 liters 7. 0.1 ounce 9. 1 milliliter 11. 385 milligrams 13. 39.6 milligrams 15. 27.5 milligrams 17. 12.5 milligrams 19. 1.7 grams 21. 315 milligrams 23. 32.4 milligrams 25. 22.5 milligrams 27. 10.3 milligrams 29. 1.4 grams 31. 38.4 milliliters

3-8. CHANGING FRACTIONS OR DECIMALS TO PERCENT FORM

If there are 3 grams of fat in a 25-gram serving of light margarine, what percent of the serving consists of fat? To answer this question, we change the ratio $\frac{3}{25}$ into percent form. There is an easy way to change a fraction into percent form.

CHANGING FRACTIONS OR DECIMALS TO PERCENT FORM

Multiply by 100%. (Multiply by 100 and insert the % sign.)

Fraction form: $\frac{3}{25} = \frac{3}{25} \times 100\% = 12\%$

Decimal form: $0.12 = 0.12 \times 100\% = 0.12\% = 12\%$

When you need percent form, immediately write the given amount $\times 100\%$. This reminds you to attach the % sign and multiply by 100 at the same time.

Examples

1. Since $100\% = \frac{100}{100} = 1$, multiplication by 100% is equivalent to multiplication by 1.
2. To find $\frac{3}{25}$ in percent form, multiply by 100%.

$$\frac{3}{25} \times 100\% = \frac{3}{\cancel{25}_{1}} \times \cancel{100}^{4}\% = 12\%$$

3. The following table illustrates the procedure for changing to percent form.

Number	*Multiply by 100%*	*Result*
$\frac{1}{2}$	$\frac{1}{2} \times 100\% = \frac{1}{\cancel{2}_{1}} \times \cancel{100}^{50}\%$	50%
0.035	0.035 × 100%	3.5%
1	1 × 100%	100%
1.5	1.5 × 100%	150%

4. Dietary guidelines advise us to limit the fat content of our food to less than 30% of calories. If a patient has an average daily total consumption of 2000 calories, and 600 of these calories come from fat, we can find the percent of his or her total daily intake that comes from fat, and decide whether this patient needs to change his or her diet.

Solution: $\frac{600}{2000} \times 100\% = \frac{6}{20} \times 100\% = \frac{6}{\cancel{20}_{1}} \times \cancel{100}^{5}\% = 30\%.$

Exercises 1–4. Express the given quantity in percent form.

SAMPLE EXERCISES

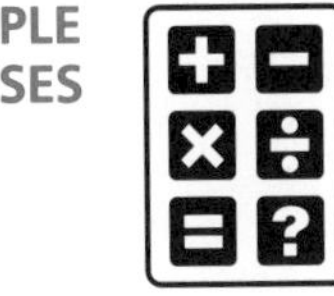

1. 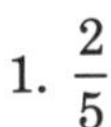 $\frac{2}{5}$
2. 0.005
3. 6
4. 27.5

ANSWERS 1. 40% 2. 0.5% 3. 600% 4. 2750%

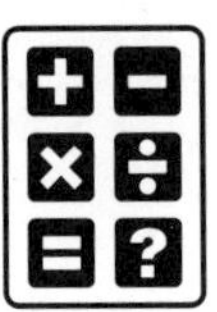

EXERCISES

Exercises 1–20. Express the given quantity in percent form. (Round to the nearest tenth wherever necessary.)

1. $\frac{1}{10}$
2. $\frac{1}{4}$
3. $\frac{1}{3}$
4. $\frac{4}{5}$
5. 2/3
6. 3/4
7. 9/10
8. 3/5
9. $\frac{1}{8}$
10. $1\frac{5}{8}$
11. 0.01
12. 0.2
13. 0.5
14. 0.64
15. 0.98
16. 1.35
17. 12.5
18. 0.009
19. 0.236
20. 0.5438
21. In a portion of turkey (100 grams), there are 23 grams of protein and 4 grams of fat. What percent of the portion is (a) protein? (b) fat?
22. If a person with an average daily total consumption of 3000 calories has about 450 calories for breakfast, what percent of his or her total daily intake is consumed at breakfast?
23. If a National Association for Nurses achievement test contains 130 questions and you answer 122 correctly, what is your score, as a percent?
24. If there are 4 grams of stannous fluoride in 1000 grams of gel, what percent of the total is stannous fluoride?

ANSWERS 1. 10% 3. 33.3% 5. 66.7% 7. 90% 9. 12.5% 11. 1% 13. 50% 15. 98% 17. 1250% 19. 23.6% 21. 23% protein, 4% fat 23. 94%

3-9. AVOID ERRORS: TABULATE, ESTIMATE, COMPUTE, AND CHECK (TECC)

When we are in a hurry, under pressure, we are tempted to do a fast computation and to ignore safety measures in the problem solving process. Unfortunately, serious errors occur. We can improve our chances of being right by using tables, estimates, and checks. These safety measures not only diminish errors and save lives but also improve our "number sense" and enable us to solve problems whose solutions elude us at first.

Every computation (except the very simplest) should be accompanied by a table, an estimate, and a check. A table presents the given data in a concise and organized way, making it easy to focus on the essentials of a problem. An estimate, made with easy numbers, quickly gives a "feel" for the size of the result. After computing, we check to evaluate our result. The estimate and check remind us **never** to use a result without thinking "Is this result **reasonable**?" or "Does this answer **make sense**?"

SAFETY MEASURES FOR COMPUTATIONS
Tabulate, Estimate, Compute, and Check (TECC)

SAMPLE EXERCISES

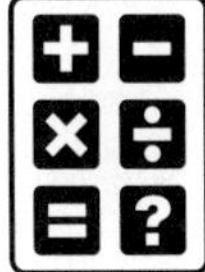

1. A can of tuna (6.5 ounces) provides 98 grams of protein. How many grams of protein are provided per ounce?

Tabulate (T):

	Protein (Grams)	*Tuna (Ounces)*
(A)	x	1
(B)	98	6.5

Estimate (E): About 20 grams/ounce

Compute (C): 15.1 grams/ounce (reasonable in light of estimate)

Check (C): Does $\frac{15.1}{98} = \frac{1}{6.5}$?

Yes, 0.15 = 0.15

2. If an IV pump delivers medication at a constant rate of 20 milligrams/hour, how many hours does it take to deliver 190 milligrams?

Tabulate:

Hours	*Medication (Milligrams)*
x	190
1	20

Estimate: About 10 hours

Compute: 9.5 hours to deliver 190 milligrams (close to estimate)

Check: $9.5 \times 20 = 190$

3. Assume that the rate of inflation is \$0.05 per dollar. On a salary of \$24,000, how much of an increase does a nurse need to keep up with the rate of inflation?

Tabulate:

Increase	*Base Amount*
\$$x$	\$24,000.00
0.05	1.00

Estimate: \$1000

Compute: \$1200

Check: $\frac{1200}{24,000} = 0.05$

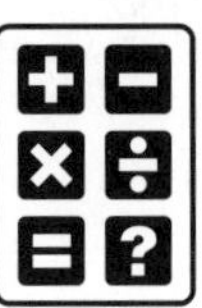

EXERCISES

Round to the nearest tenth wherever necessary.

Exercises 1–2. Assume that low-fat milk contains 11 grams of carbohydrate per ounce.

1. If a child drinks a quart (32 ounces) every day, how many grams of carbohydrate is she receiving each day from the milk?
2. To receive 319 grams of carbohydrates from milk, how much milk must the child drink?

Exercises 3–4. A certain box of crackers ($6\frac{2}{3}$ ounces) provides 65 calories.

3. How many calories are provided per ounce?
4. If the box contains 12 crackers, how many calories are there in each cracker, and how much does each cracker weigh?

Exercises 5–6. One can of sardines ($3\frac{3}{4}$ ounces) contains 42 grams of fat. How many grams of fat are contained in the following amount of sardines?

5. 1 ounce
6. 2.25 ounces

Exercises 7–8. Assume $\frac{2}{3}$ cup of oatmeal provides 87 calories.

7. How much oatmeal do we need for 65 calories?
8. How many calories does 1 cup of oatmeal provide?

Exercises 9–10. A patient is receiving medication from an IV pump at a rate of 12 milligrams/hour.

9. How many hours (correct to the nearest tenth) does it take for him to receive a total of 80 milligrams?
10. How many milligrams has he received after 7.25 hours?

Exercises 11–12. An IV pump delivers medication at a constant rate of 22 milligrams/hour.

11. How many hours does it take to deliver 75 milligrams?
12. How many milligrams have been delivered in 9.75 hours?
13. Assume that the rate of inflation is 6 cents per dollar. On a salary of $32,000, how much of an increase does a nurse need to keep up with the rate of inflation?
14. Assume that the rate of inflation is 4.5%. On a salary of $28,000, how much of an increase does a nurse need to keep up with the rate of inflation?

Exercises 15–16. To work off 70 calories, Gloria S. needs to walk for about 18 minutes.

15. How long does it take her to work off 100 calories?
16. If she walks at the same rate for 15 minutes, how many calories are used?

Exercises 17–18. A set of 24 brand A rubber gloves costs $4.95. Brand B sells the same quality rubber gloves at 30 gloves for $6.35.

17. Which brand is more economical?
18. How much should 40 brand A gloves cost?

Exercises 19–20. Assuming that a 2.7-ounce porkchop contains 305 calories, answer the following questions.

19. How many calories are in a 2.2-ounce porkchop?

20. How many ounces of porkchop correspond to 338.9 calories?

Exercises 21–22. A $\frac{1}{4}$-pound hamburger on a roll provides 418 calories.

21. Find the weight corresponding to 350 calories.

22. Find the number of calories corresponding to 6 ounces.

ANSWERS

1. *Tabulate:*

Carbohydrates	Milk
x grams	32 ounces
11 grams	1 ounce

Estimate: 300

Compute: 352 grams of carbohydrates (reasonable)

Check: $11 \times 32 = 352$

3. 9.8 calories 5. 11.2 grams 7. 0.5 cup 9. 6.7 hours

11. 3.4 hours 13. $1920 15. 25.7 minutes

17. brand A 19. 248.5 calories 21. 0.2 pound

3-10. SUMMARY

1. A ratio of two quantities is a comparison of these quantities by division, and is symbolized in fraction or colon form. A pure ratio is a ratio of numbers without units. If both terms of a ratio have identical units, the units may be omitted.

Examples

(a) $\dfrac{8}{4} = 8:4$

(b) $5 \text{ inches} : 12 \text{ inches} = \dfrac{5 \cancel{\text{inches}}}{12 \cancel{\text{inches}}} = \dfrac{5}{12}$

2. A rate is a ratio comparing two different types of measurements whose units must be shown.

Examples

(a) $\dfrac{15 \text{ inches}}{2 \text{ feet}}$

(b) 72 beats/minute

3. To simplify a ratio, divide as indicated and reduce to lowest terms.

Examples

(a) $\dfrac{1/6}{1/3} = \dfrac{1}{6} \div \dfrac{1}{3}$

$= \dfrac{1}{6} \times \dfrac{3}{1}$

$= \dfrac{1}{2}$

(b) 15 inches : 2 feet = 15 ~~inches~~ : 24 ~~inches~~

$= \dfrac{15}{24} = \dfrac{5}{8}$

4. A proportion is the equality of two ratios.

Examples

(a) $\dfrac{1}{2} = \dfrac{4}{8}$ or $1:2 = 4:8$

"1 is to 2 as 4 is to 8."

(b) 15 inches : 2 feet = 30 inches : 4 feet

"15 inches is to 2 feet as 30 inches is to 4 feet"

5. In every proportion, the cross products are equal. To find the cross products, multiply the numerator of each ratio by the denominator of the other ratio.

Example

$$\frac{1}{2} = \frac{2}{4} \qquad 1 \times 4 = 2 \times 2$$

To solve a proportion, set the cross products equal, and divide by the multiplier (coefficient) of x.

$$\frac{x}{4} = \frac{3}{10}$$

$$x \times 10 = 4 \times 3$$

$$10x = 12$$

$$x = \frac{12}{10} = \frac{6}{5}, \text{ or } 1\tfrac{1}{5}, \text{ or } 1.2$$

6. To solve a rate problem, set up a table, write and solve the proportion, then state the result with units.

Example

Tablets of ascorbic acid are labeled "100 milligrams per tablet." To find how many tablets to give for a dose of 250 milligrams we use x to represent the number of tablets.

Table:

	Number of Tablets	*Dose (Milligrams)*
(A)	x	250
(B)	1	100

Proportion:	$\frac{x}{1} = \frac{250}{100}$
Cross multiply:	$100 \times x = 250 \times 1$
	$100x = 250$
Divide:	$x = \frac{250}{100} = 2.5$
Result:	2.5 tablets

7. Percent means a ratio whose denominator is 100. The percent sign means "divided by 100." To change from percent to another form, divide by 100 and delete the % sign.

Examples

$99\% = \frac{99}{100}$ (Fraction form)

$99\% = 0.99$ (Decimal form)

8. To find a percent of a quantity, change percent form to decimal or fraction form and multiply.

Examples

$$5\% \text{ of } 325 \text{ milligrams} = 0.05 \times 325 \text{ milligrams} = 16.25 \text{ milligrams}$$

$$50\% \text{ of } 400 \text{ grams} = \frac{1}{2} \times 400 \text{ grams} = 200 \text{ grams}$$

9. To change to percent form, multiply by 100% (multiply by 100 and insert %).

Examples

Decimal form: $0.03 = 0.03 \times 100\% = 0.03\% = 3\%$

Fraction form: $\frac{3}{100} = \frac{3}{\cancel{100}_1} \times \cancel{100}^1\% = 3\%$

10. Safety measures for computations: tabulate, estimate, compute, and check (TECC).

Example

In 2 ounces of fat, there are about 500 calories. How many calories are there in 3 ounces of fat?

Tabulate (T):

Calories	*Fat (Ounces)*
x	3
500	2

Estimate (E): Between 500 and 1000

Compute (C): 750 calories

Check (C): Does $\frac{750}{500} = \frac{3}{2}$?

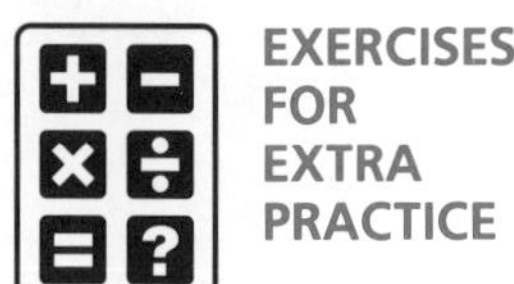

EXERCISES FOR EXTRA PRACTICE

Exercises 1–6. Write the given ratio as a pure ratio (without units), reduced to lowest terms.

1. 1 day to 1 week
2. 1 month to 1 year
3. 30 seconds to 2 minutes
4. 9 inches to 3 feet
5. $\frac{1}{2}$ pound to 5 ounces
6. 3 quarters to 7 dimes

Exercises 7–14. Solve the proportion. (Round to tenths wherever necessary.)

7. $\frac{x}{100} = \frac{33}{10}$
8. $\frac{x}{30} = \frac{60}{100}$
9. $\frac{x}{2000} = \frac{15}{100}$
10. $\frac{20}{100} = \frac{x}{8}$
11. $\frac{2}{x} = \frac{25}{100}$
12. $\frac{16}{5} = \frac{5}{x}$
13. $\frac{4}{x} = \frac{15}{100}$
14. $\frac{3}{4} = \frac{x}{100}$

Exercises 15–24. Change from percent form to decimal form.

15. 18%
16. 5%
17. 480%
18. 1000%
19. 0.25%
20. $\frac{1}{4}$%
21. $3\frac{1}{2}$%
22. 350%
23. 3.5%
24. 0.9%

Exercises 25–34. Find the indicated quantity.

25. 5% of 8 ounces
26. 20% of 10 ounces
27. 25% of 2 grams
28. 15% of 4 liters
29. 40% of 10 pounds
30. 200% of $3
31. 1/2% of 10 inches
32. 1/4% of $1200
33. 0.9 of 1%
34. 0.1 of 1%

Exercises 35–44. Change to percent form.

35. 0.57
36. 4.8
37. 1
38. 100
39. $\frac{1}{2}$
40. 3 1/2
41. $\frac{3}{4}$
42. $\frac{5}{8}$
43. $\frac{2}{5}$
44. $\frac{3}{20}$

45. Low-fat cottage cheese has 23 calories per ounce. How many calories are there in a 7-ounce portion?

46. If intravenous medication is intended to flow at 60 drops/minute, and we count 15 drops in 10 seconds, is the intravenous medication flowing as intended?

47. If a patient receives 800 milligrams of intravenous medication in 9.5 hours, what is the rate in milligrams per hour?

48. In any group of 100 nurses, we expect to find 44 nurses who plan to specialize. In a class of 325, how many nurses can we expect to find who plan to specialize?

49. Some RNs receive $36,000 in base pay; in addition, the hospital contributes about $2000 to the pension fund in their name. What percent of base pay is this pension contribution?

50. Mrs. K. is concerned that her 2-day-old infant has lost too much weight. The baby weighed 7 pounds at birth and has lost 1/2 pound. What percent of the birth weight has the baby lost?

51. If the minimum daily requirement (MDR) for iron is 14 milligrams, and breakfast furnishes 2 milligrams, what percent of the MDR should be furnished by the other meals?

52. If a high-potency tablet provides 240 milligrams of vitamin C, for which the recommended daily allowance (RDA) is 60 milligrams, find the percent of the RDA supplied by the tablet.

ANSWERS 1. $\frac{1}{7}$ 3. $\frac{1}{4}$ 5. $\frac{8}{5}$ 7. 330 9. 300 11. 8
13. 26.7 15. 0.18 17. 4.8 19. 0.0025 21. 0.035
23. 0.035 25. 0.4 ounce 27. 0.5 gram 29. 4 pounds
31. 0.05 inch 33. 0.009 35. 57% 37. 100% 39. 50%
41. 75% 43. 40% 45. 161 calories 47. 84.2 milligrams/hour
49. 5.6% 51. 85.7%

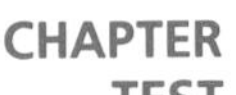

1. Find the pure ratio of 9 inches to 2 feet. 1. ________
2. Simplify the ratio 5:1/3. 2. ________
3. Find x, if $5:100 = x:2000$. 3. ________
4. Find x, if $\frac{250}{x} = \frac{5}{20}$. 4. ________
5. Change 1/6 to percent form, correct to the nearest tenth. 5. ________
6. Change 0.002 to percent form. 6. ________
7. Change 0.52% to decimal form. 7. ________
8. Of $7420 in savings, 80% will be spent. How much will be left? 8. ________
9. A 60-gram tube of nitroglycerin ointment contains 1.2 grams of nitroglycerin. What percent of the ointment is nitroglycerin? 9. ________

10. The label on a certain package of bread says "2 grams of fiber per 8/10 ounce serving." How many grams of fiber are there in 2.1 ounces of this bread?

10. ________

ANSWERS 1. $\frac{3}{8} = 0.375$ 2. 15 3. 100 4. 1000 5. 16.7% 6. 0.2% 7. 0.0052 8. $1484 9. 2% 10. 5.25 grams

FOUR

Measurement: The International System of Units (SI)

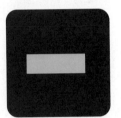

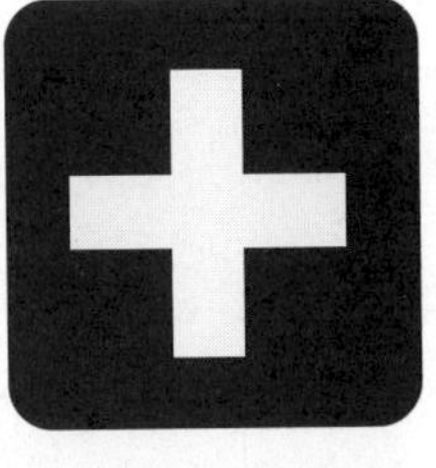

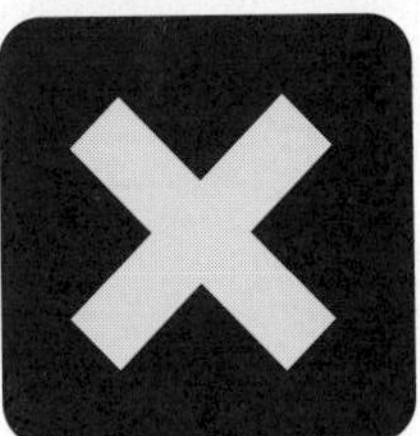
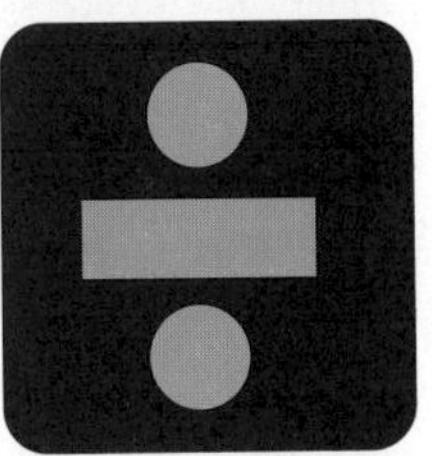

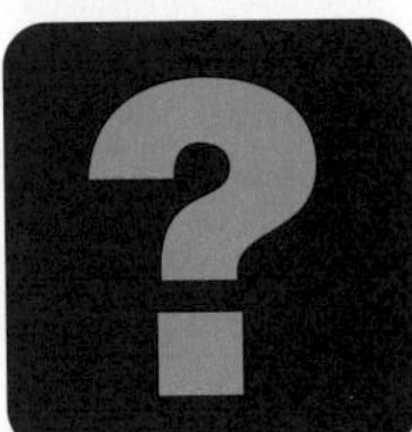

▶ OUTLINE

4-1. INTRODUCTION
4-2. LENGTH, AREA, AND VOLUME
4-3. CONVERSIONS BETWEEN UNITS OF LENGTH
4-4. LIQUID CAPACITY (VOLUME)
4-5. CONVERSIONS BETWEEN UNITS OF LIQUID CAPACITY
4-6. WEIGHT
4-7. SUBSTANCE
4-8. PROPORTIONS APPLIED TO CONVERSIONS
4-9. AVOIDING ERRORS: USING MENTAL IMAGES
4-10. SUMMARY

▶ OBJECTIVES

After studying this section, you will be able to:

1. Interpret and express measurements of length, capacity, weight, and substance in terms of SI units.
2. Convert from one unit to another.

4-1. INTRODUCTION

What is the International System of Units (SI)*? This system is a set of basic units for weighing and measuring, with rules for notation and use. It is a modernized version of the metric system, which was first adopted in France in 1799. Now the official system of measurement in most developed countries, SI is controlled by an international treaty organization and used throughout the world. Scientists and medical professionals find SI indispensable to their work. In the United States, we still use the older English system for some measurements, but the yard and pound are now defined in terms of SI units. Characteristics of SI that make it the preferred system of measurement include a decimal structure for ease of computation and a method of attaching prefixes to basic units to create multiples and subdivisions.

How do nurses use SI? The International System of Units is the major system of measurement in health care. Nurses use SI to prepare or check medications. They report given doses on medical records, and other SI measurements made in daily care. Also, to understand current medical literature, SI units must be mastered.

Examples

1. A tablet for angina may contain 150 micrograms (μg) of nitroglycerin.
2. A medication is ordered in a daily dosage of 15.25 milligrams (mg) per kilogram (kg) of the patient's body weight.
3. A liter (L) of infant formula contains 175 mg of salt.
4. Normal triglyceride levels are 0.45–1.80 millimole/liter (mmol/L) of blood.
5. A normal white blood cell count ranges between 5000 and 10,000 cells per cubic millimeter (mm^3) of blood.
6. On the average, the height of an 8-year-old girl is 127 centimeters (cm).

Proficiency Gauge

You may already have mastered the use of SI units and be able to skip Chapter 4. Gauge your proficiency by working out the following exercises. Check your answers with those given below only after you have answered all the questions.

1. What is the basic SI unit of length? 1. ____________
2. What is the basic SI unit for amount of substance? 2. ____________

Exercises 3–7. Convert as indicated.

3. 42 cm to m 3. ____________
4. 120 cc to mL 4. ____________
5. 2.3 L to mL 5. ____________

* The symbol SI stands for the French title *Système International d'Unités.*

6. 2504 g to kg 6. ____________
7. 79.2 μmol to mmol 7. ____________
8. Which tablet weighs more, A (1 g) or B (225.5 mg)? 8. ____________
9. If 500 units of vitamin A is added to every 250 mL of milk, how much vitamin A is added to 1 L of milk? 9. ____________
10. Counting 9 calories for every gram of fat, approximately how many calories are in 700 mg of fat? 10. ____________

ANSWERS 1. the meter (m) 2. the mole (mol) 3. 0.42 m 4. 120 mL 5. 2300 mL 6. 2.504 kg 7. 0.0792 mmol 8. A 9. 2000 units 10. 6 calories

---

4-2. LENGTH, AREA, AND VOLUME

Four basic SI measures of importance to the nurse are the **meter, liter, gram,** and **mole,** which measure length, liquid capacity, weight, and substance, respectively. (See Appendix 2 for a complete presentation of SI.)

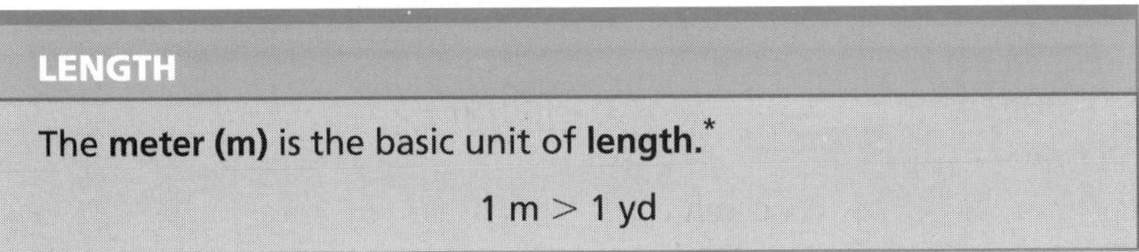

LENGTH

The **meter (m)** is the basic unit of **length.***

1 m > 1 yd

Length

Examples

1. The meter (m) is approximately 39 inches (in.), or about 3 in. longer than the yard. (The yard is a unit of the English system.)

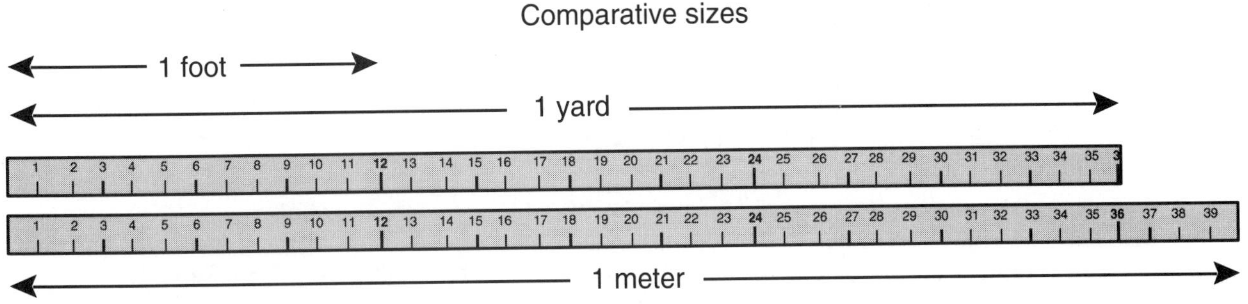

2. The meter is about 3 feet (ft) 3 in. long.

---

* The technical definition of the meter is the length of the path traveled by light in a vacuum during a time interval of 1/299,792,458 of a second.

3. The distance from the floor to a doorknob is often about 1 m.
4. Radiation intensity at a distance of 4 m from the source of exposure is only $\frac{1}{16}$ of the intensity at a distance of 1 m.

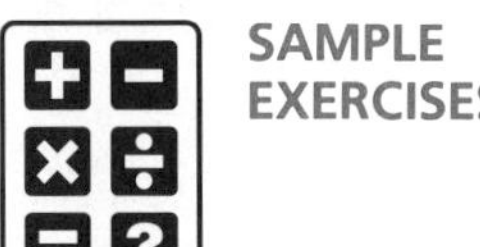

SAMPLE EXERCISES

1. Can an outstretched arm reach an object that is at a distance of 3 m?
2. To make a dress (requiring about $3\frac{1}{4}$ yards), how many meters of fabric would we need?

ANSWERS 1. No, a distance of 3 m is about the length of 5 outstretched arms. 2. 3

Standard Prefixes

One of the advantages of SI is its use of **prefixes** to denote **multiples** and **subdivisions** of basic measures. The following table shows how the prefixes are used for units of length.

Prefix	*Meaning*	*Combined Form (with Meter)*	*Relationships*
kilo (k)	1000	kilometer (km)	1 km = 1000 m 1 m = 0.001 km
deci (d)	0.1	decimeter (dm)	1 dm = 0.1 m 1 m = 10 dm
centi (c)	0.01	centimeter (cm)	1 cm = 0.01 m 1 m = 100 cm
milli (m)	0.001	millimeter (mm)	1 mm = 0.001 m 1 m = 1000 mm

The symbols m, dm, cm, and mm and all the other symbols of the SI system are not abbreviations, and no periods are used after them except at the end of a sentence. (As we will show in subsequent sections, these symbols tell us which decimal fraction to apply to the appended unit, whatever that unit may be.)

Examples

1. Each subdivision of the meter (dm, cm, and mm) is 0.1 of the previous unit, as follows.
   If we divide:

   1 m into 10 parts, each part is 1 dm (0.1 m);
   1 dm into 10 parts, each part is 1 cm (0.01 m);
   1 cm into 10 parts, each part is 1 mm (0.001 m).

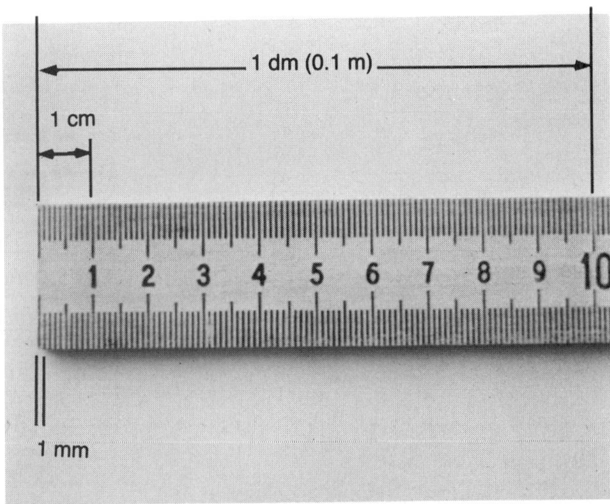

Comparative sizes

2. A standard ruler shows centimeters and millimeters. 1 in. is about 2.5 cm.

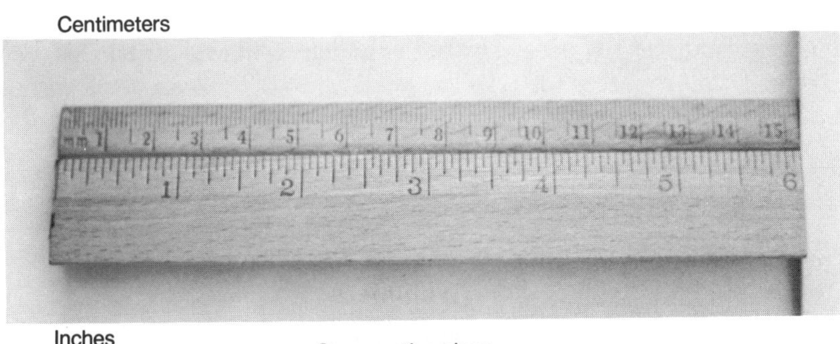

Comparative sizes

3. One type of standard paper clip is 1 cm wide and 5 cm long and is made of wire 1 mm in diameter.

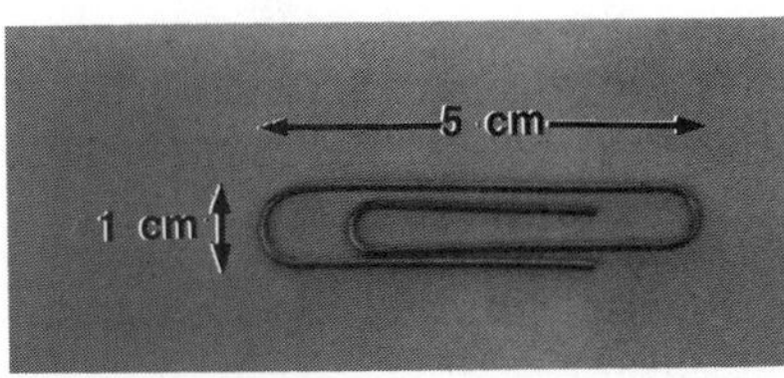

4. Wound-dressing pads come in different lengths, such as 5 cm, 7.5 cm, 10 cm, or 20 cm.
5. If gallbladder stones are less than 20 mm in diameter, medication rather than surgery may be used to treat them.

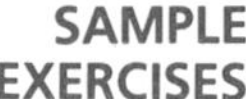

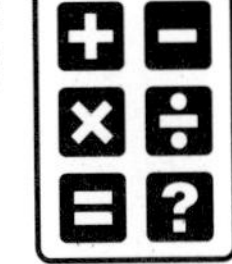

1. Use a ruler (that has centimeter markings) to find the approximate length of your thumbnail in centimeters.
2. What is the approximate length of your paper clip? The width?
3. Use the ruler to find the approximate thickness of a dime.

ANSWERS 1. Close to 1 cm? 2. Similar to the dimensions shown in Example 3 above? 3. 1 mm

Area

A square meter is a unit of surface area. Many drugs are dispensed according to the body surface area of the patient.

> **AREA**
>
> A **square meter (m^2)** is a unit of **area** of **two-dimensional** space. Each dimension is 1 m.
>
> $$1\ m^2 = 1\ m \times 1\ m$$

Examples

1. A scarf may be 1 square yard (yd^2), which would be a little less than 1 square meter (m^2).

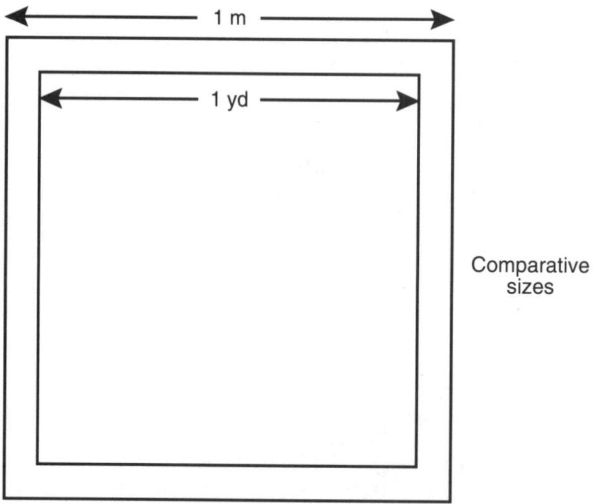

2. Suppose that a patient has a **body surface area (BSA)** of 2 m^2. To understand the meaning of this measurement, think of being tightly dressed in a leotard or a wetsuit so that the clothing comes very close to being a second skin. Then picture the fabric needed (2 m^2 or a little more than 2 square yards) to create this clothing. This gives a rough approximation of body surface area. There are scientific methods, of course, for measuring BSA more accurately.
3. To find the area of a rectangular figure, we may use the formula $A = L \times W$ (Area = Length × Width). If a typical picture post-card is 10 cm wide and 15 cm long, then its area is 10 cm × 15 cm = 150 cm^2.
4. A nitro patch that is taped onto the skin has a drug-releasing surface of 8 cm^2, as in the following diagram.

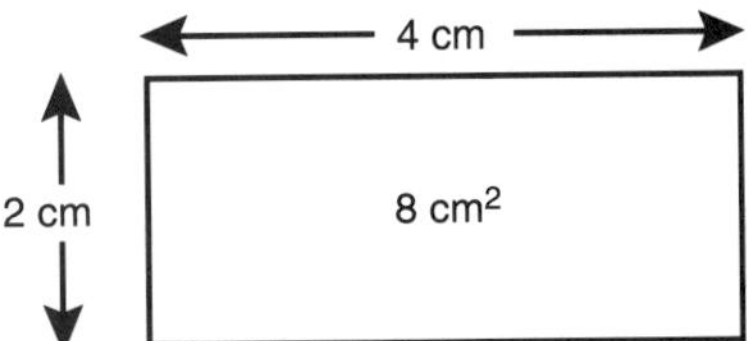

SAMPLE EXERCISES

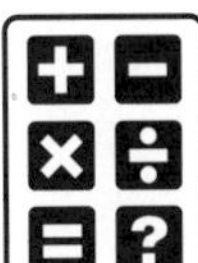

1. Find the area of a bandage that is 5 cm wide by 3 cm long.
2. For the average person, the stomach is approximately 25 cm long and 10 cm wide. Find the approximate surface area of the stomach.

ANSWERS 1. 15 cm^2 2. 250 cm^2

Volume

A normal white blood cell count ranges between 5000 and 10,000 cells per cubic millimeter of blood.

VOLUME (mm^3)

1 cubic millimeter (mm^3) is a unit of **volume** of **three-dimensional** space. Each dimension is 1 mm.

$$1\ mm^3 = 1\ mm \times 1\ mm \times 1\ mm$$

Examples

1. A cubic millimeter (mm^3) of blood is a drop of blood that could fit exactly into a space with dimensions 1 mm long, 1 mm high, and 1 mm wide. In a normal person, 1 mm^3 of blood contains between 5000 and 10,000 white blood cells.
2. Normal platelet count values range from 200,000 to 300,000/mm^3 of blood. Thus, normally, 1 mm^3 of blood contains between 200,000 and 300,000 platelets.
3. A platelet count $<$150,000/mm^3 may lead to a change in drug therapy.

SAMPLE EXERCISES

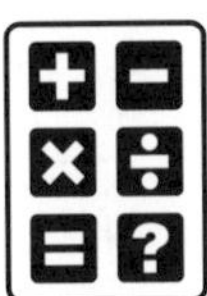

1. Give an example of a white blood cell (WBC) count within the normal limits. (See Example 1 above.)
2. Give an example of a normal platelet count. (See Example 2 above.)

ANSWERS 1. Any number between 5000/mm^3 and 10,000/mm^3, such as 6000/mm^3 2. Any number between 200,000/mm^3 and 300,000/mm^3, such as 280,000/mm^3

One cubic decimeter (dm^3) is a common unit of measure for liquid.

VOLUME (dm^3)

1 **cubic decimeter (dm^3)** is the **capacity (volume)** of a **three-dimensional** space. Each dimension is 1 dm.

$$1\ dm^3 = 1\ dm \times 1\ dm \times 1\ dm$$

Examples

1. A container whose volume is 1 dm^3 holds a little bit more than a quart (qt).
2. The quantity, 1 dm^3, is commonly called a *liter* (L).
3. The formula for the volume of a three-dimensional space is $V = L \times W \times H$ (Volume = Length × Width × Height). Thus, the volume of a container that is 8 cm long, 6 cm wide, and 10 cm high is 480 cm^3.

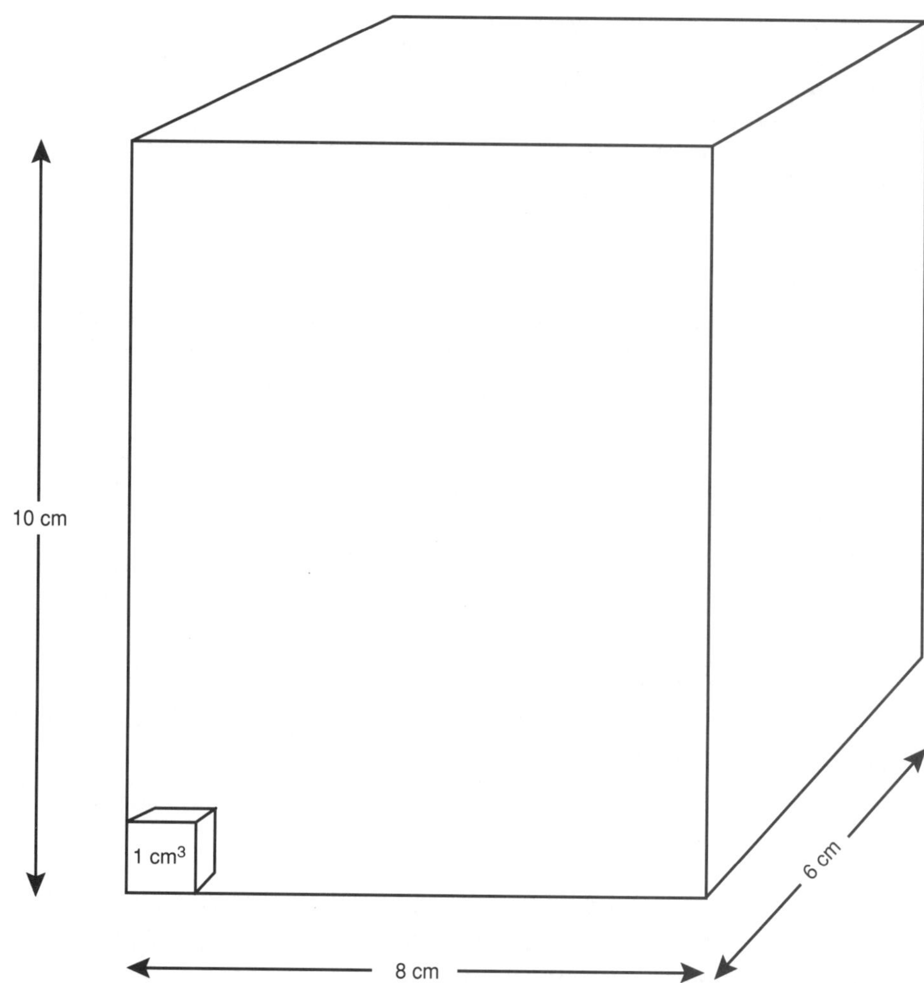

SAMPLE EXERCISES

1. About how many quarts does a 2-dm^3 container hold?
2. How many liters are there in 3.5 dm^3?
3. Find the volume of a container that is 7 cm long, 5 cm wide, and 2 cm high.

ANSWERS 1. About 2 qt 2. Exactly 3.5 L 3. 70 cm^3

EXERCISES

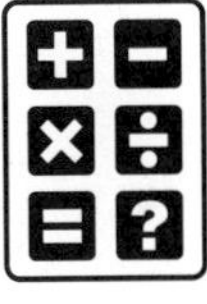

1. In yards, about how far is the fire exit from the nurses' station, if the chart shows that it is about 50 m from the station?
2. Directions to Dr. N.'s office indicate that it is about 40 yd down the hall. Give these directions, approximately, in meters.
3. According to his records, Mr. J. is 2 m tall. When you see him, will you be surprised to find that he is taller than you?
4. For her eye test, Mrs. N. is standing 6 m from the eye chart. About how many feet is the chart from the patient?

Exercises 5–8. Use the ruler to find the length (in centimeters) of the indicated item.

5. Your pen
6. Your comb
7. Your key
8. A dollar bill
9. If nails grow at a rate of about 0.1 mm/day, how much growth would you expect in 1 week?

Exercises 10–14. The diameter of the pupil of an eye changes according to its condition ("constricted," "normal," or "dilated"). If

Diameter <2 mm, the pupil is "constricted."
$=2$–6 mm, the pupil is "normal."
>6 mm, the pupil is "dilated."

Name the condition associated with each of the following measurements.

10. 4 mm
11. 6.5 mm
12. 1.5 mm
13. 5.9 mm
14. 6 mm

Exercises 15–18. Change the following ratios to pure ratios (ratios without units).

15. 1 m to 1 ft
16. 1 cm to 1 in.
17. 1 m to 1 cm
18. 1 mm to 1 m
19. On average, an ovary is approximately 3 cm by 2 cm by 1 cm. Approximately, what is the capacity of the average ovary?
20. The dimensions of the average uterus are approximately 7.5 cm by 5.0 cm by 2.5 cm. What is the capacity of this average uterus?

Exercises 21–24. If the normal range for platelets is 200,000–300,000/mm³, give examples of a platelet count value as indicated below.

21. At the midpoint of the range.

22. Normal, but closer to the lower end than to the upper end of the range.

23. Normal, but closer to the maximum than to the minimum.

24. Below the minimum.

25. About how many quarts does a 2.4-dm^3 container hold?

26. How many liters are there in a 1.5 dm^3?

ANSWERS 1. About 50 yd 3. No (unless you are over 6.5 ft tall) 5. Variable 7. Variable 9. 0.7 mm 11. Dilated 13. Normal 15. $\frac{3.3}{1}$ 17. $\frac{100}{1}$ 19. 6 cm^3 21. 250,000/mm^3 23. 260,000/mm^3, or any number between 250,000/mm^3 and 300,000/mm^3 25. About 2.4 qt

---

4-3. CONVERSIONS BETWEEN UNITS OF LENGTH

It is often necessary to convert from one unit of measurement to another. For instance, is a bandage labeled "5 cm" long enough to cover a 40-mm wound?

Converting from Larger to Smaller Units

CONVERSIONS

From	To	Relationship	Process
km m	m mm	1 km = 1000 m 1 m = 1000 mm	Multiply by 1000 (Move decimal point 3 places to right)
m	cm	1 m = 100 cm	Multiply by 100 (Move decimal point 2 places to right)
m dm cm	dm cm mm	1 m = 10 dm 1 dm = 10 cm 1 cm = 10 mm	Multiply by 10 (Move decimal point 1 place to right)

When we convert from a larger unit to a smaller one, we expect to have a larger number of the smaller units, and we move the decimal point to the right. This is just what we expect when we exchange a dollar bill for pennies. For 1 dollar, we expect 100 pennies to retain the same monetary value.

Examples

1. $2 \text{ m} = 2 \times 1000 \text{ mm} = 2000 \text{ mm}$
2. $3 \text{ m} = 3 \times 10 \text{ dm} = 30 \text{ dm}$
3. $1.5 \text{ m} = 1.5 \times 100 \text{ cm} = 150 \text{ cm}$
4. $0.125 \text{ m} = 125 \text{ mm}$
5. $\frac{1}{2} \text{ km} = \frac{1}{2} \times 1000 \text{ m} = 500 \text{ m}$
6. 4.5 cm = 45 mm (Check with the ruler.)
7. 5 cm = 50 mm. Therefore a bandage labeled 5 cm is long enough to cover a 40-mm wound.

SAMPLE EXERCISES

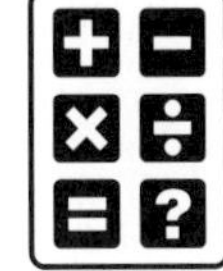

Exercises 1–5. Convert the given number of meters to centimeters.

1. 3 m
2. 5.46 m
3. 0.09 m
4. 0.482 m
5. $\frac{3}{5}$ m

Exercises 6–12. Convert as indicated.

6. 5 m to millimeters
7. 5.43 m to centimeters
8. 0.002 m to millimeters
9. 2.85 m to decimeters
10. $\frac{3}{4}$ m to centimeters
11. 7.9 cm to millimeters
12. 48 cm to millimeters

ANSWERS 1. 300 cm 2. 546 cm 3. 9 cm 4. 48.2 cm 5. 60 cm 6. 5000 mm 7. 543 cm 8. 2 mm 9. 28.5 dm 10. 75 cm 11. 79 mm 12. 480 mm

---

Converting from Smaller to Larger Units

CONVERSIONS

From	To	Relationship	Action
m mm	km m	1 m = 0.001 km 1 mm = 0.001 m	Multiply by 0.001 (Move decimal point 3 places to left)
cm	m	1 cm = 0.01 m	Multiply by 0.01 (Move decimal point 2 places to left)
dm mm	m cm	1 dm = 0.1 m 1 mm = 0.1 cm	Multiply by 0.1 (Move decimal point 1 place to left)

In other cases, we need to change from a smaller unit of measurement to a larger one, such as from 300 cm to 3 m. In these cases, we expect a smaller number of the larger units, just as we expect a small number of dollar bills when we turn in a large number of pennies.

Examples

1. 125 mm = 125 × 0.001 m = 0.125 m
2. 50 dm = 50 × 0.1 m = 5 m
3. 300 cm = 300 × 0.01 m = 3 m
4. 6200 mm = 6.2 m
5. 56.2 mm = 5.62 cm
6. One type of electrocardiograph machine uses 50-mm paper. If the paper is marked "5 cm," we know that it will fit the machine.

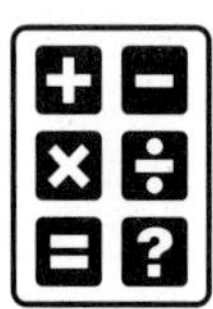

SAMPLE EXERCISES

Exercises 1–3. Convert the given number of centimeters to meters.

1. 250 cm
2. 10 cm
3. 43 cm

Exercises 4–7. Convert as indicated.

4. 2700 mm to meters
5. 380 cm to meters
6. 28.9 dm to meters
7. 14.82 mm to centimeters
8. Paper for a certain electrocardiograph machine must be 63 mm wide. Will paper marked 6.3 cm fit the requirement?

ANSWERS 1. 2.5 m 2. 0.1 m 3. 0.43 m 4. 2.7 m 5. 3.8 m 6. 2.89 m 7. 1.482 cm 8. yes

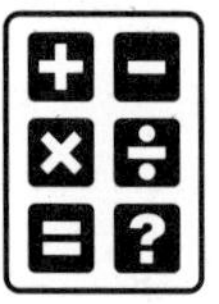

EXERCISES

Exercises 1–20. Convert as indicated.

1. 6 m to millimeters
2. 6 m to centimeters
3. 12,000 mm to meters
4. 8000 mm to meters
5. 8 m to millimeters
6. 8 m to decimeters
7. 7.25 m to millimeters
8. 85.6 m to millimeters
9. 61 dm to meters
10. 6800 mm to meters
11. 0.065 m to millimeters
12. 0.6 m to decimeters
13. 6289 mm to meters
14. 46.24 cm to meters
15. 650.6 mm to meters
16. 70.58 dm to meters
17. 979 mm to meters
18. 0.076 m to centimeters
19. 4.2 m to centimeters
20. 82.5 dm to meters

Exercises 21–24. Complete the statement.

21. To convert from meters to millimeters, multiply the number of meters by ______.
22. To convert from decimeters to meters, multiply the number of decimeters by ______.
23. To convert from millimeters to centimeters, multiply the number of millimeters by ______.
24. To convert from meters to centimeters, multiply the number of meters by ______.

ANSWERS 1. 6000 mm 3. 12 m 5. 8000 mm 7. 7250 mm
9. 6.1 m 11. 65 mm 13. 6.289 m 15. 0.6506 m
17. 0.979 m 19. 420 cm 21. 1000 23. 0.1

4-4. LIQUID CAPACITY (VOLUME)

The **liter (L)** is used to measure liquid capacity. Actually, 1 L is equal to 1 cubic decimeter (dm^3), but *liter* is a more popular term.

LIQUID CAPACITY

The **liter (L)** is a unit of **liquid capacity.**

$$1\text{ L} > 1\text{ qt}$$

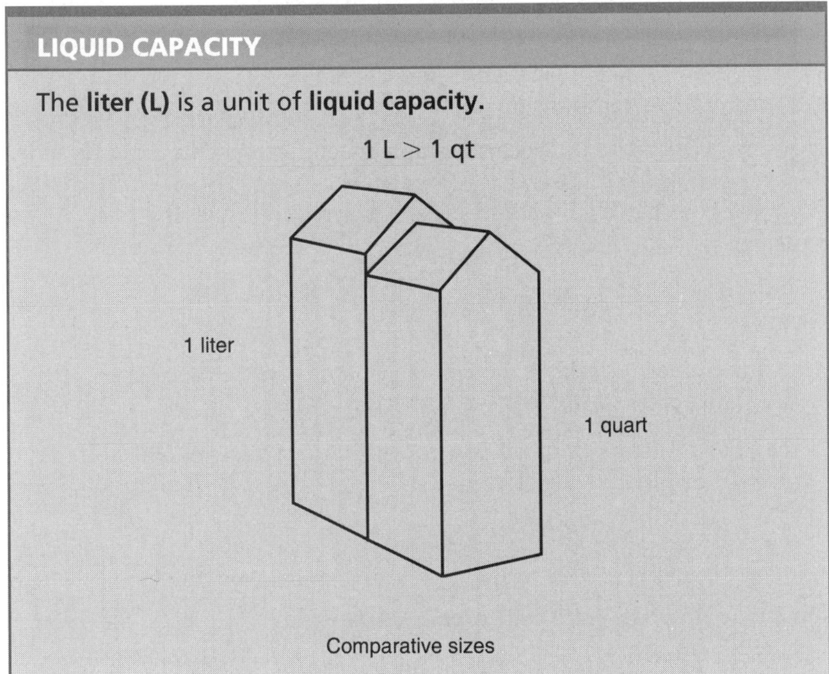

Comparative sizes

Examples

1. 1 dm^3 = 1 L. The symbol for liter is an uppercase L to avoid confusion with the numeral 1.
2. The liter is slightly greater than a quart.

$$1\text{ L} = 1.1\text{ qt (approximately)}$$

A child who drinks 7 L of milk per week is drinking a little more than 7 qt per week.

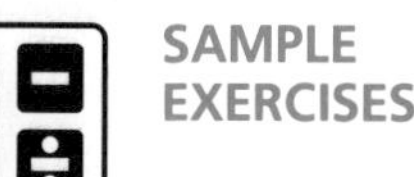

SAMPLE EXERCISES

1. A container holds 4 L of water. What quantity does the symbol 4 L represent?
2. Write eight liters in symbols:
3. Which is greater, 4 L or 4 qt?

ANSWERS 1. Four liters (a little more than 4 qt) 2. 8 L 3. 4 L

Standard Prefixes

As shown in the previous section, one of the advantages of SI is that it enables us to combine standard prefixes with different basic units. The following table shows how the same standard prefixes are combined with liter for the measurements most often used in nursing.

STANDARD PREFIXES

Prefix	Meaning	Combined Form (with Liter)	Relationships
deci (d)	0.1	deciliter (dL)	1 dL = 0.1 L 1 L = 10 dL
milli (m)	0.001	milliliter (mL)	1 mL = 0.001 L 1 L = 1000 mL

The symbols L, dL, mL, and other SI symbols involving liter all use the uppercase L.

Examples

1. A juice glass, usually 4 ounces (oz), holds a little more than 1 dL.
2. A standard teaspoon (tsp) holds about 5 mL.
3. Results of Mr. V.'s blood test for vitamin D showed 100 units (U) per dL of blood.

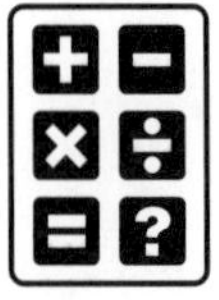

SAMPLE EXERCISES

1. How many milliliters are in a liter?
2. If a liter is divided into 10 parts, what is each part called?
3. About how many milliliters are contained in 2 standard teaspoons?

ANSWERS 1. 1000 mL 2. 1 dL 3. 10 mL

Since 1 L is equal to 1 dm^3, it follows that 1 mL is equal to 1 cm^3. The preferred SI notation for cubic centimeter, $\mathbf{cm^3}$, is replacing the old notation cc, but you will still encounter cc. Since 1 cm^3 is equivalent to 1 mL, it is common practice to use cm^3, mL, and cc interchangeably.

CUBIC CENTIMETER

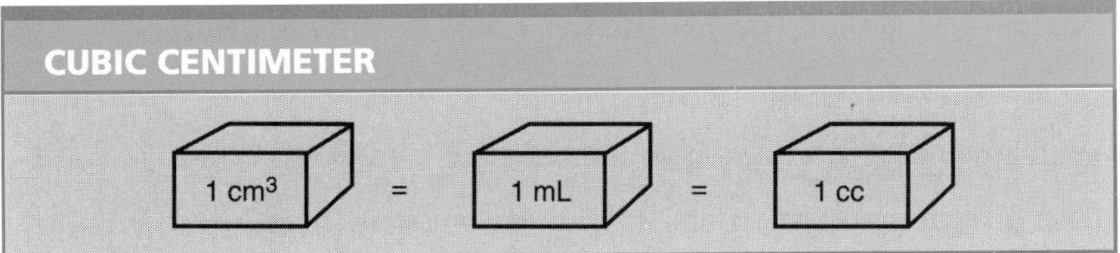

Examples

1. The capacity of the insulin syringe shown in the figure is 1 cc, which means 1 cm³, or 1 mL.

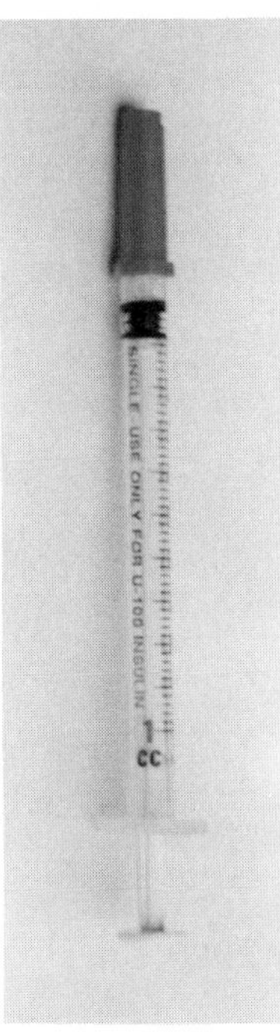

2. For injections of vitamin B, 10-cc vials are available.

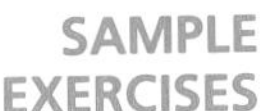

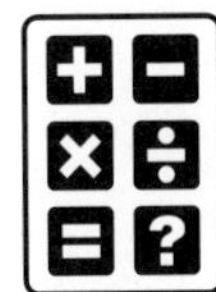

Exercises 1–4. Convert as indicated.

1. 17.6 mL to cc
2. 9 cc to cm³
3. 240 cc to mL
4. 1000 mL to cm³

ANSWERS 1. 17.6 cc 2. 9 cm³ 3. 240 mL 4. 1000 cm³

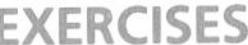

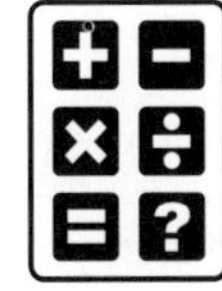

1. About how much milk (in quarts) is available if the inventory shows that there are 7 L left?
2. If 10 qt of milk have been delivered, about how many liters of milk have been delivered?

Exercises 3–4. A gallon (gal) container holds exactly 4 qt.

3. Is a gallon of gas approximately equivalent to 4 L?
4. About how many liters of milk are there in a $\frac{1}{2}$-gal container?
5. About how many quarts does a 3.5-dm^3 container hold?
6. How many liters are there in 4.2 dm^3?

Exercises 7–14. Change the following ratios to pure ratios (ratios without units).

7. $\frac{1\text{ L}}{1\text{ cL}}$

8. $\frac{1\text{ L}}{1\text{ mL}}$

9. $\frac{1\text{ mL}}{1\text{ L}}$

10. $\frac{1\text{ cL}}{1\text{ L}}$

11. 2 dm^3:1 L

12. 5.3 L:1 dm^3

13. $\frac{0.5\text{ dm}^3}{2\text{ L}}$

14. $\frac{6\text{ dm}^3}{4\text{ L}}$

Exercises 15–20. Convert as indicated.

15. 4 cm^3 to cc
16. 1 L to cc
17. 65.9 cc to mL
18. 1000 cc to dm^3
19. 2 L to cm^3
20. 4000 cm^3 to dm^3

ANSWERS 1. About 7 qt 3. 4 L > 1 gal, slightly 5. 3.5 qt
7. $\frac{100}{1}$ 9. $\frac{1}{1000} \times 0.001$ 11. $\frac{2}{1}$ 13. $\frac{0.5}{2} = 0.25 = \frac{1}{4}$
15. 4 cc 17. 65.9 mL 19. 2000 cm^3

4-5. CONVERSIONS BETWEEN UNITS OF LIQUID CAPACITY

Converting from Larger to Smaller Units

CONVERSIONS

From	To	Relationship	Action
L	dL	1 L = 10 dL	Multiply by 10 (Move decimal point 1 place to right)
dL	mL	1 dL = 100 mL	Multiply by 100 (Move decimal point 2 places to right)
L	mL	1 L = 1000 mL	Multiply by 1000 (Move decimal point 3 places to right)

Reminder: When we convert from a larger unit to a smaller one, we must have a larger number of the smaller units to retain the value of the original quantity.

Examples

1. 2 L = 2 × 1000 mL = 2000 mL
2. 3 L = 3 × 10 dL = 30 dL
3. 0.125 L = 125 mL
4. $\frac{1}{2}$ L = $\frac{1}{2}$ × 10 dL = 5 dL
5. A small container of milk may be marked 3 dL or 300 mL.

SAMPLE EXERCISES

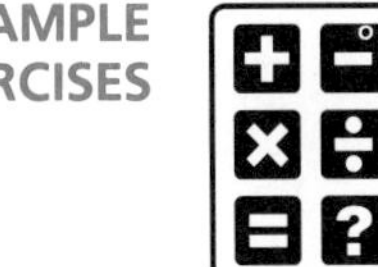

Exercises 1–5. Convert the given number of liters to milliliters.

1. 6 L
2. 1.35 L
3. 0.04 L
4. 0.375 L
5. $\frac{1}{5}$ L

Exercises 6–8. Convert as indicated.

6. 4 L to milliliters
7. 0.005 L to milliliters
8. 1.75 L to deciliters

ANSWERS 1. 6000 mL 2. 1350 mL 3. 40 mL 4. 375 mL 5. 200 mL 6. 4000 mL 7. 5 mL 8. 17.5 dL

Converting from Smaller to Larger Units

CONVERSIONS

From	To	Relationship	Action
dL	L	1 dL = 0.1 L	Multiply by 0.1 (Move decimal point 1 place to left)
mL	dL	1 mL = 0.01 dL	Multiply by 0.01 (Move decimal point 2 places to left)
mL	L	1 mL = 0.001 L	Multiply by 0.001 (Move decimal point 3 places to left)

Reminder: When we convert from a smaller unit to a larger, we must have a smaller number of the larger units.

Examples

1. 625 mL = 625 × 0.001 L = 0.625 L
2. 20 dL = 20 × 0.1 L = 2 L
3. 1200 mL = 1.2 L

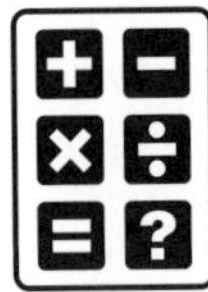

SAMPLE EXERCISES

Exercises 1–3. Convert the given number of milliliters to liters.

1. 1500 mL
2. 90 mL
3. 550 mL

Exercises 4–5. Convert as indicated.

4. 3600 mL to liters
5. 19.8 dL to liters
6. If, by sweating, Mr. G. lost 10 L of water on Thursday and absorbed a total of 9000 mL of water from food and drink that day, what was the net change (in liters) for the day?

ANSWERS 1. 1.5 L 2. 0.09 L 3. 0.55 L 4. 3.6 L 5. 1.98 L 6. 1 L

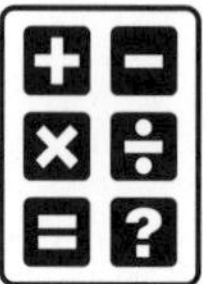

EXERCISES

Exercises 1–20. Convert as indicated.

1. 3 L to milliliters
2. 3 L to cubic centimeters
3. 9000 mL to liters
4. 5000 cc to liters
5. 5 L to cubic centimeters
6. 5 L to deciliters
7. 3.91 L to milliliters
8. 52.3 L to milliliters
9. 28 dL to liters
10. 5000 cc to liters
11. 0.032 L to milliliters
12. 0.3 L to deciliters
13. 2956 mL to liters
14. 12.91 cm^3 to liters
15. 327.3 mL to liters
16. 37.25 dL to liters
17. 646 mL to liters
18. 0.043 L to cubic centimeters
19. 1.9 L to cubic centimeters
20. 49.2 dL to liters
21. 9.35 dL to milliliters
22. 215 mL to deciliters

Exercises 23–26. Complete the statement.

23. To convert from liters to milliliters, multiply the number of liters by ______.
24. To convert from deciliters to liters, multiply the number of deciliters by ______.
25. To convert from cubic centimeters to liters, multiply the number of cubic centimeters by ______.
26. To convert from liters to cubic centimeters, multiply the number of liters by ______.

ANSWERS 1. 3000 mL 3. 9 L 5. 5000 cc 7. 3910 mL 9. 2.8 L 11. 32 mL 13. 2.956 L 15. 0.3273 L 17. 0.646 L 19. 1900 cm^3 21. 935 mL 23. 1000 25. 0.001

4-6. WEIGHT

In the SI, the gram (g) is used to measure weight.* One gram is the weight of 1 mL of ice-cold water. (Picture the amount of water in a miniature teaspoon.)

WEIGHT

The **gram (g)** is a measure of **weight.** 1 mL of liquid weighs 1 g, approximately.

The Gram

Examples

1. A typical serving of a sugar substitute weighs 1 g.
2. An ounce is about 30 times heavier than 1 g. Thus, 30 mL of water weighs about 1 oz.
3. A standard paper clip usually weighs about 1 g. A set of 30 standard clips weighs about 1 oz.
4. Each gram of protein provides 4 calories (cal). If the protein in your breakfast provided a total of 320 cal, we can determine how much protein was present. The following table summarizes the situation.

Weight (Grams)	*Calories*
x	320
1	4

Proportion: $\frac{x}{1} = \frac{320}{4}$

Result: 80 g

SAMPLE EXERCISES

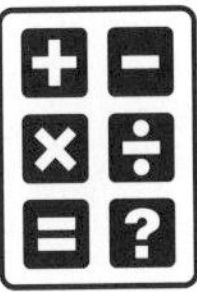

1. Each gram of fat provides 9 cal. If the fat in the patient's dinner provides a total of 1260 cal, how much fat is present?
2. If 1 oz is about 30 g, what is the weight (in grams) of a 4-oz piece of cheese?

* On earth, the terms *weight* and *mass* may be used interchangeably.

ANSWERS

1.

Weight (Grams)	*Calories*
x	1260
1	9

Proportion: $\frac{x}{1} = \frac{1260}{9}$

Result: 140 g

2.

Weight (Grams)	*Ounces*
x	4
30	1

Proportion: $\frac{x}{30} = \frac{4}{1}$

Result: 120 g

Standard Prefixes

Along with the gram, nurses often find use for the prefixes shown in the following table.

STANDARD PREFIXES

Prefix	Meaning	Combined Form (with gram)	Relationships
kilo (k)	1000	kilogram (kg)*	1 kg = 1000 g 1 g = 0.001 kg
milli (m)	0.001	milligram (mg)	1 mg = 0.001 g 1 g = 1000 mg
micro (μ)†	0.000001	microgram (μg)†	1 μg = 0.001 mg 1 mg = 1000 μg

Examples

1. Each of the units kg, g, mg, and μg is 0.001 as large as the previous unit in this list. If we divide:

   1 kg into 1000 parts, each part is 1 g (0.001 kg);
   1 g into 1000 parts, each part is 1 mg (0.001 g);
   1 mg into 1000 parts, each part is 1 μg (0.001 mg).

2. If 3 medium potatoes weigh about 1 lb, 6 such potatoes weigh about 1 kg. The kilogram is about twice as heavy as a pound.

---

* The standard for the kilogram is a cylinder of platinum–iridium alloy kept by the International Bureau of Weights and Measures in Paris. The US National Bureau of Standards keeps a duplicate.

† Special care is needed with this symbol. Sometimes μg, when handwritten, is confused with mg. Although μg is the standard SI symbol for microgram, you will sometimes see mcg instead.

3. A milligram may be pictured as the weight of a speck of dew or of a small crumb of graham cracker.
4. To see an object weighing 1 μg, we would need a microscope.
5. A glass of milk (8 oz) contains 300 mg of calcium.
6. Results of a blood test may show a normal glucose level of 60 mg/dL of blood.

SAMPLE EXERCISES

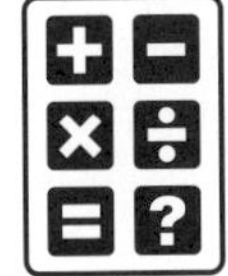

1. Would you be likely to advise a short woman weighing 100 kg to lose weight?

Exercises 2–3. Complete the statement.

2. ______ μg = 1 mg.
3. An ounce weighs about 30 g = ______ mg.

ANSWERS 1. yes, 100 kg > 200 lb 2. 1000 3. 30,000

Conversions between Units of Weight

Converting from Larger to Smaller

CONVERSIONS

From	To	Relationship	Action
kg	g	1 kg = 1000 g	Multiply by 1000 (Move decimal point 3 places to right)
g	mg	1 g = 1000 mg	
mg	µg	1 mg = 1000 µg	

Reminder: When we convert from a larger unit to a smaller, we must have a larger number of the smaller units.

Examples

1. 4 kg = 4 × 1000 g = 4000 g
2. 0.3 g = 0.3 × 1000 mg = 300 mg
3. 1.5 mg = 1.5 × 1000 μg = 1500 μg
4. 0.125 g = 125 mg
5. $1/2 \text{ kg} = \frac{1}{\not{2}_1} \times \overset{500}{\not{1000}}\text{ g} = 500 \text{ g}$

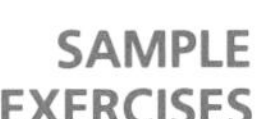

SAMPLE EXERCISES

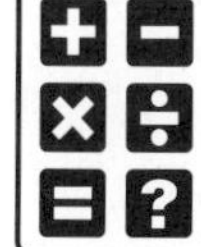

Exercises 1–4. Convert the given number of grams to milligrams.

1. 2 g
2. 57.46 g
3. 0.04 g
4. 0.482 g

Exercises 5–10. Convert as indicated.

5. 10 mg to micrograms
6. 3 g to milligrams
7. 7.42 g to milligrams
8. 0.025 mg to micrograms
9. 5.75 kg to grams
10. $\frac{3}{4}$ kg to grams
11. When Mrs. J. was pregnant, she was advised to include at least 1.5 g of calcium in her diet per day. If she actually had a total of 1800 mg of calcium per day, was she following the advice?

ANSWERS 1. 2000 mg 2. 57,460 mg 3. 40 mg 4. 482 mg 5. 10,000 μg 6. 3000 mg 7. 7420 mg 8. 25 μg 9. 5750 g 10. 750 g 11. yes

When we need to change from a smaller unit to a larger, such as from 2000 mg to 2 g, we recall that as the units increase, we need fewer of them to make up the same total weight.

Converting from Smaller to Larger

CONVERSIONS

From	To	Relationship	Action
g	kg	1 g = 0.001 kg	Multiply by 0.001 (Move decimal point 3 places to left)
mg	g	1 mg = 0.001 g	
μg	mg	1 μg = 0.001 mg	

Examples

1. 925 g = 925 × 0.001 kg = 0.925 kg
2. 600 mg = 600 × 0.001 g = 0.6 g
3. 5140 μg = 5140 × 0.001 mg = 5.14 mg
4. 13,200 mg = 13.2 g
5. A tablet of penicillin V potassium may contain 250 mg. If a patient took 4 such tablets in one day, the total dosage would be 1000 mg, or 1 g of the drug.

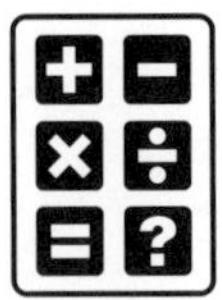

SAMPLE EXERCISES

Exercises 1–3. Convert the given number of milligrams to grams.

1. 350 mg
2. 5100 mg
3. 56 mg

Exercises 4–6. Convert as indicated.

4. 3600 μg to milligrams
5. 47,000 g to kilograms
6. 28.9 μg to milligrams

7. Mr. G., who has angina, takes 150 μg of nitroglycerin regularly. In milligrams what is this amount?
8. Find the capacity of a container that holds 1 kg of water.

ANSWERS 1. 0.35 g 2. 5.1 g 3. 0.056 g 4. 3.6 mg 5. 47 kg 6. 0.0289 mg 7. 0.15 mg 8. 1000 mL = 1 L (See Section 4-6.)

EXERCISES

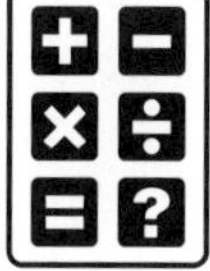

Exercises 1–20. Convert as indicated.

1. 6 kg to grams
2. 5 g to milligrams
3. 6000 mg to grams
4. 2000 μg to milligrams
5. 950 mg to micrograms
6. 145 mg to micrograms
7. 1.93 kg to grams
8. 25.3 g to milligrams
9. 528 μg to milligrams
10. 15,000 μg to milligrams
11. 0.084 mg to grams
12. 0.24 kg to grams
13. 6529 μg to milligrams
14. 1.291 kg to grams
15. 425.7 mg to grams
16. 7250 μg to milligrams
17. 658 mg to grams
18. 0.043 mg to micrograms
19. 21.9 kg to grams
20. 15,000 μg to grams

Exercises 21–24. Complete the statement.

21. To convert from grams to milligrams, multiply the number of grams by ______.
22. To convert from milligrams to grams, multiply the number of milligrams by ______.
23. To convert from micrograms to milligrams, multiply the number of micrograms by ______.
24. To convert from kilograms to grams, multiply the number of kilograms by ______.
25. Mrs. B. needs to restrict her sodium intake to <2 g/day. Records show that, during the meals and snacks of the day, her sodium intake was 200 mg, 400 mg, 250 mg, 800 mg, and 325 mg. Was the total within the maximum allowable?
26. Drug A weighs 1.04 g; drug B weighs 10.2 mg. Which drug is heavier?

Exercises 27–32. Normal serum calcium levels, measured by blood tests, range from 8.4 to 10.4 mg/dL. Determine which of the following recorded calcium levels are in the normal range.

27. 9.95 mg/dL
28. 7.85 mg/dL
29. 8.04 mg/dL
30. 0.9 mg/mL
31. 9.5 g/dL
32. 0.1 g/L

ANSWERS 1. 6000 g 3. 6 g 5. 950,000 μg 7. 1,930 g 9. 0.528 mg 11. 0.000084 g 13. 6.529 mg 15. 0.4257 g 17. 0.658 g 19. 21,900 g 21. 1000 23. 0.001 25. yes, 1975 mg < 2 g 27. yes 29. no 31. no

4-7. SUBSTANCE

The Mole

Patients take diagnostic tests to ascertain amounts of various substances in their blood. In the SI, the **mole (mol)** is used to measure the amount of a substance.

AMOUNT

The **mole (mol)** is the basic unit for the **amount** of a substance.

Examples

1. A mole is the name for a fixed number* of elements, just as a dozen is the name for a set of 12 items. One mole (mol) of a substance has the same number of atoms or *mole*cules as 1 mol of any other substance.
2. In a liter of normal blood, there may be 0.03 mol of carbon dioxide and 0.1 mol of sodium.
3. By definition, 1 mol of aspirin and 1 mol of salt have the same number* of molecules, but their weights are different, just as 1 dozen pencils weighs more than 1 dozen paper clips. The approximate weights of 1 mol of aspirin and 1 mol of salt are 180 g and 60 g, respectively.

Standard Prefixes

With the mole, nurses commonly see the following prefixes.

STANDARD PREFIXES

Prefix	Meaning	Combined Form (with mole)	Relationships
milli (m)	0.001	millimole (mmol)	1 mmol = 0.001 mol 1 mol = 1000 mmol
micro (μ)	0.000001	micromole (μmol)	1 μmol = 0.001 mmol 1 mmol = 1000 μmol
nano (n)	0.000000001	nanomole (nmol)	1 nmol = 0.001 μmol 1 μmol = 1000 nmol
pico (p)	0.000000000001	picomole (pmol)	1 pmol = 0.001 nmol 1 nmol = 1000 pmol

* The fixed number is 6.022×10^{23} = 602, 200, 000, 000, 000, 000, 000, 000.

Examples

1. Each unit is 0.001 of the next higher unit in the list. If we divide:

   1 mol into 1000 parts, each part is 1 mmol (0.001 mol);
   1 mmol into 1000 parts, each part is 1 μmol (0.001 mmol);
   1 μmol into 1000 parts, each part is 1 nmol (0.001 μmol);
   1 nmol into 1000 parts, each part is 1 pmol (0.001 nmol).

2. Blood tests may show the following results:

Substance	*Amount Normally Expected in 1 L of Blood*
Ascorbic Acid (vitamin C)	23–57 μmol
Calcitonin	<50 pmol
Carotene	0.74–3.72 mol
Cholesterol	3.9–6.5 mmol
Hemoglobin	7.4–11.2 mmol
Lead	<1.0 μmol
Progesterone	6 nmol (men) >16 nmol (women)
Testosterone	10–42 nmol (men) 1.1–3.3 nmol (women)
Triglycerides	0.45–1.80 mmol/L

SAMPLE EXERCISES

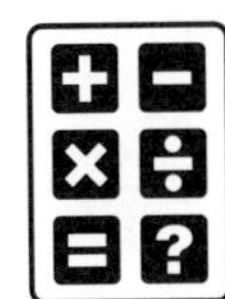

Exercises 1–4. Assess the blood test results of the patient. Use the table above for the range of normal values.

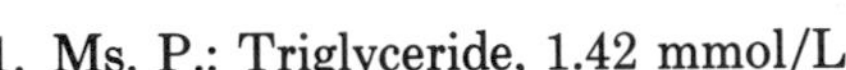

1. Ms. P.: Triglyceride, 1.42 mmol/L
2. Mr. W.: Ascorbic acid, 65.2 μmol/L
3. Mrs. V.: Calcitonin, 52.6 pmol/L
4. Prof. B.: Carotene, 0.69 mol/L

ANSWERS 1. Normal 2. Above normal 3. Above normal 4. Below normal

Conversions between Units of Substance

CONVERSIONS

From	To	Action
mol mmol μmol nmol	mmol μmol nmol pmol	Multiply by 1000 (Move decimal point 3 places to right)
mmol μmol nmol pmol	mol mmol μmol nmol	Multiply by 0.001 (Move decimal point 3 places to left)

Examples

1. $400 \text{ mol} = 400 \times 1000 \text{ mmol} = 400{,}000 \text{ mmol}$
2. $400 \text{ mmol} = 400 \times 0.001 \text{ mol} = 0.4 \text{ mol}$
3. $3.5 \text{ mmol} = 3.5 \times 1000\ \mu\text{mol} = 3500\ \mu\text{mol}$
4. $6125\ \mu\text{mol} = 6.125 \text{ mmol}$
5. Calcitonin in the blood should be <50 pmol/L, or 0.05 nmol/L.

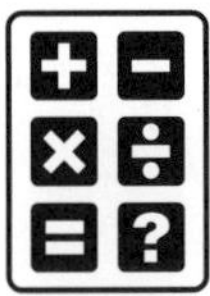

SAMPLE EXERCISES

Exercises 1–4. Convert the given number of moles to millimoles.

1. 9.5 mol
2. 2.98 mol
3. 0.06 mol
4. 0.159 mol

Exercises 5–9. Convert as indicated.

5. 9.35 mol to millimoles
6. 0.025 mol to millimoles
7. 350 mmol to moles
8. 5100 mmol to moles
9. 56 mmol to micromoles
10. A patient's blood test showed that his calcium level was 0.04 μmol in a milliliter of blood. How many nanomoles does this figure represent?

ANSWERS 1. 9500 mmol 2. 2980 mmol 3. 60 mmol 4. 159 mmol 5. 9350 mmol 6. 25 mmol 7. 0.35 mol 8. 5.1 mol 9. 56,000 μmol 10. 40 nmol

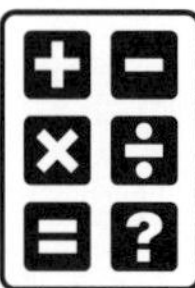

EXERCISES

Exercises 1–12. Convert as indicated.

1. 6 mol to millimoles
2. 56.1 mmol to micromoles
3. 453 pmol to nanomoles
4. 0.128 mol to millimoles
5. 32 mol to millimoles
6. 2.3 nmol to picomoles
7. 0.04 mmol to micromoles
8. 470 μmol to millimoles
9. 0.2 pmol to nanomoles
10. 0.7 nmol to micromoles
11. 87.4 μmol to nanomoles
12. 62 mmol to moles

Exercises 13–14. Complete the statement.

13. To convert from micromole to millimole, multiply the number of micromoles by ______.
14. To convert from micromole to nanomole, multiply the number of micromoles by ______.

Exercises 15–20. Normally, the carbon dioxide content of the blood is between 21 and 30 mmol/L. Are the following amounts of carbon dioxide content in the blood within the normal range?

15. 29.5 mmol/L
16. 18.9 mmol/L
17. 0.026 mol/L
18. 2.25 mmol/dL

19. 0.031 mmol/mL

20. 2500 μmol in 100 mL

Exercises 21–32. You are asked to assess the plasma cortisol level of patients on long-term therapy. Normal values are 138–635 nmol/L. For the following given recorded plasma cortisol level, what is your assessment?

21. 128 nmol/L
22. 490 nmol/L
23. 640 nmol/L
24. 630 nmol/L
25. 0.75 μmol/L
26. 0.138 nmol/L
27. 0.45 pmol/L
28. 6.35 μmol/L
29. 0.2 nmol/mL
30. 0.5 nmol/L
31. 0.99 nmol/mL
32. 265 pmol/mL

Exercises 33–36. Assess the blood test results of the patient. Use the table of normal amounts for substances found in blood in Example 2 (page 123) for the range of normal values.

33. Ms. Y.: Carotene, 950 mmol/L
34. Mr. Q.: Testosterone, 0.03 μmol/L
35. Mrs. W.: Cholesterol, 670 μmol/L
36. Prof. Z.: Calcitonin, 0.04 nmol/L

ANSWERS 1. 6000 mmol 3. 0.453 nmol 5. 32,000 mmol 7. 40 μmol 9. 0.0002 nmol 11. 87,400 nmol 13. 0.001 15. within 17. within 19. above 21. below normal 23. above normal 25. above normal 27. too low 29. normal 31. above normal 33. normal 35. below normal

---

4-8. PROPORTIONS APPLIED TO CONVERSIONS

Proportions provide a dependable, general method for conversion problems. They also serve as a strong foundation for the formulas that will be introduced in the later sections of this text and serve us well if we ever forget how to use those formulas.

General Method for Any Kind of Conversion: Proportions

Examples

1. To convert from 6.5 dL to milliliters, use the relationships:

$$1 \text{ L} = 10 \text{ dL} \quad \text{and} \quad 1 \text{ L} = 1000 \text{ mL}$$

Tabulate (T):	*Milliliters*	*Deciliters*	
(Make sure that the units match)	x	6.5	(Make the units match)
	1000	10	

Proportion: $\frac{x}{1000} = \frac{6.5}{10}$

(Use pure ratios from matching units)

Estimate (E): Between 600 and 700 mL

Compute (C): $x = \frac{6.5}{10} \times 1000$

$= 650$ (Agrees with estimate)

Result: 6.5 dL = 650 mL

Check (C): 650 mL = 6.5 dL

2. To convert 14.8 in. to centimeters, use the relationship

1 in. = 2.5 cm

Tabulate (T):

Centimeters	Inches	
x	14.8	(Make sure that the units match)
2.5	1	

Estimate (E): Between 30 and 45 cm

Proportion: $\frac{x}{2.5} = \frac{14.8}{1}$

(Use pure ratios from matching units)

Compute (C): $x = 14.8 \times 2.5 = 37$

Result: 14.8 in. = 37 cm (Agrees with estimate)

Check (C): 37 cm = 14.8 in.

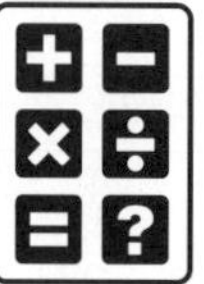

SAMPLE EXERCISES

Exercises 1–2. To answer the following questions, use the relationship 1 m = 3.3 ft.

1. Approximately how many feet are in 4.2 m?
2. Approximately how many meters are in 20.3 ft?

ANSWERS 1. 13.9 ft 2. 6.2 m

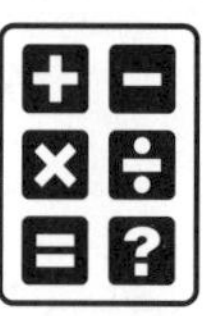

EXERCISES

Wherever rounding is appropriate, round to the nearest tenth.

Exercises 1–8. Convert as indicated. Use the relationship 1 m = 3.3 ft.

1. 4.4 m to feet
2. 14.35 ft to meters
3. 0.8 m to feet
4. 2.75 m to feet
5. 0.9 ft to meters
6. 48.5 ft to meters
7. 1.25 m to feet
8. 20.3 ft to meters

Exercises 9–16. Using the relationship 1 in. = 2.5 cm, convert as indicated.

9. 4 in. to centimeters
10. 6.5 in. to centimeters
11. 10 cm to inches
12. 6.9 cm to inches
13. 5.9 in. to millimeters
14. 22.8 mm to inches
15. 16.4 mm to inches
16. 14.8 in. to millimeters

Exercises 17–20. Convert as indicated. Where needed, use the relationship, 1 dL = 3 oz, approximately.

17. 2.5 dL to ounces
18. 2.0 oz to deciliters
19. 3.5 oz to milliliters
20. 4.2 dL to milliliters

ANSWERS 1. 13.2 ft 3. 2.6 ft 5. 0.3 m 7. 4.1 ft 9. 10 cm 11. 4 in. 13. 147.5 mm 15. 0.7 in. 17. 7.5 oz 19. 116.7 mL

4-9. AVOIDING ERRORS: USING MENTAL IMAGES

Basic Measures

To keep the basic measures (meter, liter, gram, and mole) clearly in mind, develop a special mental image for each one. Use the suggestions given below and in previous sections, and make up others that work for you.

MENTAL IMAGES FOR METER, LITER, GRAM, AND MOLE

Meter (Length): The distance from the floor to a doorknob (approximately), and a little bit more than a yard. Half the height of a very tall person.
Liter (Capacity): A little bit more than a quart.
Gram (Weight): A standard paper clip on a scale.
Mole (Amount of Substance): A fixed number of *mol*ecules.

Examples

Mental images can prevent errors.

1. If "m" is carelessly substituted for "ft," an image of the bigger distance from the floor to the doorknob clashes with the image of a foot, causing immediate correction of the error.
2. If 30 L is given as the amount of a urine sample, picturing the large amount alerts us to an error.

SAMPLE EXERCISES

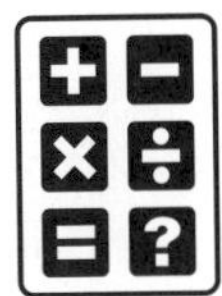

Exercises 1–4. Explain why each of the following statements must contain an error.

1. Mr. F. is 6 m tall.
2. Patty weighs 60 g.
3. Ms. C. donated 500 L of blood.
4. The premature baby weighs 2.5 g.

ANSWERS 1. Very few people are more than 2 m tall (above the top of a door). 2. Patty's weight would be no more than a box of 60 clips. 3. Ms. C. would have enough blood to fill a hot tub. 4. The baby would weigh no more than a few clips.

Conversions

For conversions from larger units to smaller, picture inserting a single dollar bill into a change machine; you expect the machine to return a handful of coins in exchange.

SUBDIVISION IMAGES

Centimeter, Millimeter: Picture the width of a paper clip and the width of its wire.
Milliliter: Picture a tiny ice cube in a liter of liquid.

Examples

Your mental images will help to prevent accidental errors such as

1. Converting 1 cm to 100 m, or 1 L to 10 mL
   or
2. Associating 1 g with 1 L.

A mental image of making change is a guide in converting from any unit to a smaller unit.

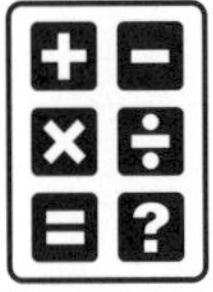

SAMPLE EXERCISES

Exercises 1–3. In each of the following cases, use a mental image as a guide in the indicated conversion.

1. 4 m to centimeters
2. 35 mL to liters
3. 0.25 mmol to micromoles

Exercises 4–5. Explain why each of the following statements must contain an error.

4. $\frac{2\text{ L}}{6\text{ mL}} = \frac{1}{3}$

5. If $\frac{2}{3}$ cup of cereal A contains 4.2 g of fiber, and $\frac{1}{3}$ cup of cereal B contains 5.9 mg of fiber, then B contains more fiber.

ANSWERS 1. 400 cm 2. 0.035 L 3. 250 μmol 4. 2 L is much larger than 6 mL; thus the fraction could not reduce to $\frac{1}{3}$. 5. Since 5.9 mg is a very small amount compared with 4.2 g, $\frac{1}{3}$ cup of B must contain less fiber.

Proportions

Keep a mental image of symmetry and balance, "everything in proportion."

$$\frac{\text{Smaller}}{\text{Larger}} = \frac{\text{Smaller}}{\text{Larger}}$$

or

$$\frac{\text{Larger}}{\text{Smaller}} = \frac{\text{Larger}}{\text{Smaller}}$$

or

$$\frac{\text{Small A}}{\text{Small B}} = \frac{\text{Large A}}{\text{Large B}}$$

Examples

1. If $\frac{x}{3} = \frac{7}{9}$, then $x < 3$, because $7 < 9$.
2. If $\frac{x \text{ mL}}{200 \text{ mL}} = \frac{10 \text{ g}}{150 \text{ g}}$, then $x < 200$, because $10 < 150$.
3. If $\frac{x \text{ mL}}{100 \text{ mL}} = \frac{200 \text{ mg}}{25 \text{ mg}}$, then $x > 100$, because $200 > 25$.

SAMPLE EXERCISES

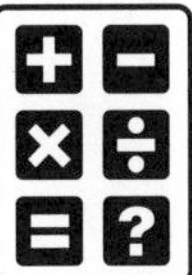

Exercises 1–2. Without computing, state why the solution for the given proportion is obviously wrong.

	Proportion	*Solution*
1.	$\frac{x}{3.27} = \frac{4.9}{12.76}$	$x = 12.6$
2.	$\frac{x \text{ mL}}{150 \text{ mL}} = \frac{500 \text{ mg}}{275 \text{ mg}}$	$x = 1.82$

ANSWERS 1. 12.6 is too big (numerator should be smaller than denominator to match the fraction on the right) 2. 1.82 is too small (numerator should be larger than denominator)

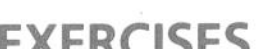

EXERCISES

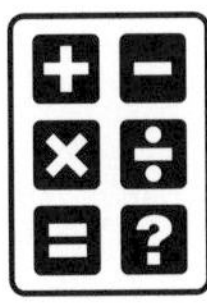

Exercises 1–8. Explain why each of the following statements must contain an error.

1. Mrs. G. is 5 m tall and weighs 120 lb.
2. Mr. J. weighs 260 g.
3. Mr. D. needed a transfusion because he lost 5 mL of blood during surgery.
4. Mrs. U.'s newborn infant drank 2 L of milk on the first day.

5. The average carrot weighs 60 mg.

6. $\dfrac{12 \text{ mL}}{4 \text{ L}} = 3$

7. A weight of 500 g is heavier than 1 kg.

8. If a piece of tape of width 2.54 cm is cut in half, each half is 127 mm wide.

Exercises 9–16. Carry out the indicated conversion, using a mental image as a guide.

9. 8.1 mm to centimeters
10. 75.4 mL to liters
11. 10.25 nmol to micromoles
12. 0.138 nmol to picomoles
13. 2.5 g to milligrams
14. 0.15 mg to micrograms
15. 70 μg to milligrams
16. 0.8 mL to deciliters

Exercises 17–20. Without computing, state why the solution for the given proportion is obviously wrong.

	Proportion	*Solution*
17.	$\dfrac{x}{23.76} = \dfrac{5.34}{93.25}$	$x = 136.1$
18.	$\dfrac{345.9}{459.2} = \dfrac{x}{32.6}$	$x = 2.46$
19.	$\dfrac{0.02}{467.24} = \dfrac{12.59}{x}$	$x = 2.94$
20.	$\dfrac{8.45}{x} = \dfrac{125.6}{39}$	$x = 262.3$

ANSWERS 1. No human is that much taller than a door. 3. No transfusion is needed for a loss of about a teaspoon. 5. 60 mg < 1 g, too little for the average carrot 7. 1 kg = 1000 g > 500 g 9. 0.81 cm 11. 0.01025 μmol 13. 2500 mg 15. 0.07 mg 17. Too large to match the right-hand fraction 19. Too small

4-10. SUMMARY

1. The International System of Units (SI) is a relatively new system of measurement, a modernized version of the metric system. The symbol SI stands for *Système International d'Unités.* Basic SI measures include:

   1 meter: A little more than a yard
   1 liter: A little more than a quart
   1 gram: About the weight of a paper clip
   1 mole: A fixed number of *mole*cules

SI UNITS

Basic Measure	Classification	Example
1 meter (m)	Length	The distance from the floor to a doorknob (about 1.1 yd)
1 liter (L)	Liquid capacity	1.1 qt
1 gram (g)	Weight	$\frac{1}{30}$ oz of ice-cold water; or the weight of a paper clip
1 mole (mol)	Amount of substance	1 mol of salt and 1 mol of aspirin have the same number of molecules but different weights
1 square meter (m^2)	Area of a two-dimensional space	A child's body surface area (BSA)

2. Prefixes denote multiples and subdivisions of the basic measures.

PREFIXES

Prefix	Symbol	Meaning	Examples
kilo	k	1000	1 km = 1000 m, about 0.6 mile 1 kg = 1000 g, about 2.2 lb
deci	d	0.1	1 dm = 0.1 m, about 4 in. 1 dL = 0.1 L, about 3 oz
centi	c	0.01	1 cm = 0.01 m, the width of a paper clip (< $\frac{1}{2}$ in.)
milli	m	0.001	1 mm = 0.001 m, diameter of paper clip wire 1 mL = 0.001 L, $\frac{1}{5}$ tsp of liquid medication 1 mg = 0.001 g, small amount of powdered drug 1 mmol = 0.001 mol, small amount of blood component
micro	µ	0.000001	1 µg = 0.001 mg 1 µmol = 0.001 mmol (Small fractions of amounts described above)
nano	n	0.000000001	1 nmol = 0.001 µmol (Small fractions of amounts described above)
pico	p	0.000000000001	1 pmol = 0.001 nmol (Small fractions of amounts described above)

3. MOST COMMON CONVERSIONS

Each unit in the following table is 1000 times as large as the unit in the column to its right. To convert from any unit in the following table, move the decimal point, in the same direction as the table indicates, 3 places for each column.

CONVERSIONS

× 1000 →	× 1000 →		← × 0.001	← × 0.001	
km	m	mm			
	L	mL			
kg	g	mg	µg		
	mol	mmol	µmol	nmol	pmol

When converting from a larger unit to a smaller one, the number of units must **increase**; when converting from a smaller unit to a larger one, the number of units must **decrease.**

Examples

	From	*To*	*Result*
(a)	3.1 g	mg	3100 mg
(b)	85.7 mg	g	0.0857 g
(c)	0.03 mmol	nmol	30,000 nmol
(d)	1234.5 nmol	mmol	0.0012345 mmol

4. MEASURES OF AREA OR CAPACITY

Unit	Classification	Example
Square centimeter (cm^2)	Area of a two-dimensional space (1 cm × 1 cm)	$< \frac{1}{4}$ in.^{2}
Cubic millimeter (mm^3)	Capacity of a three-dimensional space (1 mm × 1 mm × 1 mm)	A small amount (about $\frac{1}{5000}$ of a teaspoon)
Cubic centimeter (cm^3, cc, mL)	Capacity of a three-dimensional space (1 cm × 1 cm × 1 cm)	About $\frac{1}{5}$ of a teaspoon
Cubic decimeter (dm^3)	Capacity of a three-dimensional space (1 dm × 1 dm × 1 dm)	1.1 qt

5. GENERAL METHOD FOR CONVERSIONS: PROPORTIONS

Proportions are dependable for conversion problems, and provide the foundation for future use of formulas and shortcuts.

Example

1. To convert 11.6 in. to millimeters, use the relationship:

$$1 \text{ in.} = 2.5 \text{ cm}$$

	SI Units	*English Units*	
Tabulate (T): (Make the units match)	*x* mm	11.6 in.	(Make sure that the units match)
	25 mm		
	~~2.5 cm~~	1 in.	
Estimate (E):	Between 200 and 300 mm		

Proportion: (Use pure ratios from matching units) $\frac{x}{25} = \frac{11.6}{1}$

Compute (C): $x = 11.6 \times 25 = 290$

Result: 11.6 in. = 290 mm (Agrees with estimate)

Check (C): 290 mm = 11.6 in.

6. AVOIDING ERRORS: USING MENTAL IMAGES

Mental images can prevent errors. Use the suggestions given in the text and make up your own.

Some Reminders:

Meter (Length): The approximate distance from the floor to the doorknob
Liter (Capacity): A *lit*tle more than a quart
Gram (Weight): A paper clip
Mole (Amount of Substance): A fixed number of *mole*cules
Proportions: Symmetry and balance, "everything in proportion."

EXERCISES FOR EXTRA PRACTICE

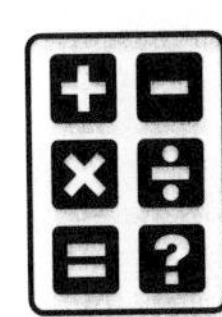

1. Instructions for preparing an injection state "Draw solution plus 0.5 cc of air into syringe." When there is 0.5 cm^3 of air in the syringe, do we have too little air, just enough, or too much?
2. A tablet for angina may contain 0.15 mg of nitroglycerin. Find the weight (in micrograms) of the nitroglycerin in 3 tablets.
3. A liter of infant formula contains 175 mg of salt. How much salt is in 10 mL?
4. Normal triglyceride levels are 0.45–1.80 mmol/L of blood. Would a measurement of 950 μmol/L be normal?
5. Jennifer, an 8-year-old girl, is 127 cm tall. Her big brother, a basketball player, is 1.9 m tall. What is the difference (in centimeters) between their heights?
6. Last month, results of Mr. V.'s blood test for vitamin D showed 100 U/dL of blood. This month the report showed 1.5 U/mL. Find the change in the number of units per deciliter of vitamin D in Mr. V.'s blood.
7. About how many milliliters are contained in 6 standard teaspoons?
8. Each gram of protein provides 4 cal. If protein in the patient's breakfast provides a total of 68 cal, how much protein is present?
9. Each gram of fat provides 9 cal. If fat in the patient's dinner provides a total of 621 cal, how much fat is present?
10. If 1 oz is about 30 g, what is the weight (in grams) of a 6.2-oz piece of cheese?
11. How many meters in a length of 562.3 cm?
12. Compare weights of 0.06 g and 48 mg.

Exercises 13–26. The table below gives the calcium content for each food listed. Use the table to answer the questions that follow.

Type of Food	Amount of Food	Amount of Calcium (Milligrams)
American cheese	30 g	175
Bok choy, cooked	8 oz	250
Broccoli, cooked	180 g	101
Cheddar cheese	60 g	410
Collard greens, cooked	4 oz	180
Sardines, with bones	3 oz	370

13. Which food has the highest calcium content?

14. Which food has the lowest calcium content?

Exercises 15–20. Find the calcium content of each quantity given below.

15. 45 g of American cheese
16. 150 g of broccoli
17. 125 g of cheddar cheese
18. 3.5 oz of sardines
19. 5 oz of bok choy
20. 5 oz of collard greens

Exercises 21–26. For each food listed below, how much is necessary to provide 500 mg of calcium?

21. sardines
22. bok choy
23. collard greens
24. broccoli
25. cheddar cheese
26. American cheese

ANSWERS 1. Just enough 3. 1.75 mg 5. 63 cm 7. 30 mL 9. 69 g 11. 5.623 m 13. Cheddar cheese 15. 262.5 mg 17. 854.2 mg 19. 156.3 mg 21. 4.1 oz 23. 11.1 oz 25. 73.2 g

CHAPTER TEST

1. What is the basic SI unit of length? 1. ______

2. What is the basic SI unit for amount of substance? 2. ______

Problems 3–5. Complete the statement.

3. 24.5 cm = ______ mm 3. ______

4. ______ g = 35.04 kg 4. ______

5. 2.3 mmol = ______ μmol 5. ______

6. Which container holds more liquid, A (5 dL) or B (50 cc)? 6. ______

Problems 7–8. Normally, serum magnesium levels range from 0.8 to 1.3 mmol/L. Convert the following blood test reports to millimoles per liter and state whether the report shows a normal level.

7. 980 μmol/L 7. ______

8. 1.35 μmol/mL 8. ____________

9. If Jacqui, a newborn infant, weighs 4.5 lb, what is her birth weight in grams? (*Reminder:* 1 kg is about 2.2 lb.) 9. ____________

10. Mr. Y., an elderly patient, is 70 in. tall. A year ago, his height was recorded as 178.8 cm. How much shorter (in centimeters) is he this year than he was last year? (*Reminder:* 1 in. is about 2.5 cm.) 10. ____________

ANSWERS 1. The meter (m) 2. The mole (mol) 3. 245 4. 35,040 5. 2300 6. A 7. 0.98 mmol/L, normal 8. 1.35 mmol/L, higher than normal 9. 2045 g 10. 3.8 cm

---

FIVE

Non-SI Measures Used in Health Care

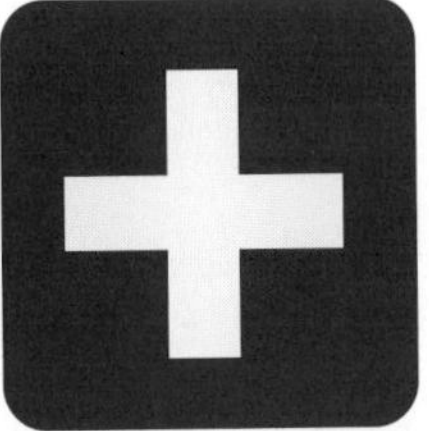
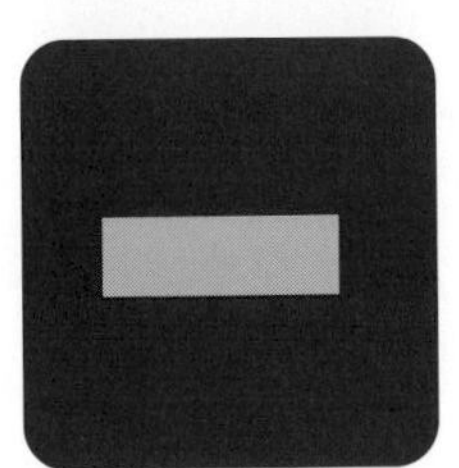
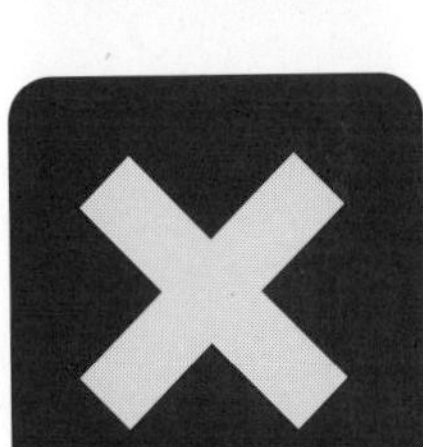
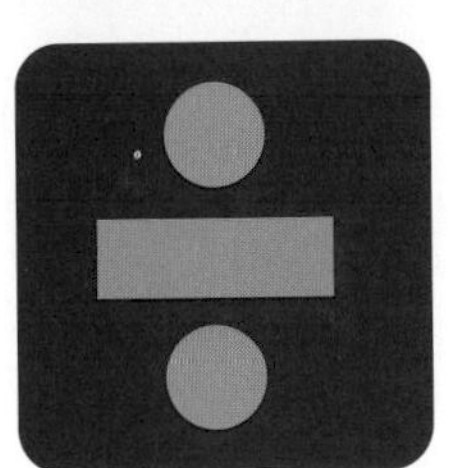
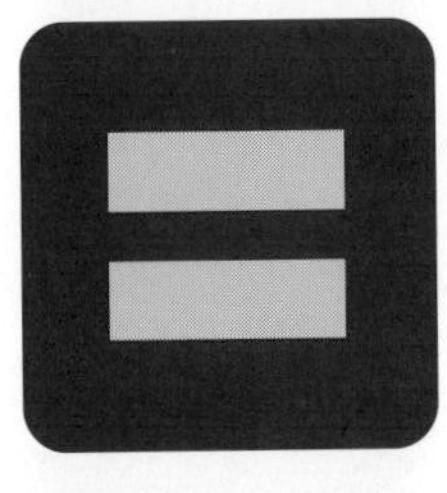
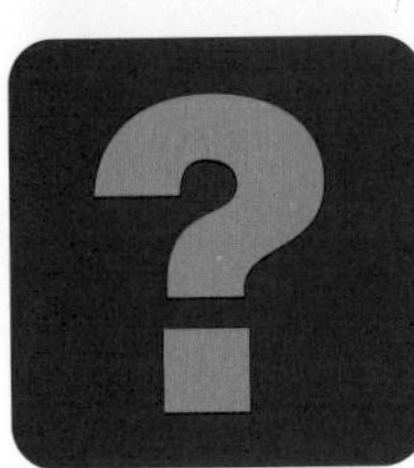

▶ OUTLINE

▶ OBJECTIVES

After studying this section, you will be able to:

1. Use the apothecaries' system and household methods of measurement for weight and fluid capacity.
2. Use a variety of approved units of potency.
3. Recognize milliequivalents as measurements of biological fluid activity.
4. Interpret and express temperature measurements on both the Celsius and Fahrenheit scales.
5. Solve problems of various types (including measurement conversions) by ratio and proportion, or by the shortcut formula, $\frac{D}{H} \times Q$.

5-1. INTRODUCTION

What non-SI measures do nurses need? Nurses need to be comfortable not only with those measures of weight and fluid capacity still in use from the old apothecaries' system or from household utensils but also with modern units of potency and measures of electrolytic activity. It is also important to know the two different temperature scales, Fahrenheit and Celsius.

Examples

1. Amount of phenobarbital in a tablet: 1 grain.
2. On hand: $\frac{1}{4}$ grain thyroid tablets; doctor's order: 30 mg.
3. The US recommended daily allowance of vitamin A: 2500 international units for children aged 2 to 4 years.
4. Doctor's order: 160,000 units of penicillin G potassium.
5. Results of a blood test: 6.5 milliequivalents of calcium per liter of blood.
6. A packet of potassium chloride powder may contain 1.5 g or 20 milliequivalents of potassium chloride.

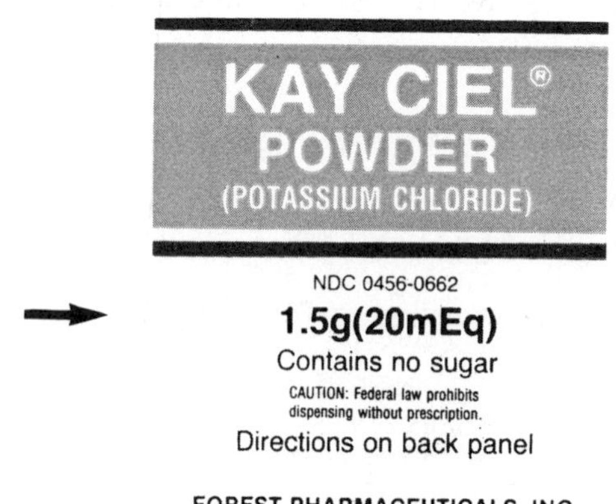

7. A baby girl's temperature: 37.5°C.

Proficiency Gauge

It is possible that you understand apothecaries' and household measures and are familiar with modern units of potency and electrolyte activity, in which case you can skip this chapter. Gauge your proficiency by working out the following exercises. Check your answers with those that follow the test only after you have answered all the questions.

1. How many $\frac{1}{4}$ grain thyroid tablets should be given to a patient if the doctor has ordered 30 mg? 1. ____________
2. How many tablespoonfuls would you use for a dose of 1 fl oz of cough syrup? 2. ____________
3. How many drops are in $\frac{1}{4}$ tsp? 3. ____________

4. How many ounces are in $\frac{1}{2}$ pt? 4. ____________
5. A container holds 4 fl oz or how many milliliters? 5. ____________
6. A patient drank $1\frac{1}{2}$ cups of milk. Record this amount in milliliters. 6. ____________
7. Convert 500 μU to mU. 7. ____________
8. The milliequivalent is what part of an equivalent? 8. ____________
9. Convert 75°F to Celsius. 9. ____________
10. Convert 37.5°C to Fahrenheit. 10. ____________

ANSWERS 1. 2 tablets 2. 2 tbsp 3. About 20 drops
4. 8 oz 5. 120 mL 6. 360 mL 7. 0.5 mU
8. 1 mEq = 0.001 Eq 9. 23.9°C 10. 99.5°F

5-2. THE APOTHECARIES' SYSTEM FOR MEASURING WEIGHT AND FLUID CAPACITY

The apothecaries' system of measurement is very old, originating in Greece, Rome, and France. By the seventeenth century, the English were using it also, and the colonists carried it to the New World. Much of this system is hardly ever used today, but we still do see the basic units, grain (for weight) and minim (for volume). Other units of this system, the ounce (oz), fluid ounce (fl oz), pint (pt), quart (qt), and gallon (gal) remain in common use in the United States. (See Appendix 3 for complete details of the apothecaries' system.)

Weight

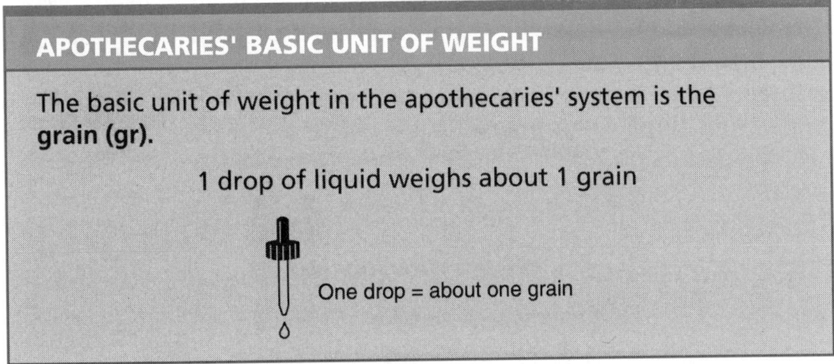

APOTHECARIES' BASIC UNIT OF WEIGHT
The basic unit of weight in the apothecaries' system is the **grain (gr).**
1 drop of liquid weighs about 1 grain
One drop = about one grain

Examples

1. A grain of wheat, a familiar farm commodity, grows in many different sizes. But, as a unit of weight of the apothecaries' system, the grain is fixed according to international standards.* The grain

---

* The grain is $\frac{1}{254.458}$ of the weight of a cubic inch of distilled water at greatest density under 30 in. of barometric pressure.

is the smallest unit of the apothecaries' system, so small that one ounce contains 480 grains.

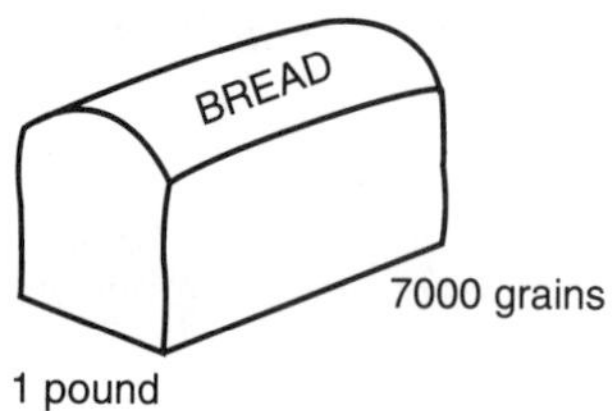

2. A sleeping pill may contain 1 grain of phenobarbital.
3. A pain tablet may contain 5 grains of aspirin.
4. The grain, a unit of the apothecaries' system, should not be confused with the SI unit, the gram. One gram (g) is about 15 times as heavy as 1 grain (gr).

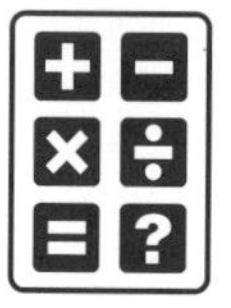

SAMPLE EXERCISES

1. If a tablet containing 1 grain of phenobarbital is dissolved and then administered in 4 equal portions, how much phenobarbital does each portion contain?
2. If Mr. Kittery has taken 2 pain tablets, each containing 5 grains of aspirin, then, in grains, what total amount of aspirin has he taken?

ANSWERS 1. $\frac{1}{4}$ grain 2. 10 grains

Symbols

Because the apothecaries' system is ancient, the symbolism is old-fashioned. In earlier times, the symbol for grain, gr, preceded the numeral: gr $\frac{1}{3}$, gr $\frac{1}{4}$, gr $\frac{1}{150}$, gr $\frac{1}{200}$, and so on. The quantity $\frac{1}{2}$ grain was written with the special symbol gr ss. To indicate 1, 2, or more grains, Roman numerals were customary: for example, gr i, gr ii, or gr v. Today, some people still write the fraction after the symbol, but the Roman numerals are not popular. (See Appendix 4 for a table of Roman numerals.)

ILLUSTRATIVE EXPRESSIONS FOR WEIGHT IN GRAINS

Amount	Symbol
$\frac{1}{2}$ grain	gr ss
$\frac{1}{4}$ grain	gr $\frac{1}{4}$
$\frac{1}{150}$ grain	gr $\frac{1}{150}$
1 grain	gr i
$1\frac{1}{2}$ grain	gr iss
3 grains	gr iii
5 grains	gr v
6 grains	gr vi
10 grains	gr x

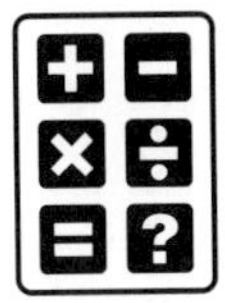

SAMPLE EXERCISES

1. If 1 tablet contains aspirin gr v, how much aspirin do 2 such tablets contain? (Use symbols.)
2. How much drug is contained in 3 tablets, if each tablet is labeled gr $\frac{1}{150}$?

ANSWERS 1. gr x 2. gr $\frac{1}{50}$

Liquid Capacity

The apothecaries' system of liquid capacity (volume) is based on the minim, a quantity of water that weighs approximately 1 grain.

APOTHECARIES' BASIC UNIT OF VOLUME

The basic unit of liquid capacity (volume) in the apothecaries' system is the **minim (♏)**.

1 minim (1 drop) of liquid weighs about 1 grain

Examples

1. The weight and volume of a drop of liquid are about 1 grain and 1 minim, respectively. Thus, 5 minims of water weighs 5 grains.
2. To prepare an injection, the nurse draws 10 minims of a medication into a syringe.

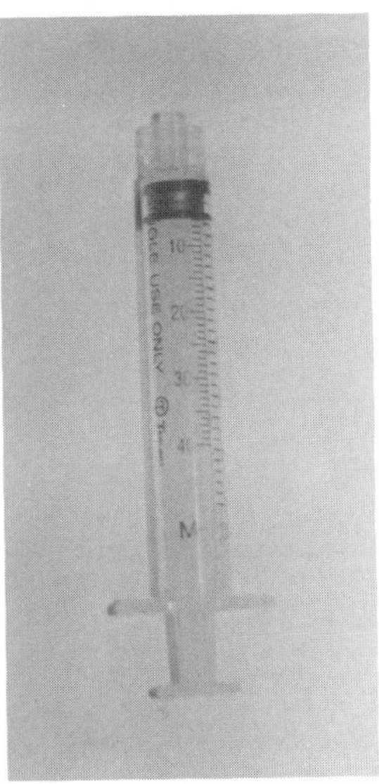

3. The minim, a unit of the apothecaries' system, should not be confused with the SI unit milliliter (mL). A volume of 1 mL is about 15 times as large as 1 minim.

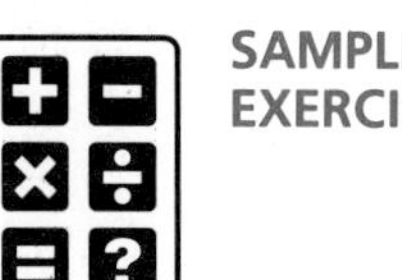

SAMPLE EXERCISES

1. What volume is associated with 3 drops of water?
2. What is the weight of 4 minims of water?

ANSWERS 1. 3 minims 2. 4 grains

As we have seen, the symbols of the apothecaries' system may be written before the numeral.

ILLUSTRATIVE EXPRESSIONS FOR LIQUID CAPACITY IN MINIMS

Amount	Symbol
1 minim	♏ i
2 minims	♏ ii
4 minims	♏ iv
8 minims	♏ viii
10 minims	♏ x
15 minims	♏ xv

The larger units of liquid capacity most often needed today are the fluid ounce, the pint, the quart, and the gallon. The following box shows the symbols for these measures and relationships between them.

LARGER UNITS OF VOLUME

1 pint (pt) = 16 fluid ounces (fl oz)
1 quart (qt) = 2 pints (pt)
1 gallon (gal) = 4 quarts (qt)

Examples

1. In $\frac{1}{2}$ pt (pt $\frac{1}{2}$), there are 8 fl oz (fl oz viii).
2. The pure ratio of 1 pt to 1 gal is

$$\frac{1 \text{ pt}}{1 \text{ gal}} = \frac{1 \text{ pt}}{4 \text{ qt}} = \frac{1 \text{ pt}}{8 \text{ pt}} = \frac{1}{8}$$

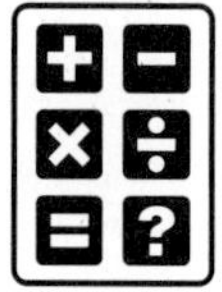

SAMPLE EXERCISES

1. What is the pure ratio of 2 pt to 3 qt?
2. How many ounces are in 3 pt?
3. How many pints are in 1 gal?

ANSWERS

1. $\frac{2 \text{ pt}}{3 \text{ qt}} = \frac{2 \text{ pt}}{6 \text{ pt}} = \frac{1}{3}$

2. *Table:*

Ounces	Pints
x	3
16	1

$$\frac{x}{16} = \frac{3}{1}$$

Result: 48 oz

3. *Table:*

x pt	1 gal (4 qt)
2 pt	1 qt

$$\frac{x}{2} = \frac{4}{1}$$

Result: 8 pt

EXERCISES

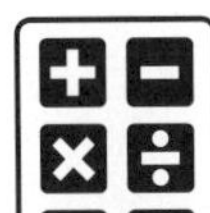

Exercises 1–8. Change each ratio indicated below to a pure ratio (a ratio without units).

1. The ratio of gr ii to gr vi
2. gr x : gr v
3. gr $\frac{1}{2}$: gr $\frac{1}{4}$
4. gr $\frac{1}{150}$ to gr $\frac{1}{200}$
5. ♏ i : ♏ viii
6. ♏ x : ♏ xv
7. $\frac{1 \text{ pt}}{1 \text{ qt}}$
8. $\frac{1 \text{ qt}}{1 \text{ gal}}$

Exercises 9–12. Answer each question.

9. How many pints are in 2.5 gal?
10. How many ounces are in 5.2 pt?
11. In 6 pt, there are how many quarts?
12. In 10 qt, there are how many gallons?

Exercises 13–16. Change each ratio indicated below to a pure ratio (a ratio without units).

13. 3 qt to 2 gal
14. 4 oz to 6 pt
15. 5 pt to 1 qt
16. 10 oz to 3 qt

Exercises 17–18. To make a holiday eggnog, Mr. K. filled a punchbowl with 4 qt of dairy eggnog, 8 oz of rum, and $1\frac{1}{2}$ pt of whipped cream. As a result:

17. How many ounces of holiday drink were in the punchbowl?
18. How many 4-oz drinks were available?

Exercises 19–20. At the neighborhood supermarket, a container of milk ($\frac{1}{2}$ gal) costs \$1.53. Consider the following.

19. At the corner delicatessen, 1 qt of milk costs \$0.99. Per quart, how much do we save by purchasing the $\frac{1}{2}$ gal at the supermarket?

20. At a luncheonette, pints of milk sell at $1.00/pt. How much do we save per pint if we buy the $\frac{1}{2}$ gallon at the supermarket?

ANSWERS 1. $\frac{1}{3}$ 3. $\frac{2}{1}$ 5. $\frac{1}{8}$ 7. $\frac{1}{2}$ 9. 20 11. 3 13. $\frac{3}{8}$ 15. $\frac{5}{2}$ 17. 160 oz 19. $0.23

5-3. HOUSEHOLD MEASURES

At home, medications are measured by the best available devices. These may range from relatively accurate measuring devices (supplied by the pharmacist), such as plastic cylinders, caps, syringes, and calibrated droppers, to kitchen measuring spoons and cups. The least accurate are the household dropper and spoons from ordinary tableware. Whatever the situation, we must do our best to administer the prescribed dose as accurately as our equipment allows.

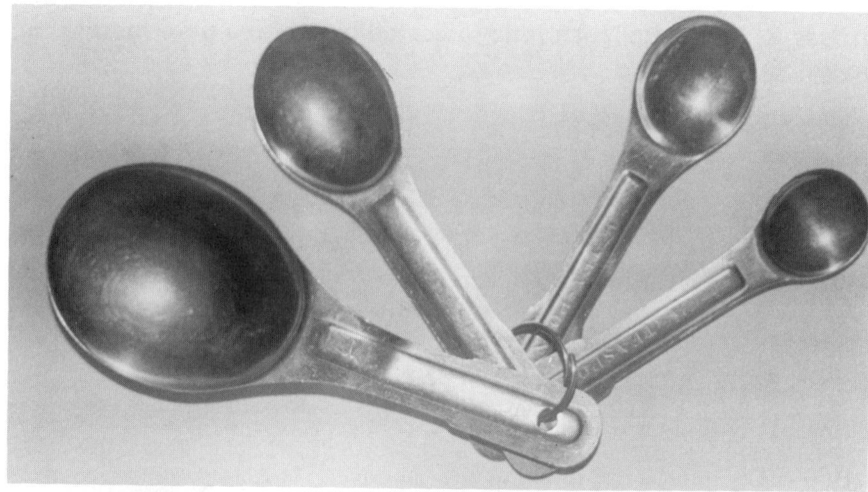

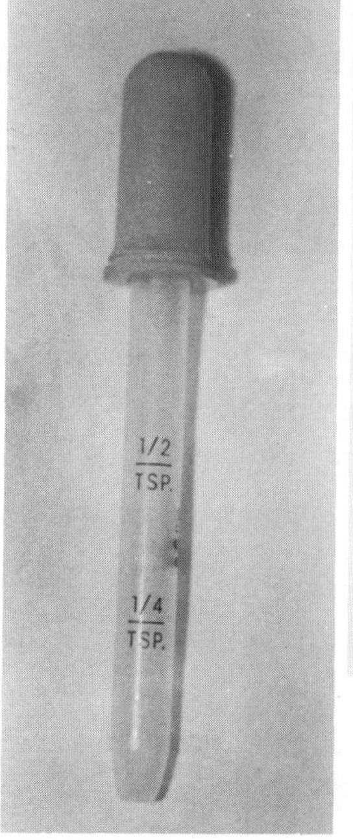

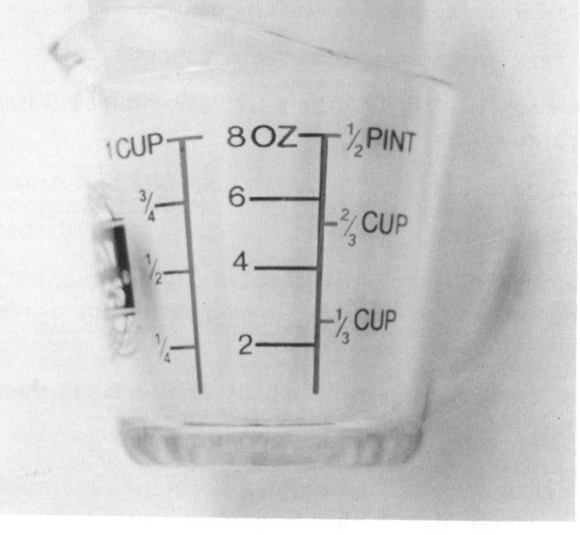

The following box shows the relationships between common household measures.

COMMON HOUSEHOLD MEASURES
1 tablespoon (tbsp) = 3 teaspoons (tsp)
2 tablespoons = 1 ounce (oz)
1 cup (glass) = 8 ounces

Examples

1. To administer $\frac{1}{2}$ oz of cough syrup, we may use 1 tbsp.
2. If Ms. Jacie has drunk a glassful of juice, we may record her intake as 8 oz.

SAMPLE EXERCISES

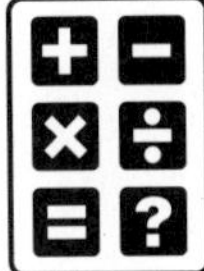

1. What household measure might be used to give 1 oz of cough syrup?
2. A cold syrup with codeine contains codeine phosphate (12 mg/tsp). If a patient takes 2 tsp 3 times per day, how many milligrams of codeine is he receiving per day?

Exercises 3–4. On some labels, you may see "Do not exceed 6 doses in 24 hours." If a child's dose is $\frac{1}{2}$ tsp, then:

3. What is the maximum number of teaspoons of medication to be received by the child in 24 hr?
4. If the medication contains 62.5 mg/tsp of antihistamine, what is the maximum amount of antihistamine to be received by the child in 24 hr?

ANSWERS 1. 2 tbsp 2. 72 mg 3. 3 tsp 4. 187.5 mg

EXERCISES

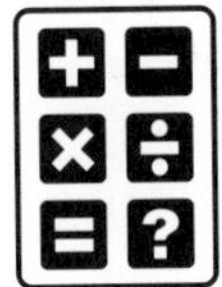

Exercises 1–8. Convert as indicated.

1. 2 tbsp to teaspoons
2. 3 oz to tablespoons
3. 2 cups to ounces
4. 0.5 tbsp to teaspoons
5. 4 oz to cups
6. 1 oz to teaspoons
7. 0.5 oz to teaspoons
8. $\frac{1}{4}$ cup to ounces

Exercises 9–18. Answer each question.

9. To stir cholestyramine resin in 2 oz of a liquid, how many tablespoons of the liquid may be used?
10. The nurse gives a child a dose of $\frac{1}{2}$ tsp of Alba-Bye. Each teaspoon contains 10 mg of vitamin B_{12}. How much vitamin B_{12} is in the dose?
11. The nurse encouraged Mr. K., a patient with diarrhea, to drink 64 oz of liquids per day. How many glassfuls does that represent?
12. When using germicidal hand rinse, dispense about 1 tsp into cupped hands. For how many rinses will a 4-oz bottle of hand rinse last?

13. If a dose of cough syrup is 2 tbsp + 1 tsp, how many ounces are in a dose?
14. From a 1-pt bottle of oral rinse, how many rinses of 0.5 oz each are available?
15. Ascorbic acid is available in a mixture of 4g/tsp of powder. In 1 tbsp of powder, there are how many grams of ascorbic acid?
16. How many doses of 1 tsp each are in a 12-oz bottle of cough syrup?
17. If no more than 3 oz of an antacid should be taken in a day, what is the maximum number of doses per day in tablespoons? (Assume that 1 dose = 1 tbsp.)
18. Mr. Y. needs to have bentiromide with 8 oz of water. Is $\frac{1}{2}$ pint of water enough?

Exercises 19–22. If 8 oz of vegetable soup provides 90 cal, 4 g of protein, and 2 g of fat, then:

19. A quart of soup contains how much fat?
20. How many ounces of soup do we need for 7 g of protein?
21. How many calories are there in a pint of soup?
22. How much protein does 1.25 cup of soup provide?

ANSWERS 1. 6 tsp 3. 16 oz 5. 0.5 cup 7. 3 tsp 9. 4 tbsp 11. 8 glassfuls 13. 1.3 oz 15. 12 g 17. 6 19. 8 g 21. 180 cal

5-4. UNITS OF POTENCY

Many vitamins, chemicals, and medications are measured in units of potency. These units may be **international units (IU), National Formulary units, United States Pharmacopeia (USP) units,** or units approved by the Food and Drug Administration (FDA) or the National Institutes of Health (NIH). The unit of potency of one drug has no relation to the unit of potency of another drug.

Although units of potency are not SI units, we use standard SI prefixes.

PREFIXES FOR UNITS OF POTENCY
1 mU = 0.001 U 1 μU = 0.001 mU

Examples

1. 5000 IU of vitamin A is 100% of the US recommended daily allowance (RDA).
2. Results of a blood test for a patient may be recorded as 5 μU/mL.
3. Penicillin may be ordered by weight in milligrams or by potency in units. If the doctor orders 160,000 U of penicillin G potassium for Ms. M., this order is equivalent to 100 mg of the drug.

4. Insulin is prepared in insulin units per milliliter.

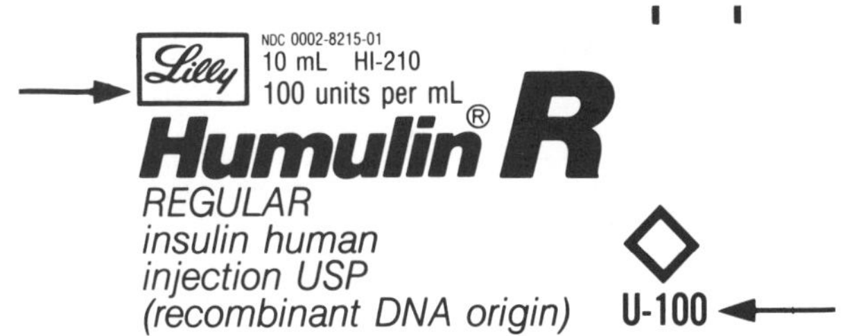

SAMPLE EXERCISES

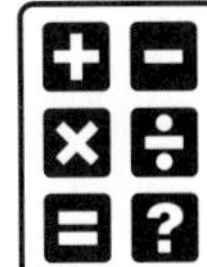

1. Complete: 5 μU/mL = _____ mU/mL.
2. If 5000 IU of vitamin A is 100% of the RDA, how much vitamin A is 60% of the RDA?

ANSWERS 1. 0.005 mU/mL 2. 3000 IU

EXERCISES

Exercises 1–4. Complete the following

1. 4000 μU/mL = _____ mU/mL
2. 25,000 μU/mL = _____ mU/mL
3. 100 μU/mL = _____ mU/mL
4. 0.05 U/L = _____ mU/L

Exercises 5–8. If 5000 IU of vitamin A is 100% of the RDA, then:

5. How much vitamin A is 10% of the RDA?
6. How much vitamin A is 75% of the RDA?
7. What percent of the RDA does 2000 IU represent?
8. What percent of the RDA does 3500 IU represent?

Exercises 9–12. If a tablet containing 20,000 U (USP) of chymotrypsin is available, then:

9. How much chymotrypsin is in 2 tablets?
10. If Mrs. Poelez takes 4 tablets/day, how much chymotrypsin does she have per day?
11. How many tablets does a patient need for a total daily supply of 60,000 U?
12. How many tablets does a patient need for a total daily supply of 80,000 U?

Exercises 13–14. The following patients are taking nystatin. Find the total amount of nystatin taken per day.

13. Mr. Kaleo takes 400,000 U, 4 times each day.
14. Mrs. Frasper takes 750,000 U, 3 times per day.

Exercises 15–18. Collagenase ointment contains 250 U/g of ointment. Therefore:

15. How many units of collagenase are in 3 g?
16. How many units of collagenase are in 224 mg?

17. How much ointment is needed for 500 U of collagenase?

18. How much ointment is needed for 125 U of collagenase?

Exercises 19–22. An enzyme ointment (Elase) contains 666.6 U/g of ointment. Therefore:

19. In 5 g of Elase, how many units are there?

20. In 3.2 g of Elase, how many units are there?

21. For 3000 U of Elase, how much ointment is needed?

22. For 500 U of Elase, how much ointment is needed?

ANSWERS 1. 4 mU/mL 3. 0.1 mU/mL 5. 500 IU 7. 40% 9. 40,000 U 11. 3 tablets 13. 1,600,000 U 15. 750 U 17. 2 g 19. 3333 U 21. 4.5 g

---

5-5. MEASUREMENTS OF ELECTROLYTES IN BODY FLUIDS

Electrolytes in body fluids are compounds that dissolve into electrically charged particles. Without electrolytes, such as sodium, potassium, calcium, and magnesium, we cannot survive.

The basic unit of measurement for electrically charged particles in liquids is the **equivalent (Eq).*** Because the quantities in body fluids are relatively small, it is the subdivision, the **milliequivalent (mEq),** that we see most often.

MILLIEQUIVALENT

The milliequivalent measures electrolytic activity in body fluids.

1 mEq = 0.001 Eq

1 Eq = 1000 mEq

A normal sodium level is 140 mEq/L.

Examples

1. A blood test of a normal adult usually shows:

   A sodium level between 135 and 145 mEq/L of blood.
   A potassium level between 3.5 and 5.5 mEq/L of blood.
   A calcium level between 4.5 and 5.5 mEq/L of blood.
   A magnesium level between 1.5 and 2.0 mEq/L of blood.

2. The amount of potassium chloride in some slow-release tablets may be given as 750 mg of drug in each tablet or as 10 mEq.

---

* One mole of electrically charged atoms of hydrogen is one equivalent.

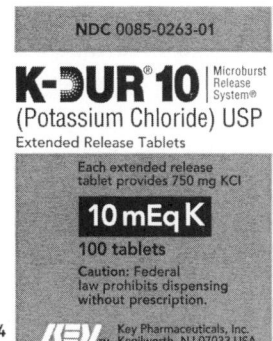

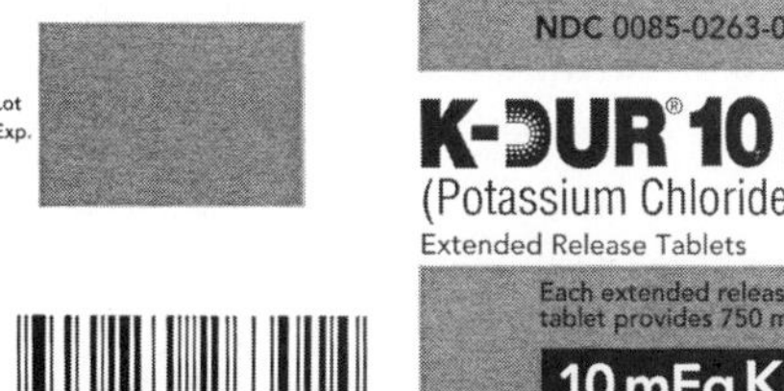
Lot
Exp.
NDC 0085-0263-01
K-DUR® 10
Microburst Release System®
(Potassium Chloride) USP
Extended Release Tablets
Each extended release tablet provides 750 mg KCl
10 mEq K
100 tablets
Caution: Federal law prohibits dispensing without prescription.
Key Pharmaceuticals, Inc. Kenilworth, NJ 07033 USA
N 3 0085-0263-01 4
6505-01-280-3014
Usual Dose: See accompanying product information.
Dispense in tight, light-resistant container as defined in the USP.
Keep tightly closed. Store at controlled room temperature 15-30°C (59-86°F).
Copyright © 1987, 1991, Key Pharmaceuticals, Inc.
All rights reserved.
16928500 Rev. 1/91

SAMPLE EXERCISES

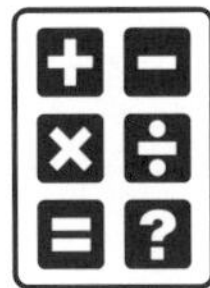

1. Refer to Example 1 above. If Mr. A.'s test results show a calcium level of 3 mEq/L, is his calcium level normal?
2. If you administer 7 potassium chloride tablets (as described in Example 2 above) to a patient per week, what is the total amount (in milligrams and in milliequivalents) of potassium chloride administered per week?

ANSWERS

1. No, too low, 3 mEq/L < 4.5 mEq/L
2. *Table:*

Milligrams	Tablets
x	7
750	1

or

Milliequivalents	Tablets
x	7
10	1

$$\frac{x}{750} = \frac{7}{1} \qquad \frac{x}{10} = \frac{7}{1}$$

Results: 5250 mg or 70 mEq

EXERCISES

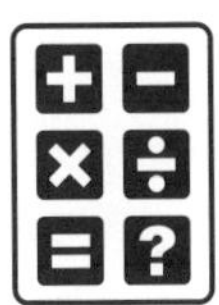

Exercises 1–4. For the following exercises, assume that the amount of potassium is

16.12 mEq in 1 medium banana.
6.42 mEq in 1 cantaloupe.
9.21 mEq in 1 medium orange.

1. Find the total amount of potassium provided by $\frac{1}{2}$ banana and $\frac{1}{4}$ cantaloupe.
2. Find the total amount of potassium provided by 2 bananas, $\frac{1}{2}$ cantaloupe, and $2\frac{1}{2}$ oranges.
3. How would you provide 30 mEq of potassium?
4. How would you provide 40 mEq of potassium?

Exercises 5–8. Mrs. L.C. takes lithium carbonate. She has her blood level checked regularly in order to maintain the recommended level of lithium carbonate (0.5–1.5 mEq/L). Which of the following satisfy the requirement?

5. 0.6 mEq/L
6. 1.2 mEq/mL
7. 1.4 Eq/L
8. 0.0009 mEq/mL

Exercises 9–12. Lithium carbonate solution contains 8 mEq/5 mL. Complete each statement.

9. Lithium carbonate solution contains _____ mEq/mL.
10. Lithium carbonate solution contains 24 mEq in _____ mL.
11. Lithium carbonate solution contains 80 mEq in _____ mL.
12. _____ mEq of lithium carbonate are contained in 10 mL.

Exercises 13–16. The nurse is to administer sodium bicarbonate to Mr. S.B. if his blood test shows a potassium level >6.5 mEq/L. For which of the following potassium levels should the nurse administer the sodium bicarbonate?

13. 6.15 mEq/L
14. 0.007 mEq/mL
15. 0.62 mEq/100 mL
16. 0.25 mEq/50 mL

Exercises 17–20. Available forms of potassium bicarbonate include an oral solution containing 2.375 mEq/5 mL, an elixir, 6.7 mEq/5 mL, and a tablet of 5 mEq. How much potassium bicarbonate is in:

17. 10 mL of the oral solution?
18. 10 mL of the elixir
19. 2 tablets?
20. 1 mL of the oral solution?
21. Sodium polystyrene sulfonate contains 65 mEq sodium/60 mL. How much sodium is in 30 mL?
22. How much ammonium chloride may be found in 1.5 mL of an ammonium chloride preparation containing 5 mEq/mL?

ANSWERS 1. 8.06 mEq + 1.61 mEq = 9.67 mEq 3. One possibility: Give 1 of each piece of fruit 5. yes 7. no 9. 1.6 11. 50 13. no 15. no 17. 4.75 mEq 19. 10 mEq 21. 32.5 mEq

---

5-6. TEMPERATURE SCALES

In the United States, two temperature scales are in common use: Celsius* and Fahrenheit. The more modern **Celsius (°C)** scale is preferred, especially for scientific data, but many weather reports, thermometers, and sets of instructions still utilize the **Fahrenheit (°F)** scale. Because instructions may refer to one scale but the available instruments may use the other scale, the nurse must be able to convert from one to the other.

* Formerly known as centigrade.

Examples

1. On a mild winter day, the weather forecaster may report a temperature of 50 degrees Fahrenheit (°F).
2. A patient may be hospitalized with a temperature of 39.8 degrees Celsius (°C).
3. Many drugs are required to be stored at 15–30°C.
4. From the Tagamet label: "Store at controlled room temperature (59°–86°F)."

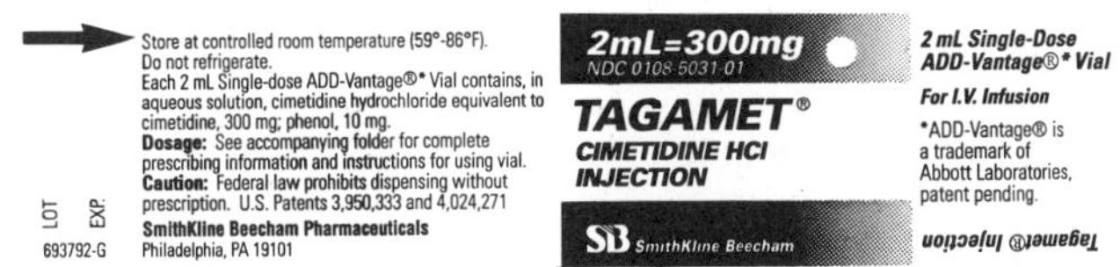

FAMILIAR TEMPERATURES ON BOTH SCALES

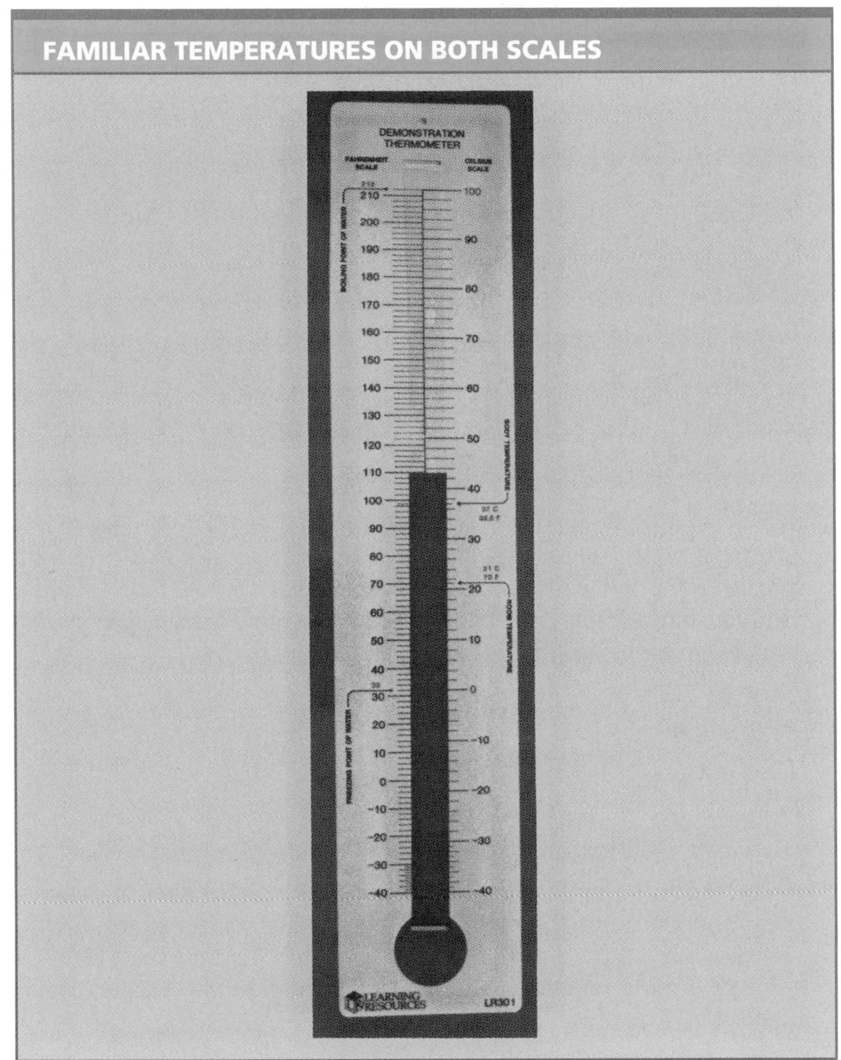

Note that for each temperature above −40°C, °C < °F.*

* For all temperatures above −40°F, °C < °F, but −40°C = −40°F, and below −40°F, °C > °F.

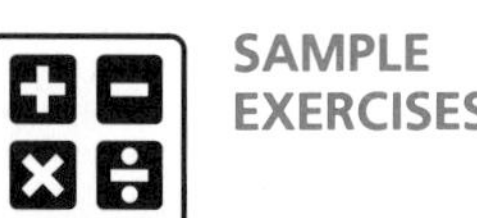

SAMPLE EXERCISES

1. On the Celsius scale, how much warmer than room temperature is body temperature?
2. On the Fahrenheit scale, what is the difference between freezing point and boiling point?
3. On the Celsius scale, what is the difference between freezing point and boiling point?

ANSWERS 1. 16°C 2. 180°F 3. 100°C

Conversion Formulas

Based on ratio and proportion, formulas enable us to convert from Celsius values to Fahrenheit values and vice versa.

CONVERSION FORMULAS

1. From °C **up** to °F:

$$°F = 1.8 \times °C + 32$$

First **multiply** °C by 1.8; then **add** 32.

2. From °F **down** to °C:

$$°C = \frac{°F - 32}{1.8}$$

First **subtract** 32 from °F; then **divide** by 1.8.

Examples

1. If a label states that the required minimum storage temperature of a drug is 4°C, we may need to find the corresponding Fahrenheit reading that satisfies this requirement. We use Formula 1 from the conversion formula box above.

   Formula 1: From °C up to °F.

   First multiply by 1.8: $4 \times 1.8 = 7.2$

   Then add: $7.2 + 32 = 39.2$

   Result: 4°C = 39.2°F

   (*Estimate:* First multiply by 2, then add 30.)

2. According to Formula 2 above, if you know a Fahrenheit measurement and you want the corresponding Celsius measurement, first subtract 32 and then divide the result by 1.8. To find the Celsius value of a room temperature from its Fahrenheit value, 68°F, we proceed as follows.

   Formula 2: From °F down to °C.

   First subtract 32: $68 - 32 = 36$

   Then divide by 1.8: $\frac{36}{1.8} = 20$

   Result: 68°F = 20°C

   (*Estimate:* Subtract 30, then divide by 2.)

3. Let us find the Celsius temperature corresponding to 101.3°F. We have the Fahrenheit value and want to work down to the Celsius value. Thus, we use Formula 2.

First subtract 32: $101.3 - 32 = 69.3$

Then divide by 1.8: $\frac{69.3}{1.8} = 38.5$

Result: $101.3°F = 38.5°C$

(*Estimate:* Subtract 30, then divide by 2.)

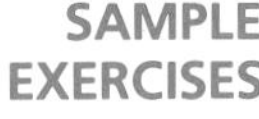

SAMPLE EXERCISES

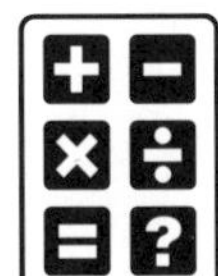

Exercises 1–2. In each of the following cases, what does a Fahrenheit thermometer read?

1. A baby girl has a temperature of 37.5°C.
2. An ice-cream freezer has a thermometer reading −10°C.

Exercises 3–4. In each of the following cases, find the corresponding Celsius temperatures.

3. Normal body temperature is 98.6°F.
4. Tagamet is stored within the temperature range of 59 to 86°F.

ANSWERS 1. $37.5 \times 1.8 + 32 = 67.5 + 32 = 99.5°F$
2. $-10 \times 1.8 + 32 = -18 + 32 = 14°F$ 3. $\frac{98.6 - 32}{1.8} = \frac{66.6}{1.8} = 37°C$
4. 15–30°C

EXERCISES

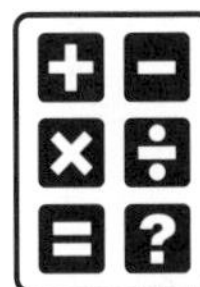

Exercises 1–4. What is the first step in each conversion?

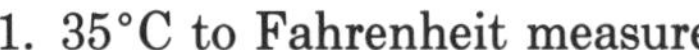

1. 35°C to Fahrenheit measure
2. 35°F to Celsius measure
3. 50°F to Celsius measure
4. 39.8°C to Fahrenheit measure

Exercises 5–8. Carry out the above conversions.

Exercises 9–12. Answer the questions below:

9. To convert from Celsius to Fahrenheit measure, multiply by 1.8. What is the next step?
10. To convert from Fahrenheit to Celsius measure, subtract 32. What is the next step?
11. An IV solution was to be stored at less than 46°F. On the Celsius scale, what temperature was this?
12. An IV solution was to be stored at less than 6°C. On the Fahrenheit scale, what temperature was this?

Exercises 13–16. Change the given temperature in the statements below to the corresponding Celsius value.

13. Do not expose albuterol to temperatures >86°F.
14. If Mrs. G.'s temperature >104°F, check for internal bleeding.
15. Reduce dosage of clofazimine when Mrs. P.'s temperature <101°F.
16. Store poliovirus vaccine at 7°F.

Exercises 17–20. Change the given temperature in the statements below to the corresponding Fahrenheit value.

17. Demerol contains a crystalline substance with a melting point of about 186°C.
18. Store Septra suspension within the temperature range of 15 to 25°C.
19. Store measles virus vaccine at 4°C.
20. Ocusert systems should be stored between 2 and 8°C.

ANSWERS 1. Multiply by 1.8 3. Subtract 32 5. 95°F 7. 10°C 9. Add 32 11. 7.8°C 13. 30°C 15. 38.3°C 17. 366.8°F 19. 39.2°F

5-7. CONVERSIONS BETWEEN SI AND NON-SI MEASURES

For many reasons, it is important to be skillful with conversions. For instance, we need to compare known amounts, such as the intake of liquids (in ounces) and the output of urine (in milliliters). Sometimes we need to convert a doctor's order from the apothecaries' system to SI units. For convenience, clarity, and safety, the use of proportions for conversions is most dependable.

The basis for conversions is a set of equivalents. Note that these "equivalents" are just approximations and may differ according to how accurate we need to be. For great accuracy, many decimal places may be needed, beyond our normal ability to measure physically. The following table gives the most commonly used approximate equivalents.

COMMONLY USED *APPROXIMATE* EQUIVALENTS

Household	Apothecaries'	SI
1 drop (gtt)	1 grain	60 mg
15 gtt	15 grains	1 g
	15 minims	1 mL
1 tsp		5 mL
1 tbsp		15 mL
2 tbsp	1 oz	30 mL
1 cup	8 oz	240 mL
1 pt	16 oz	480–500 mL
1 qt	32 oz	1 L

Examples

1. To give 10 mL of cough syrup, we might use 2 tsp.
2. A cold syrup contains acetaminophen (120 mg/5mL). This is the same as 120 mg/tsp. The doctor has ordered 2 tsp for Ms. Delaw. Thus, Ms. Delaw receives 240 mg of acetaminophen.
3. At dinner, Ramon had 200 mL of juice, a cup of soup, and a pint of milk. To record his intake of liquids, we convert and find the sum:

$$\begin{aligned} \text{milk, 1 pt} &= 480 \text{ mL} \\ \text{soup, 1 cup} &= 240 \text{ mL} \\ \text{juice} &= \underline{200 \text{ mL}} \\ \text{total intake} &= 920 \text{ mL} \end{aligned}$$

4. The doctor has ordered an atropine sulfate injection containing gr $\frac{1}{150}$ of atropine sulfate. To convert this amount to milligrams, we use a table and a proportion.

Table:

Milligrams	Grains
x	$\frac{1}{150}$
60	1

$$\frac{x}{60} = \frac{1}{150}$$

Result: 0.4 mg

SAMPLE EXERCISES

Exercises 1–4. Convert as indicated.

1. 3 drops (gtt) to milligrams
2. gr $\frac{1}{200}$ to milligrams
3. 4 tsp to milliliters
4. 200 mL to ounces

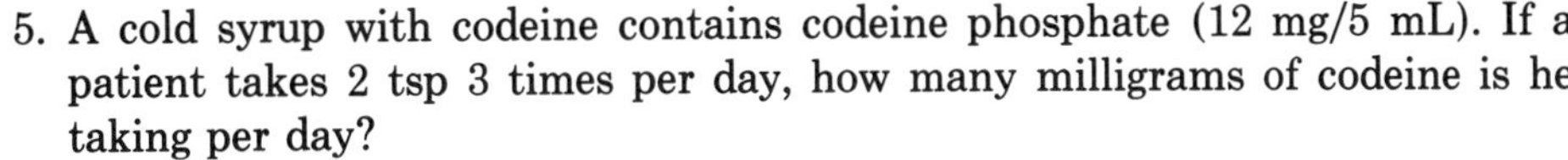

5. A cold syrup with codeine contains codeine phosphate (12 mg/5 mL). If a patient takes 2 tsp 3 times per day, how many milligrams of codeine is he taking per day?
6. Find, in milliliters, Ramon's total intake of liquids at lunch, if he had 4 oz of juice, a glass of water, and a half-pint of milk.

ANSWERS

1. *Table:*

Milligrams	Drops
x	3
60	1

$$\frac{x}{60} = \frac{3}{1}$$

Result: 180 mg

2. *Table:*

Milligrams	Grains
x	$\frac{1}{200}$
60	1

$$\frac{x}{60} = \frac{1}{200}$$

Result: 0.3 mg

3. 20 mL
4. *Table:*

Ounces	Milliliters
x	200
1	30

$$\frac{x}{1} = \frac{200}{30}$$

Result: 6.7 oz

5. *Table:*

x mg	6 tsp
	1 tsp
12 mg	~~5 mL~~

$$\frac{x}{12} = \frac{6}{1}$$

Result: 72 mg

6. juice, 4 oz = 120 mL
water, 1 glass = 240 mL
milk, $\frac{1}{2}$ pt = 240 mL
total intake = 600 mL

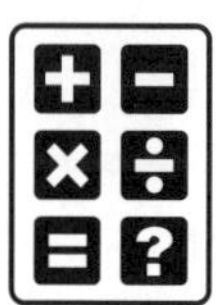

EXERCISES

Exercises 1–10. Convert as indicated.

1. 4 drops (gtt) to milligrams
2. gr $\frac{1}{300}$ to milligrams
3. 5 tsp to milliliters
4. 300 mL to ounces
5. $\frac{1}{4}$ cup to milliliters
6. 10 oz to milliliters
7. $\frac{2}{3}$ pt to milliliters
8. 3 oz to milliliters
9. gr $\frac{1}{500}$ to milligrams
10. 0.3 mL to minims

Exercises 11–16. Each of the following patients has drunk the amount shown. In each case, record, in milliliters, the amount that has been drunk.

11. Ms. A., 3 tbsp
12. Mrs. B., $\frac{1}{3}$ cup
13. Mr. C., $\frac{3}{4}$ pt
14. Dr. D., $\frac{7}{8}$ glassful
15. Prof. E., 5 oz
16. Jerry, 9 oz

Exercises 17–20. Answer each question below:

17. The nurse encouraged Mr. K., a patient with diarrhea, to drink 2000 mL of liquids per day. How many glassfuls is correct?
18. At 2:00 PM, on the day before surgery, Ms. H. is to receive $\frac{3}{4}$ oz of senna (in powdered form) dissolved in 2.5 oz of liquid. Restate the instructions in SI units.
19. If a dose of cough syrup is 2 tbsp + 1 tsp, how many milliliters are in a dose?
20. In order to give 2 mL of vitamin syrup, how many minims are administered?
21. If no more than 90 mL of an antacid should be taken in a day, what is the maximum number of doses per day? (Assume that 1 dose = 1 tbsp.)
22. How many doses (1 tsp each) are in a 300-mL bottle of cough syrup?
23. Mr. Y. needs to have bentiromide with 8 oz of water. Is 200 mL of water enough?
24. The doctor has recommended that Prof. N. drink 1 pint of fluid at each meal and at bedtime. How many liters must be available for the week (assuming 3 meals/day)?

Exercises 25–28. Penicillin may be ordered by weight in milligrams or by potency in units. A doctor's order for 160,000 U of penicillin G potassium for Ms. M. is equivalent to 100 mg of the drug. Express each of the following orders for penicillin G potassium in units.

25. 200 mg
26. 350 mg
27. 275 mg
28. 125 mg

ANSWERS 1. 240 mg 3. 25 mL 5. 60 mL 7. 320 mL 9. 0.12 mg 11. 45 mL 13. 360 mL 15. 150 mL 17. 8.3 glassfuls 19. 35 mL 21. 6 doses 23. No, Mr. Y. needs 240 mL 25. 320,000 U 27. 440,000 U

5-8. SHORTCUT FORMULA: $\frac{\text{DESIRED}}{\text{HAVE}} \times$ QUANTITY, OR $\frac{D}{H} \times Q$

The last steps of the ratio and proportion method provide an efficient shortcut for a variety of calculations, including conversions. To clarify the formula, and to see how we can shorten the problem solving process, let us look carefully at the details of the following problem. Convert 14.8 in. to centimeters. (*Reminder:* 2.5 cm = 1 in.)

Table:

Centimeters	Inches
x	14.8
2.5	1

Proportion:

$$\frac{x}{2.5} = \frac{14.8}{1}$$

Calculation:

$$x = \frac{14.8 \times 2.5}{1}$$

Rewrite the calculation as:

$$\frac{14.8}{1} \times 2.5$$

or form a ratio from the right side of the table and multiply by the bottom number on the left.

As an introduction to the shortcut, insert labels in the table as follows:

Tabulate:

	Centimeters	Inches	
	x	14.8	Desired (D)
(Q) Quantity:	2.5	1	Have (H)

Bypassing the proportion, we may immediately put the calculation into the form

$$\frac{\textbf{Desired}}{\textbf{Have}} \times \textbf{Quantity}$$

or

$$\frac{\mathbf{D}}{\mathbf{H}} \times \mathbf{Q}$$

$$\frac{14.8}{1} \times 2.5$$

Result: 37 cm

Note that $\frac{\mathbf{D}}{\mathbf{H}}$ must be a **pure ratio** (units must **match**).

Examples

1. At \$59 for every 4 hr worked, how long does it take to earn \$2500?

Tabulate:

	Hours	Earnings (\$)	
	x	2500	D
Q	4	59	H

Formula: $\frac{D}{H} \times Q = \frac{2500}{59} \times 4 = 169.5$

Result: 169.5 hr

2. Tablets of ascorbic acid are labeled 100 mg/tablet. How many tablets do we give for a dose of 250 mg?

Table:

Number of Tablets	Dose
x	250 mg
1	100 mg

Formula: $\frac{D}{H} \times Q = \frac{250}{100} \times 1 = 2.5$

Result: 2.5 tablets

3. Suppose that 4 tbsp of syrup are mixed into 1 cup of liquid. To find the number of teaspoons of syrup in 1 oz of the liquid, the procedure is the same, *except* that we must first change to **identical units.** (*Reminder:* 3 tsp = 1 tbsp; 8 oz = 1 cup)

Table:

Teaspoons	Ounces
x	1
12	8

Formula: $\frac{D}{H} \times Q = \frac{1}{8} \times 12 = 1.5$

Result: 1.5 tsp

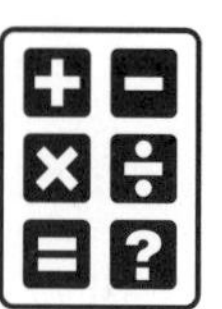

SAMPLE EXERCISES

Use $\frac{\mathbf{D}}{\mathbf{H}} \times \mathbf{Q}$ to solve the following problems. (Make sure that $\frac{D}{H}$ is a pure ratio.) Include an estimate before the calculation and a check after.

Exercises 1–2. Given that in 4 oz of protein there are 448 cal.

1. How many calories are there in 6.5 oz of protein?
2. How much protein do we need for 325 cal?

Exercises 3–4. If 5000 IU of vitamin A is 100% of the RDA, then:

3. How much vitamin A is 20% of the RDA?
4. What percent of the RDA does 2500 IU represent?
5. A medication available for injection is labeled 5 mg/mL. If a patient needs 6.75 mg, how many milliliters should you give?

ANSWERS

1. *Table:*

Calories	Ounces of Protein
x	6.5
448	4

Formula: $\frac{D}{H} \times Q = \frac{6.5}{4} \times 448 = 728$

(An estimate = 800)

Check: $448 \times 6.5 = 728 \times 4$

Result: 728 cal in 6.5 oz of protein

2. *Table:*

Ounces of Protein	Calories
x	325
4	448

Formula: $\frac{D}{H} \times Q = \frac{325}{448} \times 4 = 2.9$

(An estimate = 3)

Check: $4 \times 325 = 2.9 \times 448$

Result: 2.9 oz of protein needed for 325 cal

3. *Table:*

IU	%
x	20
5000	100

Formula: $\frac{D}{H} \times Q = \frac{20}{100} \times 5000 = 1000$

Check: $5000 \times 20 = 1000 \times 100$

Result: 1000 IU

4. *Table:*

%	IU
x	2500
100	5000

Formula: $\frac{D}{H} \times Q = \frac{2500}{5000} \times 100 = 50$

Check: $100 \times 2500 = 50 \times 5000$

Result: 50%

5. $\frac{D}{H} \times Q = \frac{6.75}{5} \times 1 = 1.35$ mL, or 1.4 mL (rounded to tenths)

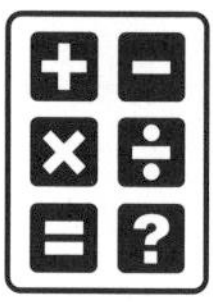

EXERCISES

Use the formula $\frac{D}{H} \times Q$ to solve the following problems. Include an estimate and a check. Wherever rounding is appropriate, round to the nearest tenth.

Exercises 1–14. Convert as indicated.

1. 6.2 in. to centimeters
2. 34.8 cm to inches
3. 12.5 cc to teaspoons
4. 180 mL to glassfuls
5. 4.2 oz to milliliters
6. 0.8 L to ounces
7. 43 mL to ounces
8. 2 gal to pints
9. 75 mL to tablespoons
10. 12 oz to teaspoons
11. 3.5 dL to milliliters
12. 160 mL to deciliters
13. gr $\frac{1}{100}$ to milligrams
14. 0.7 mL to minims
15. At $110 for every 7 hr worked, how long does it take to earn $3000?
16. Certain tablets are labeled 60 mg/tablet. How many tablets need we give for a dose of 0.15 g?
17. An oral medication is labeled 125 mg/oz. If a patient needs 575 mg, how many ounces should you give?
18. Suppose that 3 tsp of syrup are mixed into 1 cup of liquid. Find the number of tablespoons of syrup in 2 oz of the liquid.

Exercises 19–20. If milk contains 291 mg of calcium/glassful, then:

19. How much calcium is in 28 oz of milk?
20. How many ounces of milk contain 850 mg of calcium?

Exercises 21–24. If 9.5 oz of vegetable soup provides 90 cal, 16 g of carbohydrates, 1100 mg of sodium, and 360 mg of potassium, then:

21. How much potassium is there in 6 oz of soup?
22. How much sodium is there in a pint of soup?
23. How much carbohydrate is there in 12 oz of soup?
24. About how many cups of soup do we need for 136 cal?

Exercises 25–26. Express in units each of the following orders for penicillin G potassium. Assume that 160,000 U = 100 mg.

25. 175 mg
26. 325 mg

Exercises 27–28. If 5000 IU of vitamin A is 100% of the RDA, then:

27. How much vitamin A is 85% of the RDA?
28. What percent of the RDA does 4500 IU represent?

Exercises 29–30. Available forms of potassium bicarbonate include an oral solution containing 2.375 mEq/5 mL and an elixir containing 6.7 mEq/5 mL. How much potassium bicarbonate is in:

29. 7.5 mL of the oral solution?
30. 7.5 mL of the elixir?

ANSWERS (Some answers may differ because of approximations.)

1. 15.5 cm 3. 2.5 tsp 5. 126 mL 7. 1.4 oz 9. 5 tbsp
11. 350 mL 13. 0.6 mg 15. 190.9 hr 17. 4.6 oz
19. 1018.5 mg 21. 227.4 mg 23. 20.2 g 25. 280,000 U
27. 4250 IU 29. 3.6 mEq

5-9. AVOIDING ERRORS: AVOIDING THE APOTHECARIES' SYSTEM AND NON-STANDARD MEASURES

"Don't let the apothecary system put your patient at risk."* The apothecaries' system is gradually being phased out, but sometimes we are forced into using it because it is put before us (in a doctor's order, for instance). Then it is often best to **convert** the given measurements to the SI. See Appendix 3.

Don't let non-standard measures put your patient at risk either. If reference is made to 1 tsp, think instead 5 mL. One glassful means 240 mL. Household teaspoons, cups, and glasses come in a wide variety of sizes and are not reliable measuring devices. See Appendix 1.

It is wise to check with a reference table whenever an unfamiliar unit, or one that we do not use regularly, appears. Whatever the situation, always write out the calculations, because mental computations are not sufficiently dependable.

EXERCISES

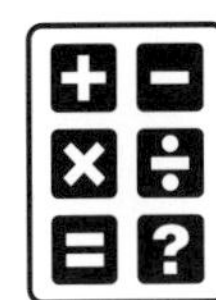

Exercises 1–14. Convert as indicated. Use the appendix where necessary.

1. gr iii to milligrams
2. gr vii to milligrams
3. gr ix to grams
4. gr xii to grams
5. gr $\frac{1}{3}$ to milligrams
6. gr $\frac{1}{5}$ to milligrams
7. gr $\frac{1}{100}$ to micrograms
8. gr $\frac{1}{250}$ to micrograms
9. 1.5 glassfuls to milliliters
10. 2.5 cups to milliliters
11. 1 dram to grains
12. 8 drams to ounces
13. 1 dram to grams
14. 15 minims to milliliters

Exercises 15–18. Change the following instructions to SI measures.

15. Administer amoxicillin on an empty stomach with a full glass of water.
16. Mix the sodium biphosphate solution with 4 oz cold water.
17. Dissolve the antacid tablet in 6 oz of water.
18. Stir Colestid in 2 oz of beverage.

Exercises 19–20. Ascorbic acid is available in a mixture of 4 g/tsp of powder. How many grams of ascorbic acid are there:

19. In $1\frac{1}{4}$ tsp?
20. $\frac{1}{2}$ tbsp

* Cohen MR: *200 Medication Errors and How to Avoid Them.* Springhouse, PA: Springhouse Corporation, 1991:iii.

ANSWERS 1. 180 mg 3. 0.5 g 5. 20 mg 7. 600 μg 9. 360 mL 11. 60 grains 13. 3.8 g 15. 240 mL 17. 180 mL 19. 5 g

5-10. SUMMARY

1. APOTHECARIES' SYSTEM: BASIC MEASURES

   Weight: the grain (gr).
   Liquid (fluid) capacity: fluid ounce (fl oz, oz), pint (pt), quart (qt), and gallon (gal).

2. APOTHECARIES' SYSTEM: NOTATION

   The symbol for grain (gr) precedes the quantity, which is shown in fractions or Roman numerals.

   Examples

   gr $\frac{1}{3}$, gr i, gr ii, gr v

3. SOME COMMONLY USED APPROXIMATE EQUIVALENTS

Household	Apothecaries'	SI
1 drop (gtt)	1 grain	60 mg
	15 grains	1 g
15 drops (gtt)	15 minims	1 mL
1 tsp		5 mL
1 tbsp		15 mL
2 tbsp	1 oz	30 mL
	1 oz	30 g
1 cup	8 oz	240 mL
1 pint	16 oz	480–500 mL
1 quart	32 oz	1 L

4. UNITS OF POTENCY

   Potency is classified using international units (IU), National Formulary units, United States Pharmacopeia (USP) units, or units approved by the Food and Drug Administration or the National Institutes of Health, or by other qualified agencies.

   Examples

   (a) 1 mg of penicillin G sodium contains about 1667 penicillin units.
   (b) Insulin is prepared in units per milliliter.
   (c) In IV therapy, a heparin-lock flush solution with strength 100 USP units/mL may be used to keep catheters clear.

5. The **equivalent** (Eq) and **milliequivalent** (mEq) are units of measurement for concentrations of electrically charged particles in biological fluids.

   Example

   A blood test for calcium is considered normal if it shows any result between 4.5 and 5.5 mEq per liter.

6. FAHRENHEIT AND CELSIUS TEMPERATURE SCALES

These are related as follows:

(a) $C = \frac{(F - 32)}{1.8}$

To convert from °F to °C, first subtract 32, then divide by 1.8.

(b) $F = 1.8\ C + 32$

To convert from °C to °F, first multiply by 1.8, then add 32.

Examples

(a) To convert 100°F to Celsius,

Subtract: $100 - 32 = 68$

Then divide: $\frac{68}{1.8} = 37.8$

Result: 100°F = 37.8°C

(b) To convert 40°C to Fahrenheit,

Multiply: $40 \times 1.8 = 72$

Then add: $72 + 32 = 104$

Result: 40°C = 104°F

7. SHORTCUT FORMULA

$$\frac{\text{DESIRED}}{\text{HAVE}} \times \text{QUANTITY}$$

or

$$\frac{D}{H} \times Q$$

On the basis of the last steps of the ratio and proportion method, $\frac{D}{H} \times Q$ takes us from our table of data to a quick solution of a problem.

Table:

x	*D*(ESIRED)
Q(UANTITY)	*H*(AVE)

$$x = \frac{D}{H} \times Q$$

Make sure that $\frac{D}{H}$ is a pure ratio (units must match).

Examples

(a) A can of tuna (6.5 oz) provides 98 g of protein. How many grams of protein are provided per ounce?

Table:

Protein (g)	Tuna (oz)
x	1
98	6.5

Formula: $\frac{D}{H} \times Q = \frac{1}{6.5} \times 98$

Estimate: about 20 g

Result: 15.1 g

Check: $98 \times 1 = 15.1 \times 6.5$

(b) If a pump delivers medication at a constant rate of 20 mg/hr, how many hours does it take to deliver 190 mg?

Table:

Hours	Milligrams
x	190
1	20

Formula: $\frac{D}{H} \times Q = \frac{190}{20} \times 1$

Estimate: About 10 hr

Result: 9.5 hr

Check: $9.5 \times 20 = 190$

8. To prevent errors, **avoid** the **apothecaries' system** and **non-standard measures.** Convert to SI measures as much as possible.

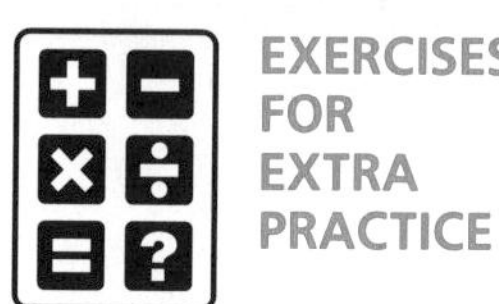

EXERCISES FOR EXTRA PRACTICE

Wherever rounding is appropriate, round to the nearest tenth.

Exercises 1–18. Convert as indicated.

1. 14.5 ft to meters
2. 1.75 m to feet
3. 5.4 in. to centimeters
4. 20.4 cm to inches
5. 2.7 in. to millimeters
6. 26.4 mm to inches
7. 3.1 dL to ounces
8. 7.3 oz to deciliters
9. 32 mL to teaspoons
10. 1.6 oz to tablespoons
11. 52°F to Celsius
12. 26°C to Fahrenheit
13. 0.3 oz to milliliters
14. 20 mL to ounces
15. 14 oz to milliliters
16. 2.2 L to pints
17. gr viii to milligrams
18. gr xiv to grams

Exercises 19–22. Normal blood chemistry values are given in the following table:

Test	Normal Values (mEq/L)
Chlorides	100–106
Potassium	3.6–5.6
Sodium	138–148

Determine which, if any, of the following quantities are within the normal range:

19. Potassium: 37 mEq/L
20. Potassium: 0.49 mEq/L
21. Chlorides: 1 mEq/mL
22. Sodium: 0.14 mEq/mL

Exercises 23–28. Answer the following questions.

23. A blood test for a patient shows 45 U/L. This is the same ratio as ______ mU/mL.
24. To stir colestipol hydrochloride in 4 oz of a liquid, how many tablespoons of the liquid are needed?

25. Ben is to take methadone in 120 mL of orange juice. How many ounces of juice should be in the glass?

26. A low-calorie diet has been prescribed for Carla. For lunch, she has a tuna salad made with 57 g of tuna. This is ______ ounces of tuna.

27. A doctor may order 320,000 U of penicillin G potassium for a patient. This is equivalent to about 200 mg of the drug. What is the weight of the drug if 240,000 U are ordered?

28. My gas tank holds 19 gal. Will it hold 40 L?

Exercises 29–30. If a patient is receiving medication at a rate of 12 mg/hr, then:

29. How many hours does it take for her to receive a total of 65 mg?

30. How many milligrams has she received after 6.45 hr?

31. Each gram of protein provides 4 cal. If protein in breakfast provides a total of 280 cal, how much protein was present?

32. Each gram of fat provides 9 cal. If fat in dinner provides a total of 1050 cal, how much fat was present?

Exercises 33–34. Convert each Fahrenheit temperature to a Celsius temperature.

33. Store calcitonin at no higher than 77°F.

34. The concentrated stock solution must be used within 24 hr if stored at a room temperature of 70–75°F or within 72 hr if kept under refrigeration at 40°F.

ANSWERS 1. 4.4 m 3. 13.5 cm 5. 67.5 mm 7. 10.3 oz 9. 6.4 tsp 11. 11.1°C 13. 9 mL 15. 420 mL 17. 480 mg 19. 37 mEq/L, too high 21. 1 mEq/mL = 1000 mEq/L, too high 23. 45 mU/mL 25. 4-oz glass 27. 150 mg 29. 5.4 hr 31. 70 g 33. 25°C

CHAPTER TEST

1. The milliequivalent is what part of an equivalent? 1. ______

2. Convert gr v to SI units. 2. ______

3. How many teaspoonfuls do you use for a dose of $\frac{1}{2}$ oz of cough syrup? 3. ______

4. How many milliliters are in $\frac{1}{2}$ tsp? 4. ______

Problems 5–8. Complete the statement.

5. A ratio of 800 U/L is equal to ______ U/mL. 5. ______

6. A container that holds 120 mL holds ______ oz. 6. ______

7. 39.8°F = ______ °C. 7. ______

8. 17.5°C = ______ °F. 8. ______

9. What is the doctor's order, in units, if 300 mg of penicillin G potassium is needed? Assume that 160,000 U = 100 mg. 9. ________

10. How much ammonium chloride may be found in 2.4 mL of a solution containing 5 mEq/mL? 10. ________

ANSWERS 1. 0.001 2. 0.3 g, or 300 mg 3. 3 tsp 4. 2.5 mL 5. 0.8 U/mL 6. 4 7. 4.3°C 8. 63.5°F 9. 480,000 U 10. 12 mEq

---

SIX

Dosage and Administration with Applications to Oral Medications

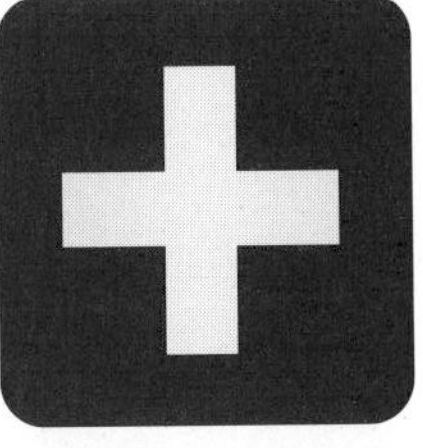

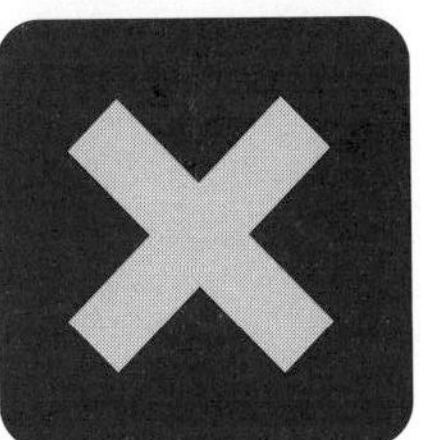

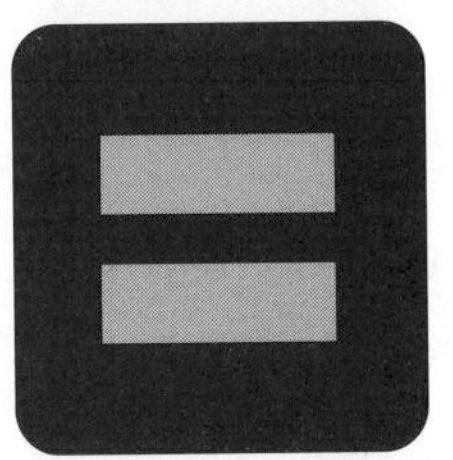

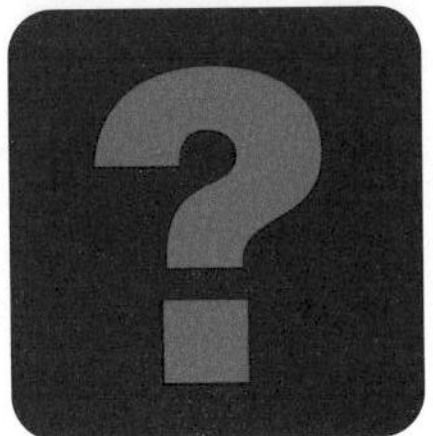

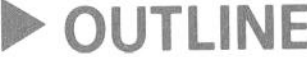

▶ OUTLINE

▶ OBJECTIVES

After studying this chapter, you will be able to:

1. Interpret and write medical symbols.
2. Compute oral doses.
3. Read labels.
4. Interpret safety limits for doses.

6-1. INTRODUCTION

Why must nurses know anything about dosage? In a typical health care center, the pharmacist prepares most doses of medication. But no matter who prepares a dose, it is the nurse who administers it to the client and is thus the last person who can detect an error. The nurse has the legal responsibility for administering the appropriate amount.

What must nurses know about dosage? To know whether a dose is appropriate, nurses need the latest information about therapeutic agents. They must be able to read and write medical symbols, interpret manufacturer's and doctor's dosage instructions, and record administered doses accurately. Although the pharmacy prepares most doses, nurses must have the basic computational skills to prepare a dose when necessary or guard against errors if the dose is already prepared.

Proficiency Gauge

It is possible that you are experienced with computing dosages and can skip Chapter 6. Gauge your proficiency by working out the following exercises. Check your answers with those that follow the test only after you have answered all the questions.

1. Interpret these instructions: "Do not administer IM or IV." 1. ______
2. Explain the following item from a doctor's order: bethanechol 2.5 mg SC q6h. 2. ______

Exercises 3–5. Find the number of tablets needed for each of the following doses.

	Dose Required	Strength of Scored Tablets Available	
3.	10 mg	20 mg	3. ______
4.	60 mg	0.02 g	4. ______
5.	0.3 mg	120 μg	5. ______

6. On hand: Unit dose packets of digoxin like the one pictured here. For a dose of 0.25 mg, how many tablets should be administered? 6. ______

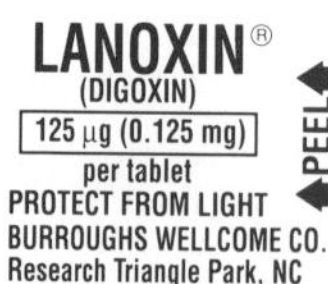

LANOXIN®
(DIGOXIN)
125 μg (0.125 mg)
per tablet
PROTECT FROM LIGHT
BURROUGHS WELLCOME CO.
Research Triangle Park, NC
PEEL

Exercises 7–10. In each of the following cases, find the amount (in milliliters) of liquid medication to be administered per dose.

	Doctor's Order	Label on Container	
7.	6000 U stat	20,000 U/mL	7. ______
8.	80 mg stat	50 mg in 2 cc	8. ______
9.	100 mg	0.5 g/1.8 mL	9. ______
10.	3 mg bid	See label on p. 169.	10. ______

16 fl. oz. (1 pint)

Proventil®

brand of albuterol sulfate

Syrup

Usual Dose: See package insert

Each teaspoonful (5 mL) contains:
2 mg albuterol as the sulfate.

Read accompanying directions carefully.

Store between 2° and 30°C (36° and 86°F).

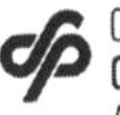

Copyright © 1987, 1990, **Schering Corporation,** Kenilworth, NJ 07033 USA. All rights reserved.

16194620 Rev. 10/90

6505-01-256-4997

SCHERING NDC-0085-0315-02

16 fl. oz. (1 pint)

Proventil®

brand of albuterol sulfate

Syrup

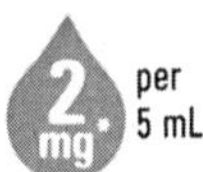

per 5 mL

*Potency expressed as albuterol.

Caution: Federal law prohibits dispensing without prescription.

ANSWERS 1. Do not use either the intravenous or intramuscular routes of administration. 2. Administer subcutaneously 2.5 mg of bethanechol every 6 hr. 3. 1/2 tablet 4. 3 tablets 5. 2.5 tablets 6. 2 tablets 7. 0.3 mL 8. 3.2 mL 9. 0.4 mL 10. 7.5 mL

6-2. MEDICAL SYMBOLS FOR DOSAGE INSTRUCTIONS

Doses and Dosage

What is a dose? A **dose** is the amount of medication given at a single time.

What do we mean by dosage? **Dosage** means more than just the amount of medication at any given time. By dosage we mean a **course of treatment,** prescribed by the doctor, detailing not only the amount of medication, but also the type of medication, and how it is to be administered over a specified period of time.

DOSAGE INSTRUCTIONS

Dosage instructions include:

What	drug to administer (name)
Why	the drug has been chosen (rationale)
How	to administer (method or route)
How Much	to administer (dose)
How Often	to administer (frequency)
How Long	to continue (length of time)

Examples

1. The phrase "intravenous infusion" tells how to administer the medication to the patient and is an example of **route** of administration, or the **method** by which the patient receives the medication.
2. The **frequency** of administration of cough medicine may be "four times per day."

Frequency of Administration

Symbols for Frequency of Administration

Per Day
bid = 2 times per day (two times in 24 hr)
tid = 3 times per day (three times in 24 hr)
qid = 4 times per day (four times in 24 hr)
qd = every day
qam = every morning
qpm = every evening

Every ____ Hours

qh = every hour	q2h = every 2 hours
q3h = every 3 hours	q4h = every 4 hours
q6h = every 6 hours	q8h = every 8 hours

stat: immediately
prn: whenever necessary
ac = before meals   pc = after meals
hs = before sleep

Examples

1. To indicate the frequency "every 12 hours," we write q12h.
2. The frequency qid means four times a day, but the exact schedule of administration of the four doses may be determined by the doctor, nurse, or pharmacist. Sometimes qid means "q6h"; sometimes qid is used for four doses given during waking hours only.

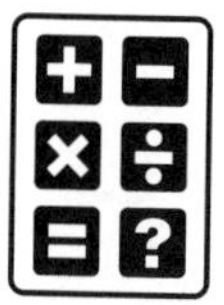

SAMPLE EXERCISES

1. Milk of magnesia is often given pc and hs. Explain the symbols.
2. Write symbols to indicate two times per day.
3. tid stands for what frequency?

ANSWERS 1. After meals and at bedtime 2. bid (think of *2* wheels on a *bi*cycle 3. 3 times per day (think of *3* wheels on a *tri*cycle)

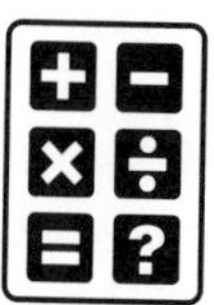

EXERCISES

1. Some clients with hypertension take captopril, 25 mg tid. How often is this?
2. The doctor wrote, "Administer erythromycin 250 mg q6h." How often is erythromycin to be administered?

Exercises 3–10. Match the symbols on the left with the correct expression on the right.

3. bid	a. at 12:00 noon
4. qd	b. every morning
5. ac	c. at bedtime
6. q12h	d. immediately
7. q2h	e. two times per day
8. hs	f. every day
9. qam	g. every 2 hours
10. stat	h. before meals
	i. every 12 hours

Exercises 11–18. Match the symbols on the left with the correct expression on the right.

11. pc	a. three times each day
12. prn	b. every 4 hours
13. qpm	c. pronto
14. qid	d. every 3 hours
15. q4h	e. after meals
16. tid	f. every hour
17. qh	g. whenever necessary
18. q3h	h. four times per day
	i. every evening

Exercises 19–28. Replace the indicated expression with symbols.

19. before meals
20. every day
21. at bedtime
22. three times per day
23. immediately
24. every morning
25. every 2 hours
26. whenever necessary
27. twice each day
28. after meals

ANSWERS 1. three times a day 3. e 5. h 7. g 9. b 11. e 13. i 15. b 17. f 19. ac 21. hs 23. stat 25. q2h 27. bid

---

6-3. ROUTE OF ADMINISTRATION

If a tablet is to be swallowed, the route of administration is **oral**. If the tablet is placed under the tongue, to dissolve there, the route of administration is called **sublingual.** Another route of administration, called **parenteral,** includes injection into a muscle or a vein and injection into tissue under the skin. The following table shows the most common symbols for route (or method) of administration of drugs.

SYMBOLS FOR ROUTE OF ADMINISTRATION

PO: oral (by mouth)
IM: intramuscular
IV: intravenous
SC: subcutaneous (under the skin)
SL: sublingual (under the tongue)

Examples

1. A doctor's order, "butorphanol tartrate 2 mg IM q3h" means "Give 2 mg of butorphanol tartrate by intramuscular injection every 3 hours."
2. The instructions, "captopril 25 mg PO bid" means that the patient is to take 25 mg of captopril orally (by mouth) twice each day.
3. A dosage of chlorpheniramine 5 mg SC qd means that 5 mg of chlorpheniramine is to be administered subcutaneously every day.

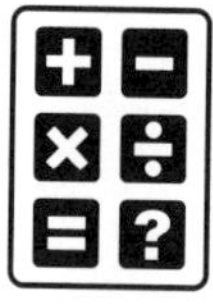

SAMPLE EXERCISES

Exercises 1–3. Interpret the following doctor's orders.

1. nitroglycerin gr 1/150 SL prn
2. milk of magnesia 5 mL qid pc and hs
3. betaxolol hydrochloride 1 gtt in each eye bid

ANSWERS 1. 1/150 grain of nitroglycerin may be taken under the tongue whenever necessary 2. Administer 5 milliliters of milk of magnesia 4 times each day, after meals and at bedtime. 3. Administer 1 drop of betaxolol hydrochloride in each eye twice each day.

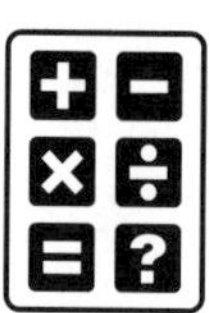

EXERCISES

Exercises 1–6. In each of the following cases, give the frequency and route of administration.

1. 4 mg PO qid
2. 30 mg SC daily
3. 12 mg PO tid
4. 10 mg SL q6h
5. gr 1/10 IM qh
6. gr 1/50 SC stat

Exercises 7–12. Explain the following items from medication administration records.

Medication	Amount	Frequency	Route
7. bethanechol	2.5 mg	q6h	SC
8. aluminum hydroxide	600 mg	1 h pc and hs	PO
9. acebutolol	1 g/d	bid	PO
10. butorphanol tartrate	500 mcg	q3h	IV

11. atropine sulfate	gr 1/100	before anesthesia	IM
12. morphine sulfate	gr 1/4	q4h	SC

Exercises 13–20. Interpret the symbols for dosage and administration.

13. cholestyramine 4 g PO ac and hs, not to exceed 32 g daily.

14. Nubain 20 mg IM q6h prn

15. rifampin 600 mg/d PO as single dose 1 h ac or 2 h pc

16. isoproterenol HCl 20 mg SL q8h

17. Desferal 2 g SC over 24 h

18. ergoloid mesylate 1 mg SL tid

19. Pima syrup saturated solution 0.25 mL PO qid

20. ACTH 40 U IM q12h

Exercises 21–24. Interpret the symbols for dosage and administration in the doctor's orders shown in Figure 6–1 on page 174.

25. Write symbols to use in filling out the hospital's medication administration record (MAR) for the patient to whom you have been giving the following medications: 650 milligrams of aspirin per day, orally; and 400,000 units of penicillin every 8 hours by intravenous administration.

26. If 300,000 units of penicillin are given four times each day by intramuscular injection, how would you record this in symbols?

ANSWERS 1. Four times each day, orally 3. three times per day, orally 5. every hour, intramuscularly 7. 2.5 mg every 6 hours, subcutaneously 9. 1 g each day, divided into two doses of 0.5 g each, orally 11. 1/100 grain before anesthesia, intramuscularly 13. cholestyramine orally, 4 g, before meals and at bedtime, not to exceed 32 g/day 15. rifampin, 600 mg/day, in a single oral dose 1 hour before a meal or 2 hours after a meal 17. Desferal, 2 g, subcutaneously, over 24 hours 19. Pima syrup, oral doses, 0.25 mL saturated solution each dose, four times a day 21. Rocephin, 1 g, intramuscularly, every 12 hours, for 7 days 23. cholestyramine, 4 g, orally, before meals and at bedtime 25. aspirin, 650 mg PO qd; penicillin 400,000 U IV q8h

---

6-4. DOSES FROM TABLETS OR CAPSULES

One of the most important methods of providing drug therapy is oral administration of tablets, capsules, or liquids. A typical computation requires no new mathematical techniques. We can find the quantity of tablets, capsules, or liquid to give for the required dosage, or information about ingredients, by using (1) proportions, or (2) the shortcut formula, $\frac{D}{H} \times Q$. Let us first consider tablets and capsules.

Utopia Health Care Center

PHYSICIANS ORDERS

AUTHORIZATION IS GIVEN FOR THE DISPENSING AND ADMINISTERING OF THE SAME MEDICATION OR ONE OF IDENTICAL STRENGTH, DOSAGE FORM AND CONTENT OF ACTIVE THERAPEUTIC INGREDIENT UNLESS DRUG IS CIRCLED.

Date Order Written	Time Order Written	ORDERS PHYSICIAN SIGN ON LINE DIRECTLY UNDER LAST ORDER ON A SECTION	Time Order Noted	Nurses Signature	DRAW RED LINE THROUGH DISCONTINUED ORDERS
		Rocephin 1g IM q12h x 7 days for pneumonia W. R. Smith, M.D.			Height / Weight / Drug Allergy
		IBUPROFEN 300 MG PO TID FOR ARTHRITIC PAIN C. Mitchell, M.D.			Height / Weight / Drug Allergy
		Cholestyramine 4g PO ac and hs for diarrhea K. Johnson, M.D.			Height / Weight / Drug Allergy
		Cephalothin sodium 500 mg IV q4h for bacterial peritonitis V. Allen, M.D.			Height / Weight / Drug Allergy

Figure 6–1 Physicians' orders for Exercises 21–24. *21*: Rocephin; *22*: ibuprofen; *23*: cholestyramine; *24*: cephalothin sodium.

SOLVING DOSAGE PROBLEMS

Use:

1. Proportions

or

2. $\frac{D}{H} \times Q$

Examples

1. A tablet is solid; a capsule is usually a gelatin container filled with medication, which may be solid or liquid. Each is small enough to swallow whole, but some tablets may be scored for subdivision, whereas the capsule is not made to be subdivided.

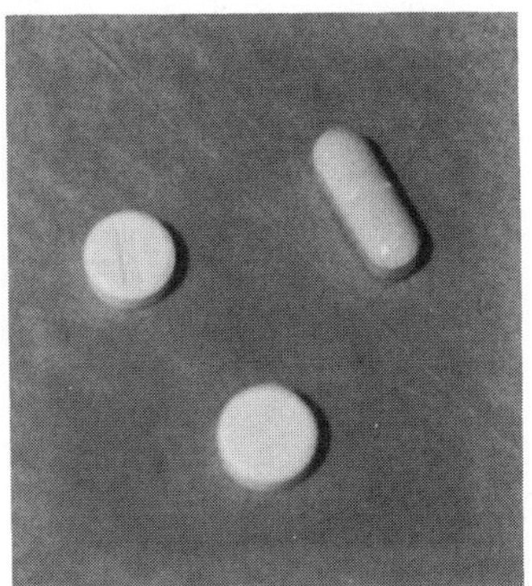

2. Tofranil (imipramine hydrochloride) is available in tablets of 25 mg. Mr. Debrew needs a dose of 75 mg. How many tablets do you give him?

   Table: x tab for a 75-mg dose (*D*esired information)
   1 tab for a 25-mg dose (Information we *H*ave)

   (Make sure the units match.)

   Proportion: $\frac{x}{1} = \frac{75}{25}$

   or

   Formula: $\frac{D}{H} \times Q = \frac{75}{25} \times 1 \text{ tab}$

   Result: 3 tablets

3. According to the doctor's orders, Prof. Delsom should be taking 250 mg of amoxicillin q8h. The label on her packet of tablets reads 125 mg/tablet. To find how many tablets she should be taking for each dose, consider the following table.

   Table: x tab for a 250-mg dose (*D*esired information)
   1 tab for a 125-mg dose (Information we *H*ave)

   Proportion: $\frac{x}{1} = \frac{250}{125}$

   or

   Formula: $\frac{D}{H} \times Q = \frac{250}{125} \times 1 \text{ tablet}$

Result: 2 tablets

Check: $125 \times 2 = 250$

4. "When administering ibuprofen tablets, do not exceed 2.4 g total daily dosage." Therefore, per day, the maximum number of 400-mg tablets is six. Here are the details:

   Table:

   x tab for ~~2.4 g~~ 2400 mg (*Desired* information)
   1 tab for 400 mg (Information we *Have*)

   (Convert 2.4 g to 2400 mg to make the units match.)

   Proportion: $\frac{x}{1} = \frac{2400}{400}$

   or

   Formula: $\frac{D}{H} \times Q = \frac{2400}{400} \times 1 \text{ tab}$

   Result: 6 tablets

   Check: 6 tab × 400 mg/tab = 2400 mg = 2.4 g

5. Product information shows that an antacid contains an acid-neutralizing capacity of 17 mEq/2 tablets. How much acid-neutralizing capacity is there in 5 tablets?

   Table:

   x mEq in 5 tab
   17 mEq in 2 tab

   Proportion: $\frac{x}{17} = \frac{5}{2}$

   or

   Formula: $\frac{D}{H} \times Q = \frac{5}{2} \times 17 \text{ mEq}$

   Result: 42.5 mEq

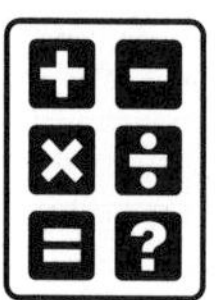

SAMPLE EXERCISES

Exercises 1–2. Mrs. Petromalla needs a certain drug; the order calls for 0.375 mg tid. Scored 0.25-mg tablets will be used. Then:

1. How many tablets do you expect the pharmacy to provide per dose?
2. How many doses per day?
3. The doctor has prescribed 7.5 mg of minoxidil for Mr. Kolsen. On hand are scored tablets 2.5 mg and 10 mg. Which would you use and how many would you give?

ANSWERS 1. $\frac{0.375}{0.25} \times 1$ tablet = 1.5 tablets for each dose

2. 3 doses per day 3. $\frac{7.5}{2.5} \times 1$ tablet = 3 tablets of 2.5 mg or, alternatively, 1 tablet of 2.5 mg and 1/2 tablet of 10 mg = 2.5 mg + 5 mg = 7.5 mg

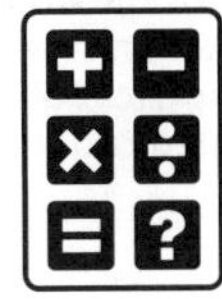

Exercises 1–12. How many tablets do you give per day?

Doctor's Order (*Desired*)	On Hand (*Have*)
1. captopril 12.5 mg PO tid	tab 12.5 mg
2. captopril 0.025 g PO bid	tab 12.5 mg
3. fenoprofen calcium 600 mg qid	cap 0.6 g
4. erythromycin 333 mg PO q6h	tab 333 mg
5. temazepam 30 mg PO hs	tab 0.03 g
6. conjugated estrogens 1.25 mg PO qd	tab 625 μg
7. levothyroxine sodium 100 μg PO qd	tab 0.05 mg
8. levothyroxine sodium 0.2 mg qd	tab 200 μg
9. clorazepate dipotassium 7.5 mg/day	tab 3.75 mg
10. alprazolam 500 μg tid	tab 0.25 mg
11. Nembutal 3 gr stat	cap 100 mg
12. Tylenol gr xv qid	tab 325 mg

Exercises 13–24. How many tablets will you give for the indicated dose?

Doctor's Order (*Desired*)	Scored Tablets on Hand (*Have*)
13. sulindac 0.2 g	200 mg
14. nadolol 0.06 g	120 mg
15. Coumadin 15 mg	10 mg
16. Lasix 60 mg	40 mg
17. hydrochlorothiazide 25 mg	0.05 g
18. Inderal 25 mg	0.01 g
19. Isordil 15 mg	0.01 g
20. digoxin 0.187 mg	125 μg
21. fenoprofen calcium 0.3 g	600 mg
22. levothyroxine sodium 0.25 mg	100 μg
23. acetaminophen 162.5 mg	325 mg
24. acetaminophen 487.5 mg	325 mg

ANSWERS 1. 3 tablets/day (1 tablet dose) 3. 4 capsules 5. 1 tablet 7. 2 tablets 9. 2 tablets 11. 2 capsules 13. 1 tablet 15. 1.5 tablets 17. 0.5 tablet 19. 1.5 tablets 21. 0.5 tablet 23. 0.5 tablet

6-5. DOSES FROM LIQUIDS

As indicated in Section 6-4, a typical problem in oral administration requires no new mathematical techniques. Whether we administer tablets or liquids, we can compute the quantity to give for the required dosage, or information about ingredients, by using (1) proportions, or (2) the shortcut formula, $\frac{D}{H} \times Q$.

Examples

1. You are to give Mr. W. a morning dose of 80 mg of Lasix. On hand you have Lasix oral liquid, 10 mg/mL. How many milliliters do you give him?

   Table: x mL for 80 mg (Desired information)
   1 mL for 10 mg (Information we *Have*)
   (Check that units match.)

   Proportion: $\frac{x}{1} = \frac{80}{10}$

   or

   Formula: $\frac{D}{H} \times Q = \frac{80}{10} \times 1 \text{ mL}$

   Result: 8 mL

   Check: 8 mL × 10 mg/mL = 80 mg

2. For a systemic infection, Ms. G is taking amoxicillin suspension 0.5 g tid. If amoxicillin suspension, 125 mg/5 mL, is available, how many milliliters should she receive for each dose?

   Table: x mL for a ~~0.5 g~~ 500 mg dose (Desired information)
   5 mL for a 125 mg dose (Information we *Have*)
   (Convert 0.5 g to 500 mg so that units match.)

   Proportion: $\frac{x}{5} = \frac{500}{125}$

   or

   Formula: $\frac{D}{H} \times Q = \frac{500}{125} \times 5 \text{ mL}$

   Result: 20 mL

3. The doctor ordered a ferrous sulfate elixir (325 mg bid) for Mrs. L. The elixir on hand contains 220 mg/5 mL. How many milliliters should be administered to Mrs. L. per dose?

   Table: x mL for 325 mg (Desired information)
   5 mL for 220 mg (Information we *Have*)

   Proportion: $\frac{x}{5} = \frac{325}{220}$

   or

   Formula: $\frac{D}{H} \times Q = \frac{325}{220} \times 5 \text{ mL}$

   Result: 7.4 mL

4. An order reads "Trilisate liquid, 1000 mg bid." If Trilisate liquid 500 mg/5 mL is available, the nurse needs to administer 10 mL.

SAMPLE EXERCISES

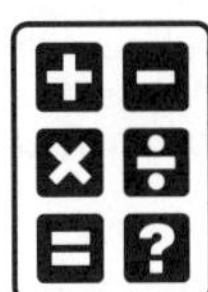

1. The doctor ordered 1 tbsp of lactulose syrup 3.33 g/5 mL for Johnny S. How much lactulose is contained in 1 tbsp of syrup?
2. Give Trilisate liquid 1500 mg bid. If Trilisate liquid 500 mg/5 mL is available, how many milliliters do you give per dose?

ANSWERS 1. $\frac{\overset{15\text{ mL}}{\cancel{1\text{ tbsp}}}}{5\text{ mL}} \times 3.33\text{ g} = 9.99\text{ g}$

2. $\frac{1500}{500} \times 5\text{ mL} = 15\text{ mL}$

EXERCISES

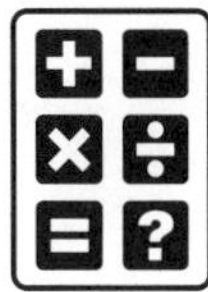

Exercises 1–12. Find the number of milliliters to give for the indicated dose.

	Doctor's Order (*D*esired)	On Hand (*H*ave)
1.	pyrantel pamoate oral suspension 700 mg	50 mg/mL
2.	Elixophyllin suspension 330 mg	100 mg/5 mL
3.	Elixophyllin liquid 220 mg	160 mg/15 mL
4.	Elixophyllin elixir 100 mg	80 mg/tbsp
5.	Amicar syrup 1 g	250 mg/mL
6.	Trilisate liquid 2 g	500 mg/tsp
7.	Trilisate liquid 600 mg	500 mg/tsp
8.	Trilisate liquid 600 mg	870 mg/5 mL
9.	Erythromycin suspension 250 mg	200 mg/5 mL
10.	Erythromycin suspension 333 mg	200 mg/5 mL
11.	Erythromycin suspension 333 mg	400 mg/5 mL
12.	Erythromycin suspension 250 mg	400 mg/5 mL

Exercises 13–18. Find the number of milligrams of drug in the indicated dose.

13. 2 tsp of lactulose syrup 3.33 g/5 mL
14. 20 mL of oxacillin sodium 250 mg/5 mL
15. 0.5 tsp cephalexin 250 mg/tsp
16. 7.5 mL of erythromycin suspension 400 mg/5 mL
17. 1.5 tsp of Mylanta 200 mg/5 mL
18. 2 mL of amoxicillin suspension 125 mg/5 mL

Exercises 19–24. Corresponding to each order, find the number of milliliters per dose.

Ordered	Available
19. Zantac syrup 75 mg bid	Zantac syrup 15 mg/mL
20. Trilisate liquid 1.5 g bid	Trilisate liquid 500 mg/5 mL
21. amoxicillin suspension 0.25 g each day	amoxicillin suspension 250 mg/5 mL
22. Ceclor suspension 125 mg tid	Ceclor suspension 125 mg/tsp
23. Pepcid 20 mg qid	Pepcid 40 mg/5 mL
24. naproxen sodium 0.275 g qid	naproxen sodium 125 mg/5 mL

ANSWERS 1. 14 mL 3. 20.6 mL 5. 4 mL 7. 6 mL 9. 6.25 mL 11. 4.2 mL 13. 6660 mg 15. 125 mg 17. 300 mg 19. 5 mL 21. 5 mL 23. 2.5 mL

6-6. READING LABELS

Information on the Label

Docusate sodium (a stool softener) 100 mg has been ordered by the doctor for a client. To find the correct medication and to ensure the correct dose, it is important to read labels carefully (Fig. 6–2A).

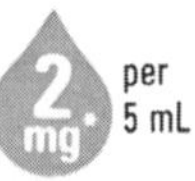

Figure 6–2 (A, B) Examples of labels.

RU-TUSS® Tablets

Ingredients of tablets

DESCRIPTION: Each prolonged action tablet contains.

Phenylephrine Hydrochloride .... 25 mg
Phenylpropanolamine Hydrochloride ... 50 mg
Chlorpheniramine Maleate .... 8 mg
Hyoscyamine Sulfate .... 0.19 mg
Atropine Sulfate .... 0.04 mg
Scopolamine Hydrobromide ...... 0.01 mg

Inactive Ingredients: carnauba wax, D&C Yellow No. 10 Lake, ethylcellulose, FD&C Blue No. 1 Lake, magnesium stearate, microcrystalline cellulose, povidone, sodium starch glycolate, stearic acid, talc.

RU-TUSS Tablets act continuously for 10 to 12 hours. RU-TUSS Tablets are an oral antihistaminic, nasal decongestant and anti-secretory preparation.

Expected effects

INDICATIONS AND USAGE: RU-TUSS Tablets provide relief of the symptoms resulting from irritation of sinus, nasal and upper respiratory tract tissues. Phenylephrine and phenylpropanolamine combine to exert a vasoconstrictive and decongestive action while chlorpheniramine maleate decreases the symptoms of watering eyes, post nasal drip and sneezing which may be associated with an allergic-like response. The belladonna alkaloids, hyoscyamine, atropine and scopolamine further augment the anti-secretory activity of RU-TUSS Tablets.

Contraindications

CONTRAINDICATIONS: Hypersensitivity to antihistamines or sympathomimetics. RU-TUSS Tablets are contraindicated in children under 12 years of age and in patients with glaucoma, bronchial asthma and women who are pregnant. Concomitant use of MAO inhibitors is contraindicated.

WARNINGS: RU-TUSS Tablets may cause drowsiness. Patients should be warned of possible additive effects caused by taking antihistamines with alcohol, hypnotics or tranquilizers.

PRECAUTIONS: RU-TUSS Tablets contain belladonna alkaloids, and must be administered with care to those patients with urinary bladder neck obstruction. Caution should be exercised when RU-TUSS Tablets are given to patients with hypertension, cardiac or peripheral vascular disease or hyperthyroidism. Patients should avoid driving a motor vehicle or operating dangerous machinery. (See **WARNINGS**.)

ADVERSE REACTIONS: Hypersensitivity reactions such as rash, urticaria, leukopenia, agranulocytosis, and thrombocytopenia may occur. Large overdoses may cause tachypnea, delirium, fever, stupor, coma and respiratory failure.

Gastrointestinal: nausea, vomiting, diarrhea, constipation, epigastric distress.

Genitourinary System: urinary frequency and dysuria.

Cardiovascular: tightness of the chest, palpitation, tachycardia, hypotension/hypertension.

Central Nervous System: drowsiness, giddiness, faintness, dizziness, headache, incoordination, mydriasis, hyperirritability, nervousness, and insomnia.

Metabolic/Endocrine: lassitude, anorexia.

Miscellaneous: dryness of mucous membranes, xerostomia.

Respiratory: thickening of bronchial secretions.

Special Senses: tinnitus, visual disturbances, blurred vision.

Overdosage

OVERDOSAGE: Since the action of sustained release products may continue for as long as 12 hours, treatment of overdoses directed at reversing the effects of the drug and supporting the patient should be maintained for at least that length of time. In children and infants, antihistamine overdosage may produce convulsions and death.

Dosage and administration

DOSAGE AND ADMINISTRATION: Adults and children 12 years of age and older, one tablet morning and evening. Not recommended for children under 12 years of age. Tablets are to be swallowed whole.

Available forms

HOW SUPPLIED: RU-TUSS® Tablets: elongated, light green, scored tablet debossed with BOOTS logo and "58".

Bottles of 100	NDC 0048-0058-01
Bottles of 500	NDC 0048-0058-05

Store at controlled room temperature 15°-30°C (59°-86°F).

CAUTION: Federal (USA) law prohibits dispensing without prescription.

Manufactured for
Boots Pharmaceuticals, Inc.
Lincolnshire, Illinois 60069 USA
By
Vitarine Pharmaceuticals, Inc.
Springfield Gardens, New York 11413 USA

Rev. 4/16/90 8467-01

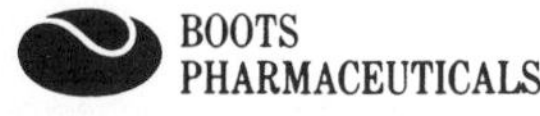

Figure 6–3 Example of a package insert.

INFORMATION ON THE LABEL

Trade Name and/or Generic Name
Form
Quantity in Container
Strength of the Medication
Manufacturer or Distributor
Instructions for Dosage and Administration (sometimes)
Suggestions for Storage (sometimes)

The **trade name** (brand name) is given by the manufacturer or distributor of the medication, whereas the **generic name** (chemical or official name) is chosen by the researcher. A drug may have several different trade names (if

ergoloid mesylates

ur´go-loyd mess-ah´lates
(Gerimal, Hydergine)

CANADIAN AVAILABILITY: Hydergine

CLASSIFICATION

PHARMACOTHERAPEUTIC: Ergot alkaloid

CLINICAL: Psychotherapeutic agent

PHARMACOKINETICS

Rapidly absorbed from GI tract. Undergoes first-pass metabolism in liver. Eliminated primarily in feces.

ACTION

Increases brain metabolism (may increase cerebral blood flow), thereby enhancing motor activity, mental alertness, appetite, sociability, orientation, recent memory; reduces fatigue, depression, confusion, anxiety/fears, dizziness.

USES

Treatment of age-related (those >60 yrs) mental capacity decline (cognitive and interpersonal skills, mood, self-care, apparent motivation).

PO ADMINISTRATION

1. Instruct pt to allow sublingual tablets to completely dissolve under tongue; do not crush or chew.
2. Do not break or chew capsule or tablet form.

INDICATIONS/DOSAGE/ROUTES

Age-related decline in mental capacity:
PO: Adults: Initially, 1 mg 3 times/day. **Range:** 1.5-12 mg/day.

PRECAUTIONS

CONTRAINDICATIONS: Acute or chronic psychosis, regardless of etiology. **CAUTIONS:** None significant.

INTERACTIONS

DRUG INTERACTIONS: None significant. **ALTERED LAB VALUES:** None significant.

SIDE EFFECTS

OCCASIONAL: GI distress, transient nausea, sublingual irritation.

ADVERSE REACTIONS/TOXIC EFFECTS

None significant.

NURSING IMPLICATIONS

BASELINE ASSESSMENT:

Exclude possibility that pt's signs and symptoms arise from a possibly reversible and treatable condition secondary to systemic disease, neurological disease, or primary disturbance of mood before administering medication.

INTERVENTION/EVALUATION:

Periodically reassess benefit of current therapy.

PATIENT/FAMILY TEACHING:

Elimination of symptoms appears gradual; results may not be noted for 3-4 wks.

ergonovine maleate

er-goe-noe´veen
(Ergotrate, Ergometrine)

Figure 6–4 Illustration of types of information to be found in a nurse's drug handbook. (From Hodgson BB, Kizior RJ, Kingdon RT: *Nurse's Drug Handbook*. Philadelphia: W.B. Saunders, 1993.)

produced by several manufacturers), but it can have only one generic name. The **strength** of a tablet (sometimes also called the dosage strength) is the weight of the drug per tablet. Sometimes the label may contain instructions for dosage and administration, as well as suggestions for storage (Fig. 6–2B); but very often these instructions are printed in accompanying literature (the package insert).

Many labels contain a reminder to consult the package insert. Often, the nurse does not have access to the package insert (the pharmacy has it), but when there is a need, you may find a copy in the *Physicians' Desk Reference.* A package insert may be a few pages long, giving more detailed information than is printed on the label, including chemical analysis, precautions, antidotes for overdoses, and recommendations for dosage and administration. A relatively simple package insert is shown in Figure 6–3.

Even more important than the package insert are the drug references prepared especially for nurses. These include not only relevant information from the package insert about each drug but also companion details about nursing procedures. Examples of such details are:

1. What changes in weight or blood pressure require a call to the doctor.
2. Suggestions for diet in support of drug therapy.
3. Methods of evaluating therapeutic responses.
4. What to teach patient and family about use of the medication (Fig. 6–4).

SAMPLE EXERCISES

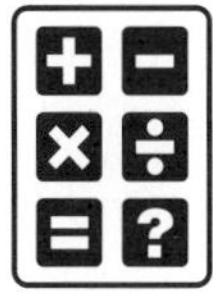

Exercises 1–6. Using the label below, fill in the required information in the blanks below.

1. Trade Name ____________________
2. Generic Name ____________________
3. Form ____________________
4. Strength ____________________
5. Manufacturer ____________________
6. Storage Instructions ____________________

N 0071-2214-20

Shake Well

Dilantin-125®

(Phenytoin Oral Suspension, USP)

125 mg per 5 mL potency

Important—Another strength available; verify unspecified prescriptions.

Caution—Federal law prohibits dispensing without prescription.

8 fl oz (237 mL)

PARKE-DAVIS ©1990
Div of Warner-Lambert Co/Morris Plains, NJ 07950 USA

Shake well before using.

Each 5 mL contains phenytoin, 125 mg with a maximum alcohol content not greater than 0.6 percent.

Usual Dosage—Adults, 1 teaspoonful three times daily; Children, see package insert.

See package insert for complete prescribing information.

Store below 30° C (86° F). Protect from freezing.

Keep this and all drugs out of the reach of children.

6505-00-890-1110

Exp date and lot

2214G014

Exercises 7–11. Using the label below, fill in the required information in the blanks below.

7. Trade Name ______________________
8. Generic Name ______________________
9. Form ______________________
10. Strength ______________________
11. Manufacturer ______________________

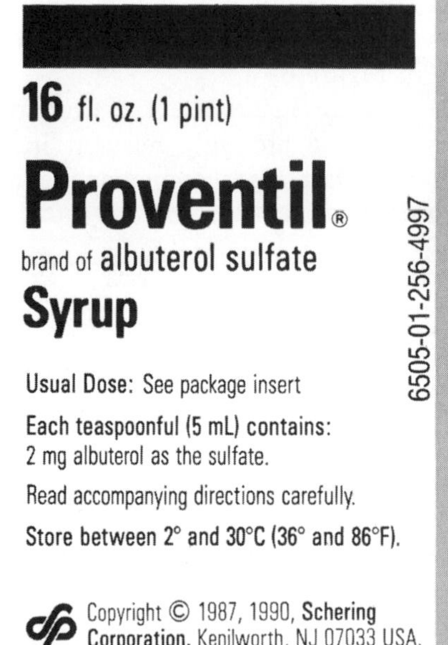

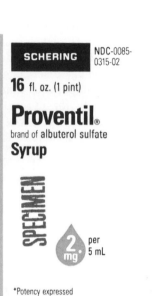

ANSWERS 1. Dilantin-125 2. phenytoin 3. oral suspension 4. 125 mg/5 mL 5. Parke-Davis 6. store below 30°C, protect from freezing 7. Proventil 8. albuterol sulfate 9. liquid (syrup) 10. 2 mg/5 mL 11. Schering

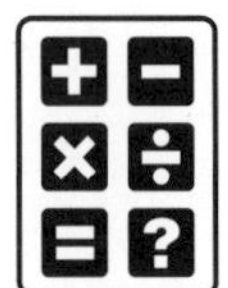

EXERCISES

Exercises 1–20. Using the appropriate label selected from the set of labels shown in Figure 6–5, fill in the required information in the blanks below.

Generic Name: potassium chloride

1. Trade Name ______________________
2. Form ______________________
3. Dosage strength ______________________
4. Quantity in packet ______________________
5. Expiration date ______________________

240 mL NDC 0081-0113-18

RETROVIR® Syrup
(ZIDOVUDINE)

Each 5 mL (1 teaspoonful) contains zidovudine 50 mg and sodium benzoate 0.2% added as a preservative.

CAUTION: Federal law prohibits dispensing without prescription.

U.S. Patent Nos. 4818538 (Product Patent); 4724232, 4833130, and 4837208 (Use Patents)

For indications, dosage, precautions, etc., see accompanying package insert.
Store at 15° to 25°C (59° to 77°F) and protect from light.
Made in U.S.A. 587016

LANOXIN®
(DIGOXIN)
125 μg (0.125 mg)
per tablet
PROTECT FROM LIGHT
BURROUGHS WELLCOME CO.
Research Triangle Park, NC
PEEL

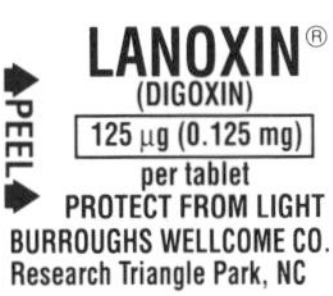

A

BURROUGHS WELLCOME CO.
Research Triangle Park, NC 27709

LOT
EXP

B

87-770
KLOTRIX®
(POTASSIUM CHLORIDE)
SLOW-RELEASE TABLET 10 mEq
BRISTOL LABORATORIES®
A Bristol-Myers Squibb Company
Evansville, IN 47721, U.S.A.
MDM53E EXP 1 MAY 93

C

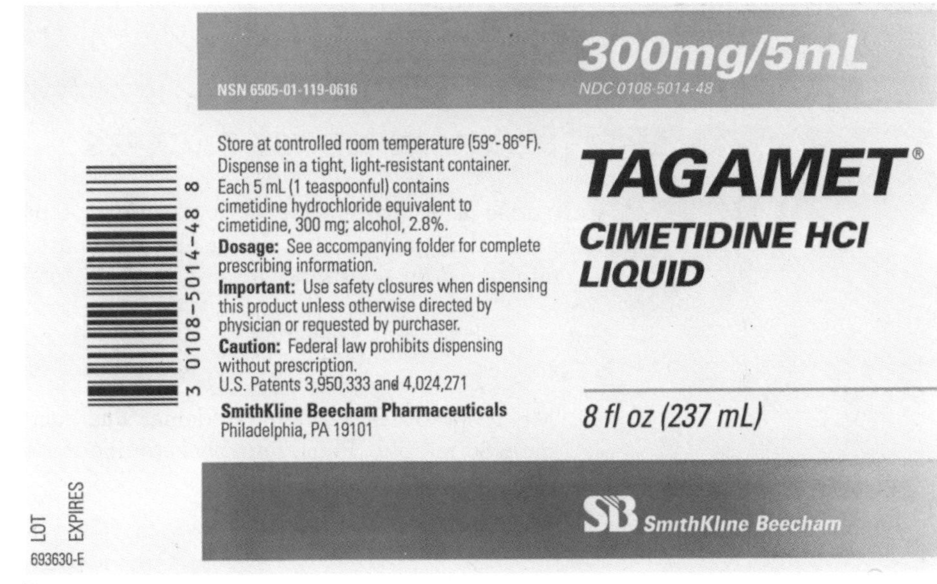

D

Figure 6–5 (A, B, C, D) Labels for Exercises 1–20.

Generic Name: digoxin

6. Trade Name ____________________

7. Form ____________________

8. Dosage strength ____________________

9. Storage ____________________

10. Manufacturer ____________________

Trade Name: Retrovir

11. Generic Name ____________________

12. Form ____________________

13. Strength ______________

14. Preservative ______________

15. Quantity ______________

Generic Name: cimetidine hydrochloride

16. Trade Name ______________

17. Form ______________

18. Strength ______________

19. Total Quantity ______________

20. Storage ______________

ANSWERS 1. Klotrix 3. 10 mEq 5. May 1, 1993 7. tablet 9. Protect from light 11. zidovudine 13. 50 mg/5 mL 15. 240 mL 17. liquid 19. 8 fl oz (237 mL)

6-7. USING UNIT DOSE PACKETS

A **unit dose** is a single dose of medication prepared by the pharmacy. In modern facilities, packets containing unit doses are sent to the nurses' station and administered by the nurses according to doctors' orders.

Examples

1. Mrs. Glotko has pulmonary edema. The doctor has ordered furosemide 80 mg bid. Thus, four packets like the one pictured are administered each day.

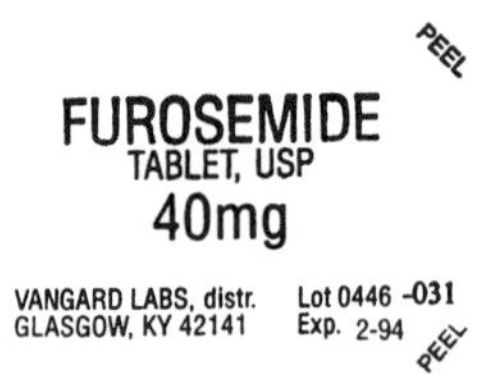

PEEL
FUROSEMIDE
TABLET, USP
40mg
VANGARD LABS, distr.
GLASGOW, KY 42141
Lot 0446 -031
Exp. 2-94
PEEL

2. For Mr. Semfur, the doctor has ordered docusate sodium, 50 mg qd, with casanthranol. The packet shown is not appropriate, because a 100-mg capsule is too large a dose. A capsule is not scored and should not be taken apart except under unusual circumstances.

PRO-SOF® PLUS
DOCUSATE SODIUM
and CASANTHRANOL
SOFTGEL CAPSULE
100mg/30mg
VANGARD LABS, distr.
GLASGOW, KY 42141
Lot 0587 -015
Exp. 12/92
PEEL

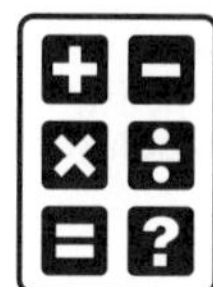

SAMPLE EXERCISES

1. A total of 300 mg/day of docusate sodium has been ordered for Mrs. Udley. How many packets does she need? (See Pro-Sof Plus label above.)
2. Doses of potassium chloride (Klotrix) for Mr. Jones should not exceed 60 mEq/day, in divided doses. What is the maximum number of packets to be administered to Mr. Jones each day?

87-770
KLOTRIX®
(POTASSIUM CHLORIDE)
SLOW-RELEASE TABLET 10 mEq
BRISTOL LABORATORIES®
A Bristol-Myers Squibb Company
Evansville, IN 47721, U.S.A.
MDM53E EXP 1 MAY 93

ANSWERS 1. 3 2. 6

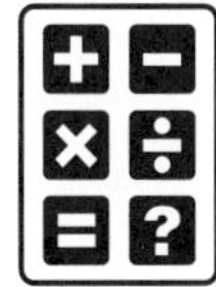

EXERCISES

Exercises 1–4. Aspirin has been ordered for patients in Utopia Hospital. For each patient, indicate the number of unit dose packets (using the label shown below) that corresponds to the ordered dosage.

PEEL
ASPIRIN TABLET 325mg
WARNING: Children and teenagers should not use this medicine for chicken pox or flu symptoms before a doctor is consulted about Reye syndrome, a rare but serious illness reported to be associated with aspirin.
WARNING: Keep this and all medicines out of children's reach. In case of accidental overdose, contact a physician immediately.
VANGARD LABS, distr. Lot 0522 -033
GLASGOW, KY 42141 Exp. 2-94
PEEL

1. For Mr. Jisone, 325 mg PO q4h prn for pain.
2. For Mrs. Foxley, 650 mg PO q6h prn for fever.
3. For Ms. Muid, gr x PO q4h prn for pain and fever.
4. For Prof. Leprol, 3.9 g/day PO in divided doses for arthritis.

Exercises 5–6. The doctor has given orders for meclizine hydrochloride tablets, USP. Using the label shown here, indicate for each client the number of tablets that corresponds to the ordered dosage.

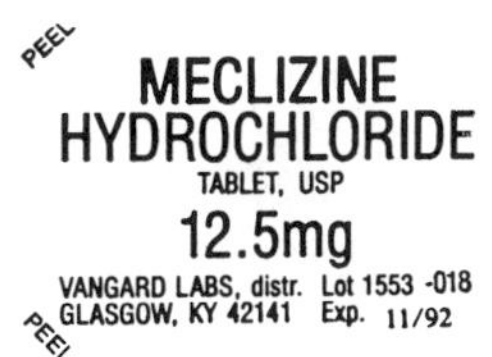

PEEL
MECLIZINE
HYDROCHLORIDE
TABLET, USP
12.5mg
VANGARD LABS, distr. Lot 1553 -018
GLASGOW, KY 42141 Exp. 11/92
PEEL

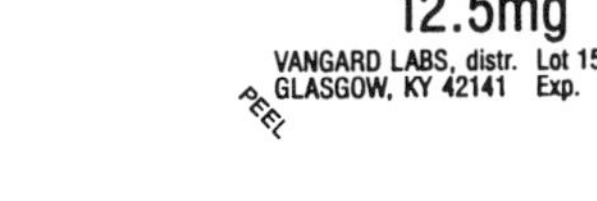

5. PO 50 mg/day for seizures
6. PO 25 mg/day for neuritic pain

Exercises 7–8. Triazolam (Halcion) is on hand for clients with insomnia. Using the label information shown here, indicate the number of unit dose packets that corresponds to each ordered dosage.

Halcion® (IV)
triazolam
0.125 mg LOT 506 HF
EXP 7/96
The Upjohn Co.
Kalamazoo, MI

7. PO 0.25 mg

8. PO 125 μg

Exercises 9–16. The nurses' station has received the unit dose packets shown in Figure 6–6. State the number of packets to be placed in the patient's bin per day for each doctor's order in Figure 6–7 on pages 190–191.

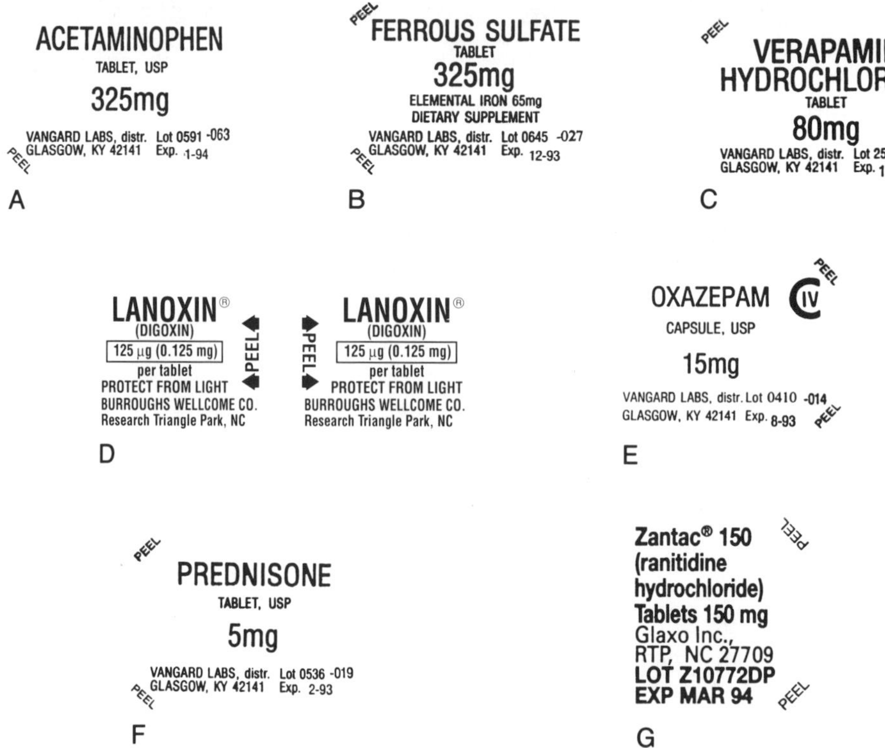

ACETAMINOPHEN
TABLET, USP
325mg
VANGARD LABS, distr. Lot 0591 -063
GLASGOW, KY 42141 Exp. 1-94
PEEL
A
PEEL
FERROUS SULFATE
TABLET
325mg
ELEMENTAL IRON 65mg
DIETARY SUPPLEMENT
VANGARD LABS, distr. Lot 0645 -027
GLASGOW, KY 42141 Exp. 12-93
PEEL
B
PEEL
VERAPAMIL HYDROCHLORIDE
TABLET
80mg
VANGARD LABS, distr. Lot 2518 -023
GLASGOW, KY 42141 Exp. 11-93
C
LANOXIN®
(DIGOXIN)
125 μg (0.125 mg)
per tablet
PROTECT FROM LIGHT
BURROUGHS WELLCOME CO.
Research Triangle Park, NC
PEEL
PEEL
LANOXIN®
(DIGOXIN)
125 μg (0.125 mg)
per tablet
PROTECT FROM LIGHT
BURROUGHS WELLCOME CO.
Research Triangle Park, NC
D
PEEL
OXAZEPAM (IV)
CAPSULE, USP
15mg
VANGARD LABS, distr. Lot 0410 -014
GLASGOW, KY 42141 Exp. 8-93
PEEL
E
PEEL
PREDNISONE
TABLET, USP
5mg
VANGARD LABS, distr. Lot 0536 -019
GLASGOW, KY 42141 Exp. 2-93
PEEL
F
Zantac® 150
(ranitidine hydrochloride)
Tablets 150 mg
Glaxo Inc.,
RTP, NC 27709
LOT Z10772DP
EXP MAR 94
PEEL
PEEL
G

Figure 6–6 (A, B, C, D, E, F, G) Unit dose packets for Exercises 9–16.

Exercises 17–18. On Monday, Mrs. Jopper called for and received a tablet for pain, propoxyphene napsylate and acetaminophen, five times. From the packet shown here, find:

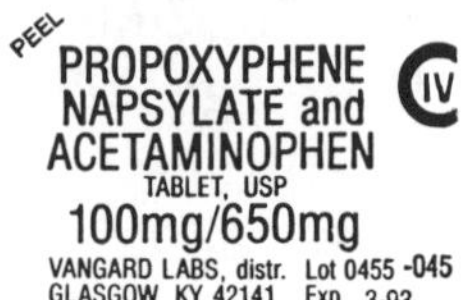

PEEL
PROPOXYPHENE NAPSYLATE and ACETAMINOPHEN (IV)
TABLET, USP
100mg/650mg
VANGARD LABS, distr. Lot 0455 -045
GLASGOW, KY 42141 Exp. 3-93

17. How much acetaminophen she received from 5 packets.
18. How much propoxyphene napsylate she received from 5 packets.

Exercises 19–20. The physician has ordered Pro-Sof Plus for Ms. Koler, who is to receive a total of 200 mg of docusate sodium per day as well as casanthranol. See label.

PRO-SOF® PLUS
DOCUSATE SODIUM
and CASANTHRANOL
SOFTGEL CAPSULE
100mg/30mg
VANGARD LABS, distr. GLASGOW, KY 42141
Lot 0587 -015
Exp. 12/92
PEEL

19. How many packets should be administered per day?
20. How much casanthranol is administered per day?

ANSWERS 1. 1 packet 3. 2 packets 5. 4 tablets 7. 2 packets 9. 4 11. 8 13. 12 15. 4 17. 3.25 g 19. 2

6-8. COMPUTING LIQUID DOSES FROM LABELS

As we have seen in Section 6-5, computing liquid oral doses involves finding the quantity (in milliliters) of liquid medication to administer. The computation depends on information printed on the label.

Examples

Refer to the labels in Figure 6–8 on pages 192–194.

1. When Mrs. Gios is to receive her next dose, 2 mg of albuterol, we note that the Proventil label states that each teaspoonful (5 mL) of syrup contains 2 mg of drug. Therefore, the dose for Mrs. Gios is 5 mL.
2. The label on Lanoxin (digoxin) pediatric elixir states that each milliliter contains 50 μg of digoxin. Therefore, to give a baby 25 μg q12h, we give 0.5 mL/dose.

SAMPLE EXERCISES

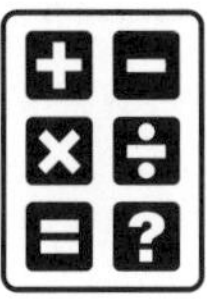

Use the labels in Figure 6–8 (pp. 192–194) to complete these exercises.

1. The doctor has ordered Tagamet liquid 1200 mg/day in divided doses for Prof. Rilk. How many milliliters do you give Prof. Rilk per day?
2. A child is to receive a dose of 75 μg of Lanoxin pediatric elixir. How many milliliters should she receive?

ANSWERS 1. $\frac{1200}{300} \times 5\text{ mL} = 20\text{ mL}$ 2. $\frac{75}{50} \times 1\text{ mL} = 1.5\text{ mL}$

Utopia Health Care Center

PHYSICIANS ORDERS

AUTHORIZATION IS GIVEN FOR THE DISPENSING AND ADMINISTERING OF THE SAME MEDICATION OR ONE OF IDENTICAL STRENGTH, DOSAGE FORM AND CONTENT OF ACTIVE THERAPEUTIC INGREDIENT UNLESS DRUG IS CIRCLED.

Date Order Written	Time Order Written	ORDERS PHYSICIAN SIGN ON LINE DIRECTLY UNDER LAST ORDER ON A SECTION	Time Order Noted	Nurses Signature	DRAW RED LINE THROUGH DISCONTINUED ORDERS
		Ranitidine hydrochloride 150 mg PO bid, 300 mg PO hs for ulcers W. Read, M.D.			Height / Weight / Drug Allergy
		Prednisone 5 mg PO qid for an inflammation A. Mazar, M.D.			Height / Weight / Drug Allergy
		Oxazepam 30 PO qid for anxiety S. Aristov, M.D.			Height / Weight / Drug Allergy
		Ferrous sulfate 0.65 g PO bid for iron deficiency C. Webb, M.D.			Height / Weight / Drug Allergy

A

Figure 6–7 (A, B) Physicians' orders for Exercises 9–16.

Utopia Health Care Center

PHYSICIANS ORDERS

AUTHORIZATION IS GIVEN FOR THE DISPENSING AND ADMINISTERING OF THE SAME MEDICATION OR ONE OF IDENTICAL STRENGTH, DOSAGE FORM AND CONTENT OF ACTIVE THERAPEUTIC INGREDIENT UNLESS DRUG IS CIRCLED.

Date Order Written	Time Order Written	ORDERS PHYSICIAN SIGN ON LINE DIRECTLY UNDER LAST ORDER ON A SECTION	Time Order Noted	Nurses Signature	DRAW RED LINE THROUGH DISCONTINUED ORDERS
		Digoxin 375 mcg PO q6h for congestive heart failure B. Richer, M.D.			Height / Weight / Drug Allergy
		Verapamil HCl 80 mg PO qid for angina pectoris B. Richer, M.D.			Height / Weight / Drug Allergy
		Verapamil HCl 320 mg/day PO in divided doses for angina pectoris B. Richer, M.D.			Height / Weight / Drug Allergy
		Acetaminophen 650 mg PO q4h prn up to 4 g/day for pain H. Kajua, M.D.			Height / Weight / Drug Allergy

B

Figure 6–7 *Continued*

BERLEX

Each 5mL (teaspoonful) contains 2mg chlorpheniramine maleate and 30mg d-pseudoephedrine HCl. Contains no alcohol or dye.
Usual Dosage: Adults and children over 12 years, 1 to 2 teaspoonfuls (5 to 10mL) 3 or 4 times daily. Children 6 to 12 years, 1/2 to 1 teaspoonful (2.5 to 5mL) 3 or 4 times daily, not to exceed 4 teaspoonfuls in 24 hours. Children 2 to 6 years, 1/2 teaspoonful (2.5mL) 3 or 4 times daily, not to exceed 2 teaspoonfuls in 24 hours. Children under 2 years, as directed by physician.
See package insert.
Store at controlled room temperature, between 15°-30°C (59°-86°F).
Bulk container — not for household use.
Dispense in tight, light-resistant container.

45287-1

NDC 50419-185-16

473mL

Deconamine®

(2mg chlorpheniramine maleate and 30mg d-pseudoephedrine HCl per 5mL)

Syrup

Caution: Federal law prohibits dispensing without prescription.

Mfd by
KV Pharmaceutical Co.
St. Louis, MO 63144
Mfd for
BERLEX
Laboratories, Inc.
Wayne, NJ 07470

A

NDC 0031-1833-25 1 Pint

SUGAR-FREE

Dimetane®-DC Cough Syrup

Bulk Container–Not for Household Dispensing
Store at Controlled Room Temperature, Between 15°C and 30°C (59°F and 86°F).
Dispense in tight, light-resistant container.

Each 5 mL (1 teaspoonful) contains:

Brompheniramine Maleate, USP	2.0 mg
Phenylpropanolamine Hydrochloride, USP	12.5 mg
Codeine Phosphate, USP	10.0 mg

Warning: May be habit forming.

Alcohol 0.95 per cent in a palatable, aromatic vehicle

CAUTION: Federal law prohibits dispensing without prescription.

For dosage and other prescribing information, see accompanying product literature.

PHARMACEUTICAL DIVISION
A. H. ROBINS COMPANY, RICHMOND, VA. 23220

A-H-ROBINS

B

Figure 6–8 (A, B, C, D, E, F) Labels for examples and Exercises 1–20.

60 mL NDC 0081-0264-27

LANOXIN®
(DIGOXIN)
ELIXIR PEDIATRIC

Each mL contains
50 μg (0.05 mg)
PLEASANTLY FLAVORED

Alcohol 10%, Methylparaben 0.1% (added as a preservative)
For indications, dosage, precautions, etc., see accompanying package insert.
Store at 15° to 25°C (59° to 77°F) and protect from light.
CAUTION: Federal law prohibits dispensing without prescription.

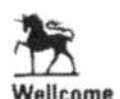

BURROUGHS WELLCOME CO.
RESEARCH TRIANGLE PARK, NC 27709
Made in U.S.A 542399

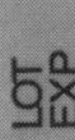

C

16 fl. oz. (1 pint)

Proventil®
brand of albuterol sulfate
Syrup

6505-01-256-4997

Usual Dose: See package insert
Each teaspoonful (5 mL) contains:
2 mg albuterol as the sulfate.
Read accompanying directions carefully.
Store between 2° and 30°C (36° and 86°F).

16194620 Rev. 10/90

SCHERING NDC-0085-0315-02

16 fl. oz. (1 pint)

Proventil®
brand of albuterol sulfate
Syrup

SPECIMEN

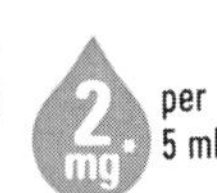

per 5 mL

*Potency expressed as albuterol.

Caution: Federal law prohibits dispensing without prescription.

D

NDC 0081-0855-96
1 pint (473 ml)

SEPTRA®
Suspension
(TRIMETHOPRIM AND SULFAMETHOXAZOLE)

*Mfd. under U.S. Patent No. 3,956,327

STORE AT 15°-25°C (59°-77°F).
SHAKE WELL.

CHERRY
FLAVOR
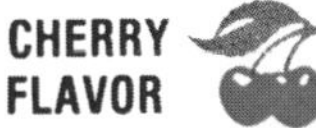

595286 Made in U.S.A.

LOT
EXP

1 pint (473 ml) NDC 0081-0855-96

SEPTRA®
Suspension
(TRIMETHOPRIM AND SULFAMETHOXAZOLE)

Each 5 ml (1 teaspoonful) contains trimethoprim* 40 mg, sulfamethoxazole 200 mg, alcohol 0.26% and added as preservatives methylparaben 0.1%, sodium benzoate 0.1%.
CAUTION: Federal law prohibits dispensing without prescription.
For indications, dosage, precautions, etc., see accompanying package insert.
Store at 15°-25°C (59°-77°F).
SHAKE WELL BEFORE USING.
Dispense in tight, light-resistant container as defined in the U.S.P.

3 0081-0855-96 9

CHERRY
FLAVOR
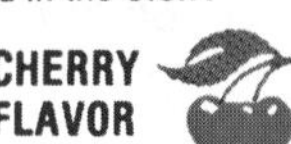

BURROUGHS WELLCOME CO.
Research Triangle Park, NC 27709
6505-01-086-7611

E

Figure 6–8 *Continued*

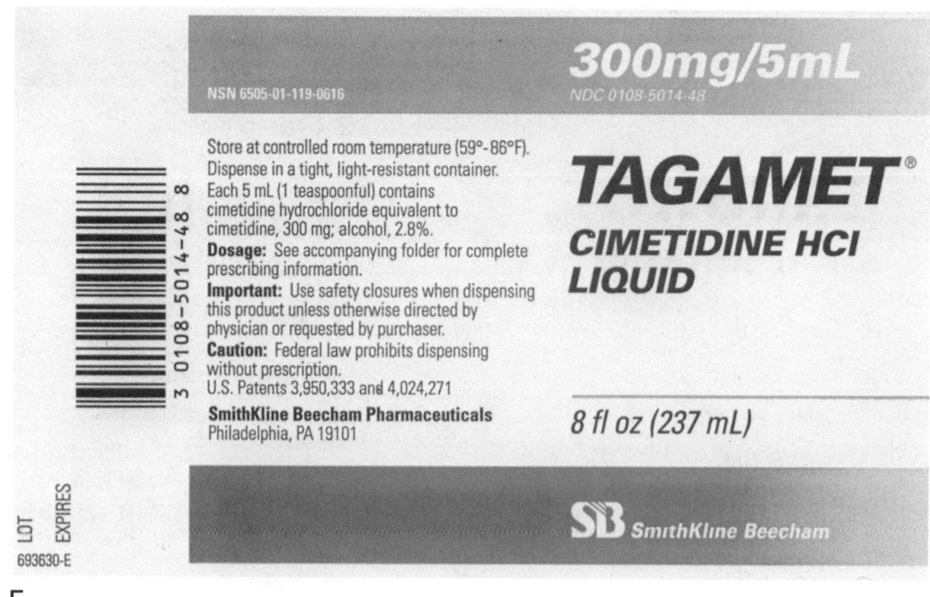

F

Figure 6–8 *Continued*

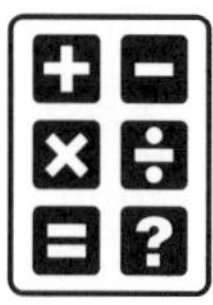

EXERCISES

Use the labels in Figure 6–8 to complete these exercises.

1. The doctor has ordered cimetidine hydrochloride 300 mg for Mr. R. at each meal. How many milliliters of Tagamet liquid do you administer at each meal?
2. The doctor has also ordered cimetidine hydrochloride 400 mg for Mr. R. at bedtime. How many milliliters of Tagamet liquid do you give him at bedtime?
3. To give a total daily dose of 16 mg of albuterol sulfate, what volume (in milliliters) of albuterol sulfate syrup is necessary per day?
4. To give a total daily dose of 12 mg of albuterol sulfate in 3 separate doses, what volume (in milliliters) of albuterol sulfate liquid is necessary per dose?

Exercises 5–12. Find the dose (in milliliters) for each client whose ordered dose is given below.

5. 0.125 mg of digoxin
6. 175 μg of digoxin.
7. cimetidine hydrochloride 180 mg
8. cimetidine hydrochloride 0.25 g
9. 1 mg of albuterol sulfate
10. 3 mg of albuterol sulfate
11. digoxin 350 μg
12. digoxin 0.3 mg

Exercises 13–20. Find the amount of the specified drug in 10 mL of the liquid medication that contains the drug.

13. cimetidine hydrochloride in Tagamet liquid
14. chlorpheniramine maleate in Deconamine syrup
15. codeine phosphate in Dimetane-DC cough syrup
16. trimethoprim in Septra suspension

17. digoxin in Lanoxin pediatric elixir
18. sulfamethoxazole in Septra suspension
19. phenylpropanolamine hydrochloride in Dimetane-DC cough syrup
20. *d*-pseudoephedrine hydrochloride in Deconamine syrup

ANSWERS 1. 5 mL 3. 40 mL 5. 2.5 mL 7. 3 mL 9. 2.5 mL 11. 7 mL 13. 600 mg 15. 20 mg 17. 500 μg 19. 25 mg

6-9. AVOIDING ERRORS: HEEDING SAFE DOSAGE INSTRUCTIONS

Safe dosage instructions are found in authoritative sources, such as package inserts that accompany the medications, nurses' drug handbooks, and the *Physicians' Desk Reference,* or other similar reference texts. (See the References at the back of the book for a complete list.)

If you have any question about a dose, call the doctor. There can be errors in intention, transcription, or computation. If a client questions a dose, be sure to verify the "five rights" of drug administration.

1. Right patient
2. Right drug
3. Right dose
4. Right time
5. Right route

Remember to use HI-TECC: *H*eed safe dosage *I*nstructions; *T*abulate, *E*stimate, *C*ompute, and *C*heck.

Examples

1. Dosage of Prozac pulvules (a type of capsule) "should not exceed 80 mg qd." Thus, the order, "Prozac pulvules (fluoxetine hydrochloride) 0.2 g bid," contains an error because the total dosage per day would be 0.4 g = 400 mg > 80 mg.
2. An order for Mrs. S calls for buspirone hydrochloride PO 5 mg tid. The package insert recommends that no dosage "exceed 60 mg/day." Mrs. S is to receive a total of 15 mg/day, which does not exceed the specified limit.

SAMPLE EXERCISES

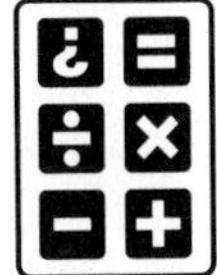

Exercises 1–3. Check each of the following dosages. Is the dosage within the given safe dosage limit?

	Dosage Ordered	Recommended Maximum Dosage Limit
1.	captopril 150 mg bid	450 mg daily
2.	alprazolam 0.5 mg tid	4 mg per day in divided doses
3.	spironolactone 200 mg tid	400 mg daily

ANSWERS 1. yes, 300 mg < 450 2. yes, 1.5 mg < 4 mg 3. no, 600 mg > 400 mg

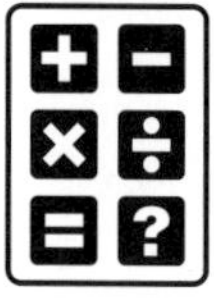

EXERCISES

Exercises 1–8. Check each of the following dosages. Is the dosage within the given safe dosage limit?

	Dosage Ordered	Recommended Maximum Daily Dosage Limit
1.	benztropine 6 mg qd	6 mg
2.	Ceclor 500 mg q8h	4 g
3.	Valium 10 mg qid	60 mg
4.	lithium carbonate 12 g q24h in 3 divided doses	3600 mg
5.	Meclomen 125 mg q6h	400 mg
6.	naproxen sodium 2.75 g tid	1475 mg
7.	penicillin V potassium 500 mg q6h	7 g
8.	quinidine 3 g qid	4000 mg

Exercises 9–16. Daily dosages of acetaminophen have been prepared for administration to a group of clients. In each case, the daily dosage should not exceed 4 g. Is the dosage for each client less than this specified maximum?

	Preparation Used	Dosage Prepared
9.	capsule 325 mg	2 capsules q4h
10.	elixir 160 mg/5 mL	elixir 10 mL q3h
11.	chewable tablet 80 mg	2 tablets qid
12.	capsule 650 mg	2 capsules qid
13.	capsule 650 mg	2 capsules tid
14.	elixir 120 mg/5 mL	elixir 15 mL q3h
15.	liquid 500 mg/15 mL	liquid 150 mL in 6 divided doses
16.	liquid 500 mg/15 mL	liquid 30 mL q4h

Exercises 17–22. Daily dosages of required medications have been prepared for administration to a group of clients. In each case, the daily dosage should not exceed the maximum allowable amount specified. Is the prepared dosage for each client less than the maximum allowable?

	Preparation Used	Maximum Allowable	Prepared Dosage
17.	Lithostat tablets 250 mg	1.5 g/day	1 tablet q6h
18.	Amicar syrup 250 mg/mL	30 g/day	6 mL qh
19.	Cytadren tablets 250 mg	2 g/day	3 tablets qid
20.	Tavist tablets 2.68 mg	8.04 mg/day	2 tablets bid

21. Tavist syrup 0.67 mg/mL	8.04 mg/day	5 mL tid
22. Seromycin capsules 250 mg	1 g/day	1 capsule q6h

ANSWERS 1. yes 3. yes 5. no 7. yes 9. yes 11. yes 13. yes 15. no 17. yes 19. no 21. no

6-10. SUMMARY

1. DOSAGE

A schedule for administration of therapeutic agents, including name of drug, amount, method, and frequency.

Example

Captopril 25 mg PO bid

2. SYMBOLS FOR FREQUENCY OF ADMINISTRATION

Times per Day	Intervals
bid = two times per day	qh = every hour
tid = three times per day	q3h = every 3 hours
qid = four times per day	q6h = every 6 hours
qd = every day	
stat = immediately	
prn = whenever necessary	
ac = before meals	
pc = after meals	
hs = before sleep	
qam = every morning	
qpm = every evening	

3. ROUTES OF ADMINISTRATION

The following symbols are commonly used.

PO: by mouth
IM: intramuscular injection
IV: intravenous administration
SC: subcutaneous, in the tissue under the skin
SL: sublingual (under the tongue)

4. SOLVING DOSAGE PROBLEMS

Use

1. Proportions

or

2. $\frac{D}{H} \times Q$

Example

Give 375 μg, using scored 250-μg tablets.

Table:

x tab for 375 μg
1 tab for 250 μg

Make sure that units match.

Proportion Method:

$$\frac{x}{1} = \frac{375}{250}$$

$$x = 1.5 \text{ tablets}$$

Formula Method:

$$\frac{D}{H} \times Q = \frac{375}{250} \times 1 \text{ tablet} = 1.5 \text{ tablets}$$

5. INFORMATION TO BE FOUND ON MEDICATION LABELS

   1. Trade Name
   2. Generic Name
   3. Form
   4. Quantity in Container
   5. Strength
   6. Expiration Date
   7. Instructions for Dosage and Administration (sometimes)
   8. Suggestions for Storage (sometimes)

   Whoever administers the drug is **legally responsible.**

6. SAFE DOSAGE RESTRICTIONS

   These are found in authoritative sources. (See References at back of the book.) If you have a question about a dose, call the doctor. *H*eed safe dosage *I*nstructions (*HI*); also *T*abulate, *E*stimate, *C*ompute, and *C*heck (*HI-TECC*).

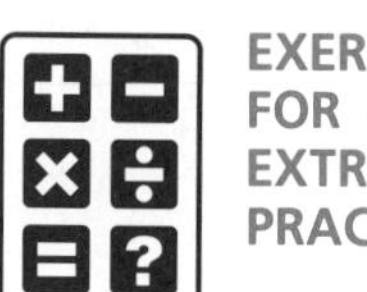

EXERCISES FOR EXTRA PRACTICE

***Reminder:* For safety, use HI-TECC!**

HI: *H*eed *I*nstructions for safe dosage
TECC: *T*abulate, *E*stimate, *C*ompute, and *C*heck

Exercises 1–6. Interpret the following medication orders.

1. hydroxyzine hydrochloride 50 mg IM q4h prn
2. morphine sulfate 15 mg SC q4h prn
3. phenobarbital sodium 200 mg IM
4. methylene Blue 150 mg IV
5. potassium chloride 400 mEq/day, slow IV infusion
6. Lithostat 0.25 g PO tid q8h

Exercises 7–12. Write the following medication orders in symbols.

7. Give 500 milligrams of Cefadyl by intramuscular injection every 4 hours.
8. Give 80 units of ACTH per day, in 4 divided doses, by subcutaneous injection.
9. Give 2 milligrams of biperiden hydrochloride every 30 minutes by intravenous infusion, whenever necessary.
10. Give 500 milligrams of aminophylline orally.

11. Give 250 milligrams of ammonium chloride orally every 2–4 hours, as needed.

12. Give 0.5 milligram of Bellafoline twice each day by subcutaneous injection.

Exercises 13–22. Find the number of tablets needed for each of the following doses.

	Dose Required	Strength of Tablets Available
13.	1 g	500 mg
14.	250 mg	500 mg
15.	40,000 U	20,000 U
16.	22.5 mg	15 mg
17.	500 μg	0.25 mg
18.	1.8 mg	0.6 mg
19.	1.2 mg	600 μg
20.	2.25 mg	0.75 mg
21.	7.5 mg	3.75 mg
22.	1,500,000 U	500,000 U

Exercises 23–32. Find the dose (in milliliters) for each doctor's order.

	Dose Required	Strength of Liquid Available
23.	3 mg	0.5 mg/5 mL
24.	0.75 mg	0.5 mg/0.5 mL
25.	0.3 mg	0.2 mg/5 mL
26.	2 mg	0.25 mg/5 mL
27.	0.4 mg	200 μg/5 mL
28.	1.5 mg	250 μg/5 mL
29.	25 mg	12.5 mg/5 mL
30.	3.3 mg	0.6 mg/5 mL
31.	600 mg	500 mg/15 mL
32.	350 mg	500 mg/15 mL

ANSWERS 1. Give 50 milligrams of hydroxyzine hydrochloride, by intramuscular injection, every 4 hours, when necessary. 3. Give 200 milligrams of phenobarbital sodium, by intramuscular injection. 5. Give 400 milliequivalents of potassium chloride per day by slow intravenous infusion. 7. Cefadyl 500 mg IM q4h 9. biperiden hydrochloride 2 mg IV q30 min prn 11. ammonium chloride 250 mg PO q2–4h prn 13. 2 tablets 15. 2 tablets 17. 2 tablets 19. 2 tablets 21. 2 tablets 23. 30 mL 25. 7.5 mL 27. 10 mL 29. 10 mL 31. 18 mL

CHAPTER TEST

Problems 1–2. Write each expression in medical symbols.

1. (a) every two hours — 1(a) ________
   (b) under the tongue — (b) ________
2. (a) four times per day — 2(a) ________
   (b) immediately — (b) ________

Interpret each item from doctors' orders.

3. (a) terbutaline sulfate 0.25 mg SC q8h — 3(a) ________
   (b) potassium iodide 1 mL PO in water tid pc — (b) ________

Problems 4–7. Find the number of tablets needed for each of the following doses.

Dose Ordered	Strength of Tablets Available	
4. 7.5 mg	5 mg	4. ________
5. 30 mg	0.01 g	5. ________
6. 0.5 mg	250 μg	6. ________
7. 0.3 g	See the label	7. ________

Problems 8–10. Find the quantity (in milliliters) needed for each of the following doses of liquid oral medication.

Dose Ordered	Strength of Liquid Available	
8. 330 mg	240 mg/5 mL	8. ________
9. 8000 U	20,000 U/mL	9. ________
10. 0.8 g	500 mg/15 mL	10. ________

ANSWERS 1. (a) q2h (b) SL 2. (a) qid (b) stat 3. (a) Give 0.25 milligram of terbutaline sulfate by subcutaneous injection every 8 hours (b) Give orally 1 milliliter of potassium iodide in water three times per day after meals. 4. 1.5 tablets 5. 3 tablets 6. 2 tablets 7. 2 tablets 8. 6.9 mL 9. 0.4 mL 10. 24 mL

SEVEN

Solutions

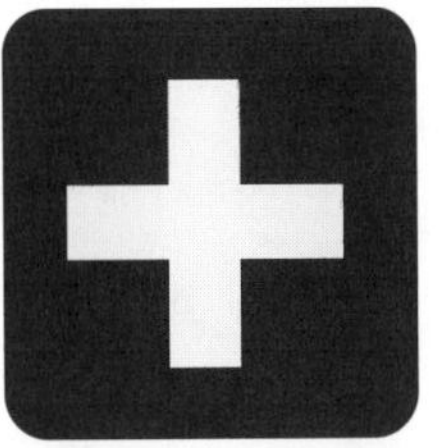

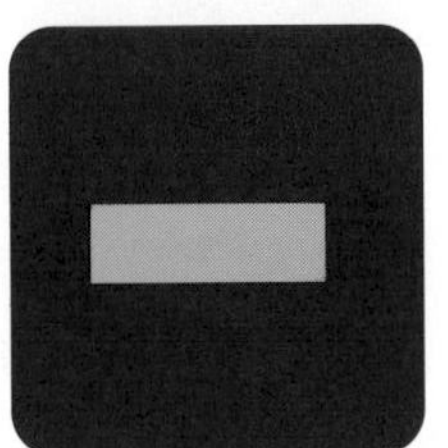

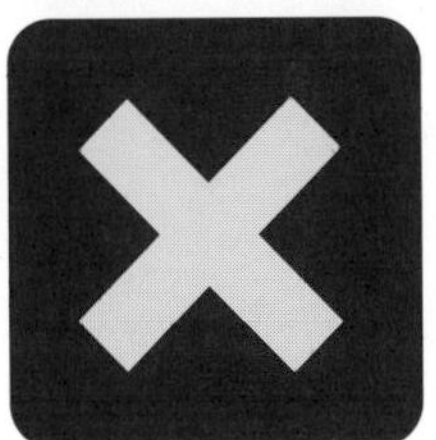

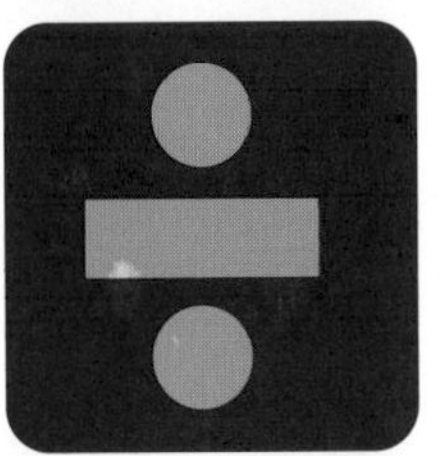

▶ OUTLINE

▶ OBJECTIVES

After studying this chapter, you will be able to:

1. Express and interpret the strength of a solution.
2. Find the amount of pure drug in a solution.
3. Find the amount of solution to use for a prescribed dose.
4. Read the scale on a syringe.
5. Apply all of the above to insulin solutions.

7-1. INTRODUCTION

What are solutions? Sometimes we dissolve a tablet in a glass of orange juice to make it more palatable. Often, a strong drug (tablet, powder, or liquid) must be dissolved in a suitable liquid before it can be administered. The resulting homogeneous mixture of drug and liquid is called a **solution;** the drug is the **solute** and the liquid is the **diluent** (or solvent).

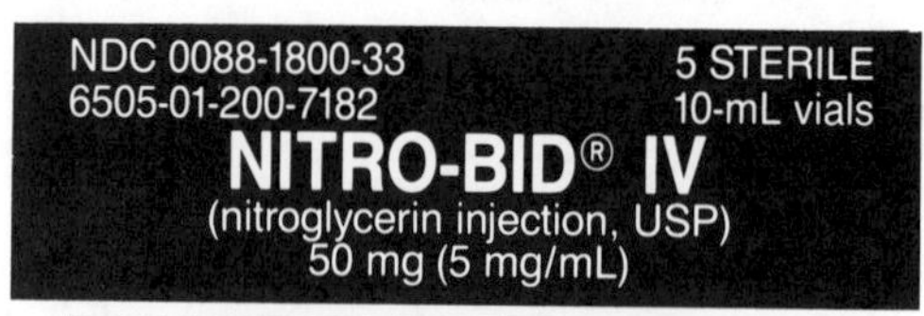

FOR INTRAVENOUS INFUSION ONLY.
NOT FOR DIRECT IV INJECTION.
→ MUST BE DILUTED BEFORE USE.
ONLY GLASS IV BOTTLES SHOULD BE USED
IN PREPARING THE IV ADMIXTURE.
SINGLE-DOSE VIAL—DISCARD UNUSED PORTION.

Mfd for 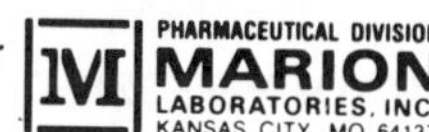

Mfd by Sterling Drug
McPherson, KS 67460

DEFINITIONS

Solution: Homogeneous mixture of two (or more) substances
Solvent: Substance present in the largest amount
Solute: Substance(s) present in smaller amount

Both the solute and the solvent may be solid, liquid, or gas. Most of the time, nurses deal with solutions made by dissolving liquid or solid solutes (such as pure drugs) in liquid solvents (such as sterile water).

Why are computations necessary when dealing with solutions? It is true that many solutions are stocked in a form ready for administration and that unit doses are available. But in some situations, fresh solutions must be prepared by the nurse just before administering an injection or intravenous therapy. Computations are often necessary to (1) ensure the right combination of diluent and drug for a desired strength, and (2) find the right amount of solution to administer.

Examples

1. Administer fibrinolysin: "After reconstituting with 10 mL of sterile NaCl solution, use only fresh solution." *
2. Dosage instructions for isoetharine hydrochloride solution include "0.5 mL diluted 1:3"† with normal saline.
3. Administer cephalothin sodium IV solution after diluting to 1 g/10 mL of D5W, normal saline, or sterile H_2O for injection.

---

* Skidmore-Roth: *Mosby's 1992 Nursing Drug Reference.* St. Louis: Mosby: 1992:421.
† Ibid., p. 521.

4. Per doctor's order: Azathioprine (Imuran) IV 70 mg

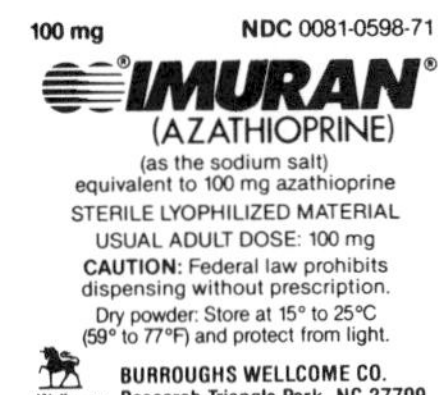

100 mg
NDC 0081-0598-71
IMURAN®
(AZATHIOPRINE)
(as the sodium salt)
equivalent to 100 mg azathioprine
STERILE LYOPHILIZED MATERIAL
USUAL ADULT DOSE: 100 mg
CAUTION: Federal law prohibits dispensing without prescription.
Dry powder: Store at 15° to 25°C (59° to 77°F) and protect from light.
BURROUGHS WELLCOME CO.
Research Triangle Park, NC 27709
Preparation of solution: Inject into the vial 10 mL Sterile Water for Injection. Swirl the vial until solution results. Use within 24 hours.
Sterile solution for intravenous use only.
For indications, dosage, precautions, etc., see accompanying package insert.
Made in U.S.A. 517055

Proficiency Gauge

You may already understand how to calculate and administer solutions, in which case you can skip Chapter 7. To evaluate your knowledge of this subject, answer the questions below. Do not look at the answers until all the questions have been answered.

---

1. A certain solution contains 0.4 mg in 2 mL. Express the strength of the solution. 1. ____________
2. What is the weight of the pure drug in 250 mL of a 1:5 w/v solution? 2. ____________
3. In 100 mL of a 0.9% w/v solution, what is the weight of the solute? 3. ____________
4. An insulin suspension is labeled U-100. What is the strength of the suspension? 4. ____________
5. Doctor's order: Calcium chloride 0.5 g IV.
   Available: Calcium chloride solution, 10%.
   How much solution should be administered? 5. ____________
6. Which is the stronger docusate calcium oral solution?
   (a) 16.7 mg/5 mL
   (b) 10 mg/1 mL 6. ____________
7. Determine the calibration of the 10-cc syringe shown in Figure 7–1. 7. ____________
8. What volume is indicated by the arrow on the syringe shown in Figure 7–1? 8. ____________
9. Locate 3.4 cc on the 10-cc syringe in Figure 7–1. 9. ____________
10. Doctor's order: Phenobarbital sodium 175 mg IM. Available: Phenobarbital sodium solution 65 mg/1 mL. Mark the dose on the 3-cc syringe in Figure 7–2. 10. ____________

Figure 7–1 Syringe for Exercises 7, 8, and 9.

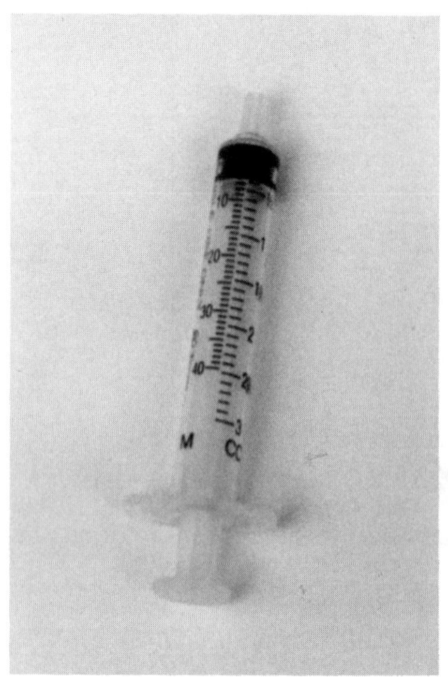

Figure 7–2 Syringe for Exercise 10.

ANSWERS 1. 0.4 mg/2 mL = 1 mg/5 mL 2. 50 g 3. 0.9 g 4. 100 U/mL 5. 5 mL 6. (b) 7. 0.2 cc 8. 7.8 cc

9.

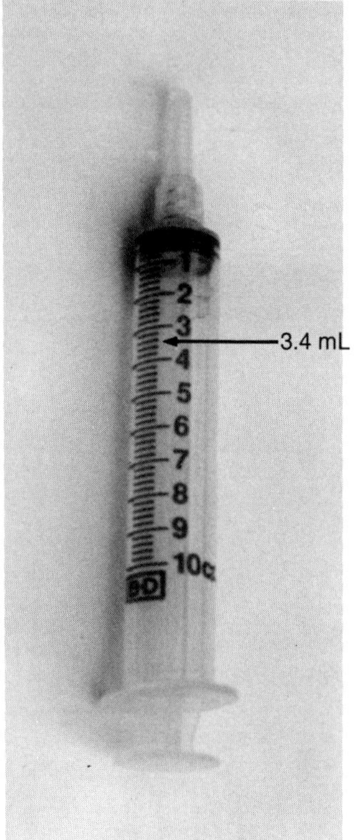

10.

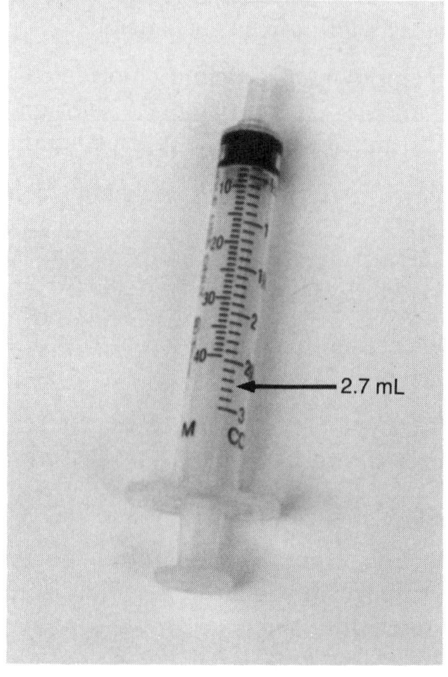

7-2. SOLUTION STRENGTH

Which is the stronger pain reliever, a morphine solution with a strength of 10 mg/5 mL or one with a strength of 20 mg/mL? Too strong a dose can be deadly; too weak a dose, useless. Thus, the nurse must pay attention to the strength of a solution. Two solutions may have the same name but different strengths.

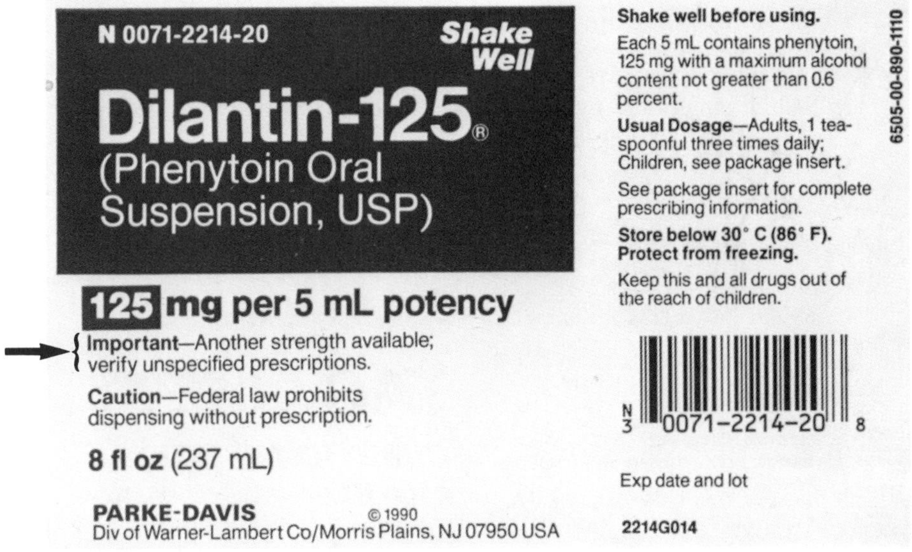

A therapeutic solution is a homogeneous mixture of at least one substance (the solute) dissolved in another substance (the diluent, or solvent). The solute is usually a powder, crystals, or a liquid; the diluent is usually liquid. The strength (concentration) of the therapeutic solution is the ratio of the amount of the drug to the volume of the solution. Because the solution is homogeneous, the strength is the same for any portion of the total solution.

STRENGTH (CONCENTRATION)

$$\frac{\text{Amount of solute (weight, volume, or other units)}}{\text{Total volume of solution (solute + diluent)}}$$

Note that the **volume** of the solution is the volume of the **combination** of solute and diluent. Sometimes, however, the amount of the solute is so small in comparison with the diluent that the difference between the volume of the diluent and the total volume of the solution is ignored.

Examples

1. Coffee lovers describe a cup of coffee as "weak" or "strong" depending on the amount of coffee used to brew the drink. The strength of a cup of coffee may be given as 1 tsp of coffee powder per cup of water. A different cup of coffee is twice as strong as the first, if instead of 1 tsp we use 2 tsp of coffee powder per cup of water. A cup of coffee is an example of a solution; the solute is coffee powder and the diluent is water.

2. Morphine solution is available in a variety of strengths, such as 10 mg/5 mL and 20 mg/mL. By 10 mg/5 mL, we understand that there are 10 mg of the drug morphine in every 5 mL (or 2 mg/mL) of this liquid medication. But a strength of 20 mg/mL means that there are 20 mg of the drug in every milliliter. Thus, the second solution, containing a higher concentration of the drug, is 10 times as strong as the first.
3. As with any ratio, strength may also be expressed in colon form.

$$10 \text{ mg}/5 \text{ mL} = 10 \text{ mg}:5 \text{ mL}$$

4. In Chapter 6, we gave many examples of oral solutions, one of which is cimetidine hydrochloride (Tagamet), which is available at a strength of 300 mg/5 mL.

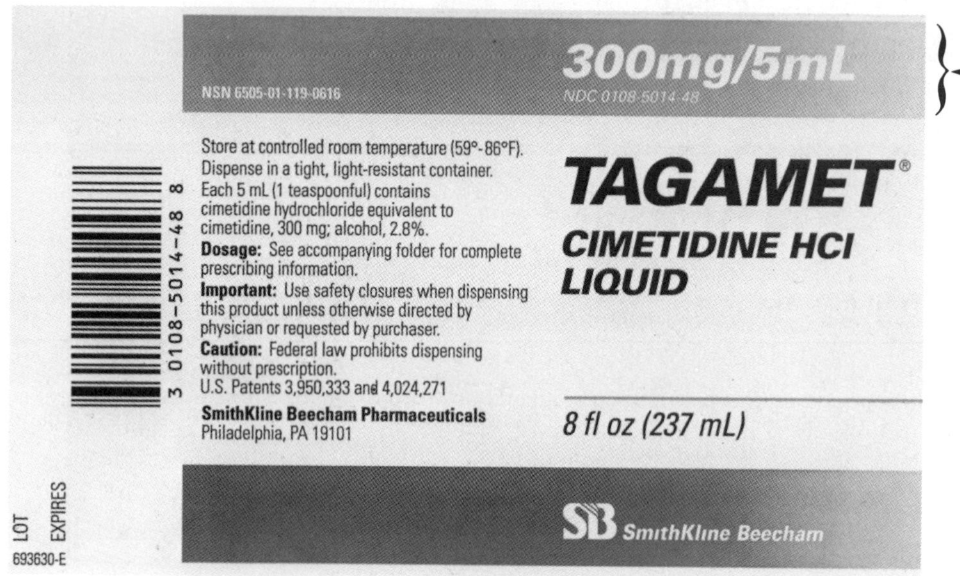

5. A magnesium solution for IV therapy comes as 20 g of magnesium sulfate in 1000 mL of diluent. The strength of the solution is given as 20 g/1000 mL, although the total volume of the solution (drug + diluent) is slightly more than 1000 mL. For practical purposes, the difference is so small that it is ignored.
6. As with all fractions, there are equivalent forms of the same ratio strength.

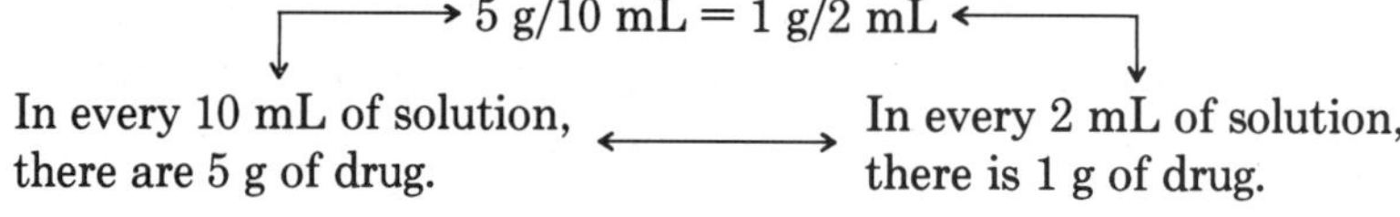

5 g/10 mL = 1 g/2 mL
In every 10 mL of solution, there are 5 g of drug.
In every 2 mL of solution, there is 1 g of drug.

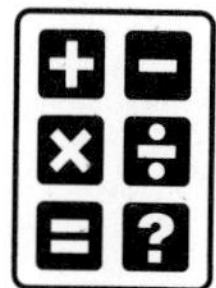

SAMPLE EXERCISES

1. A syringe containing calcium chloride solution is labeled 1 g in 10 mL. What is the strength of the calcium chloride solution?
2. You may be using an atropine sulfate solution for an injection. According to the label on the next page, what is the strength of the solution?

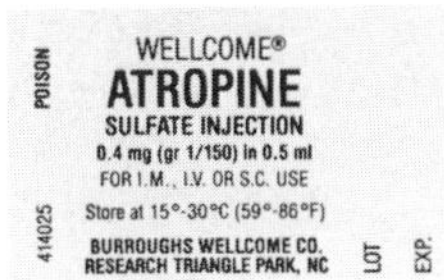

3. In every 10 mL of a solution, there is 1 mg of epinephrine. Express the ratio strength in colon form.
4. An anticough syrup has a strength of 7.5 mg/5 mL. How many milligrams of drug may be found in every milliliter of syrup?
5. Which is the stronger morphine solution?
   (a) 10 mg/5 mL
   (b) 20 mg/10 mL

ANSWERS 1. 1 g/10 mL 2. 0.4 mg/0.5 mL = 4 mg/5 mL, or 0.8 mg/mL 3. 1 mg : 10 mL 4. 1.5 mg 5. Neither; (a) and (b) are equally strong because both fractions may be simplified to 2 mg/mL.

Percent Form

A diagnostic aid, fluorescein sodium (Funduscein), is available as an injection in strengths of 10% and 25%. To interpret these percent strengths, special care must be taken, because no units are specified. With percent form or whenever units are not specified, weight is understood to be in grams only, and volume is understood to be in milliliters only.

RELATIONSHIP BETWEEN RATIO STRENGTH AND PERCENT STRENGTH

Ratio Strength	Percent Strength
$\frac{\text{Amount of solute}}{\text{Total volume of solution}}$ =	$\frac{\text{Number of grams or milliliters}}{\text{100 mL of solution}}$

Examples

1. The diagnostic aid fluorescein sodium 10% contains 10 g of pure drug in every 100 mL of solution. Another form of Funduscein (25%) contains 25 g of drug in every 100 mL of solution.
2. A common intravenous therapy solution, called D5W, consists of dextrose dissolved in water. There are 5 g of dextrose in every 100 mL of solution. Thus, D5W is also called D5%.
3. Nuromax (see label) contains not only doxacurium chloride but also "0.9% w/v benzyl alcohol," that is, 0.9 g benzyl alcohol in each 100 mL of diluent.

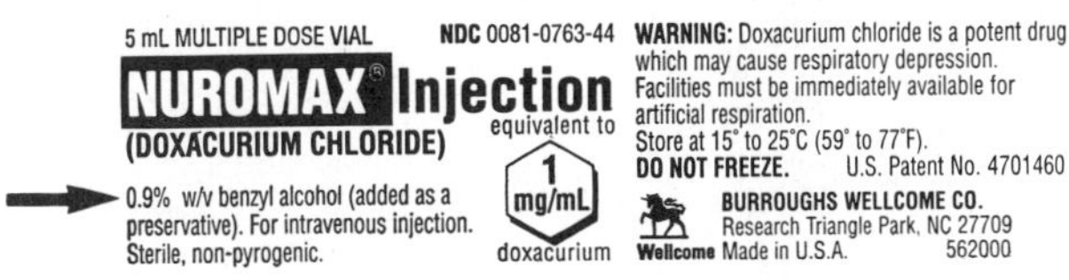

4. To eliminate decimal points, we convert to smaller units. Thus, 0.9 g/100 mL = 900 mg/100 mL = 9 mg/mL.

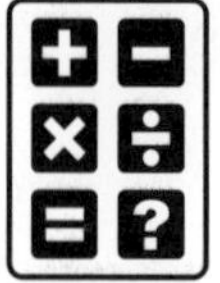

SAMPLE EXERCISES

Exercises 1–3. Express in fraction form the strength of each of the following solutions.

1. magnesium sulfate injection 50%
2. mannitol injection 15%
3. naphazoline hydrochloride (Privine) 0.1%
4. As therapy for clients with fluid or electrolyte deficiency, we may provide normal saline (NS), a 0.9% solution of sodium chloride and water. In every 100 mL of solution, how much sodium chloride is present?

ANSWERS

1. 50 g/100 mL = 1 g/2 mL, or 500 mg/mL
2. 15 g/100 mL = 3 g/20 mL, or 150 mg/mL
3. 0.1 g/100 mL = 1 mg/mL
4. 0.9 g, or 900 mg

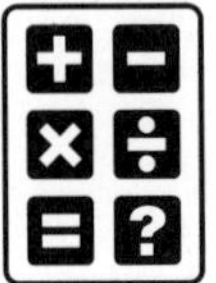

EXERCISES

Exercises 1–6. Write in fraction form the ratio strength described on the label.

1.

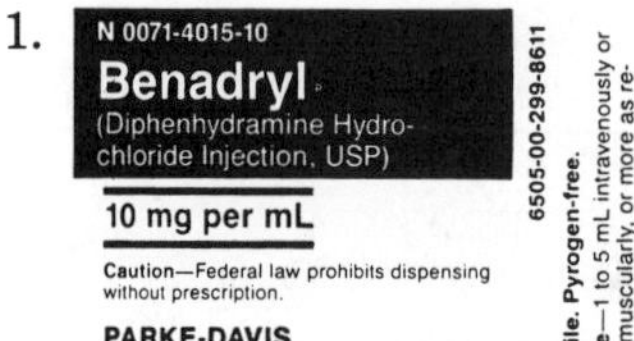

2.

N 0071-4160-10
STERI-VIAL
Pitocin
(Oxytocin Injection, USP)
Synthetic
10 units per mL
PARKE-DAVIS
Div of Warner-Lambert Co
Morris Plains, NJ 07950 USA 10 mL
Caution—Federal law prohibits dispensing without prescription.
For Intravenous Infusion or Intramuscular Injection
Dose—See package insert.
Contains 0.5% Chloretone® (chlorobutanol) (chloroform derivative) as a preservative.
Acidity adjusted with acetic acid.
Store at controlled room temperature 15°-30°C (59°-86°F).
Protect from excessive heat.
4160G252

3.

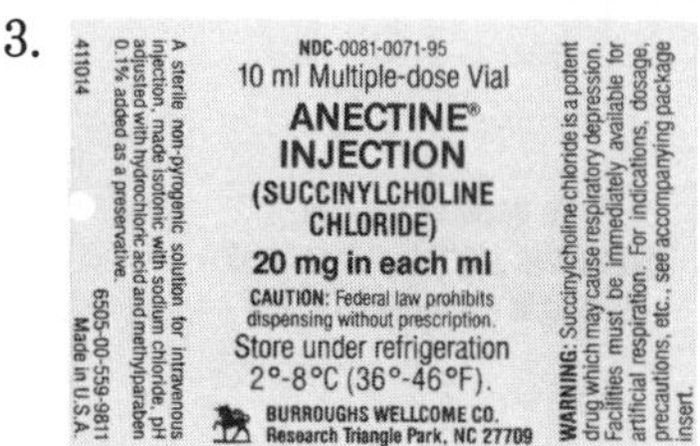

4. 20 mL Single-Use Vial NDC 0081-0107-93

RETROVIR® I.V. INFUSION Sterile

(ZIDOVUDINE) Each mL contains 10 mg zidovudine

FOR INTRAVENOUS INFUSION ONLY. MUST BE DILUTED FOR ADMINISTRATION.

Dilute with 5% Dextrose Injection to a concentration no greater than 4 mg/mL. Contains no preservative. The vehicle contains Water for Injection, qs. Hydrochloric acid and/or sodium hydroxide may have been added to adjust pH. For indications, dosage, precautions, etc., see accompanying package insert.
Store at 15° to 25°C (59° to 77°F) and protect from light.
CAUTION: Federal law prohibits dispensing without prescription.

U.S. Patent No. 4724232 (Use Patent) Other Pats. Pending

Wellcome BURROUGHS WELLCOME CO. Research Triangle Park, NC 27709 Made in U.S.A. 587012

5.

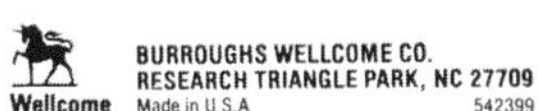

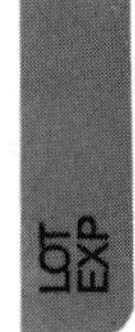

VHA +PLUS

NDC 0108-5031-77
2 ML SINGLE-DOSE
ADD-VANTAGE®* VIAL

TAGAMET®

CIMETIDINE HCl INJECTION

2 mL=300 mg

TAGAMET® INJECTION

6. 60 mL NDC 0081-0264-27

LANOXIN®

(DIGOXIN)

ELIXIR PEDIATRIC

Each mL contains
50 μg (0.05 mg)
PLEASANTLY FLAVORED

Alcohol 10%, Methylparaben 0.1% (added as a preservative)
For indications, dosage, precautions, etc., see accompanying package insert.
Store at 15° to 25°C (59° to 77°F) and protect from light.
CAUTION: Federal law prohibits dispensing without prescription.

Wellcome BURROUGHS WELLCOME CO. RESEARCH TRIANGLE PARK, NC 27709 Made in U.S.A 542399

LOT EXP

Exercises 7–12. In each case, state which medication has the greater strength.

7. dopamine injection
   (a) 0.8 mg/mL
   (b) 1.6 mg/mL
8. dicloxacillin sodium suspension
   (a) 62.5 mg/5 mL
   (b) 12.5 mg/mL
9. Benadryl syrup
   (a) 12.5 mg/5 mL
   (b) 2.5 mg/mL
10. erythromycin suspension
   (a) 100 mg/2.5 mL
   (b) 400 mg/5 mL
11. neostigmine bromide
   (a) 1:1000
   (b) 1:2000
12. neostigmine bromide
   (a) 1:4000
   (b) 1:2000

Exercises 13–18. Express in fraction form the strengths of the following solutions.

13. acetaminophen, 20%
14. Beta-2, 0.5%
15. Dilocaine, 1.5%
16. Isuprel, 0.2%
17. Echodide, 0.03%
18. ammonium chloride, 2.14%

ANSWERS 1. 10 mg/mL 3. 20 mg/mL 5. 300 mg/2 mL, or 150 mg/mL 7. (b) 9. neither, 12.5/5 = 2.5/1 11. (a), 1/1000 > 1/2000 13. 20 g/100 mL = 1 g/5 mL, or 200 mg/mL 15. 1.5 g/100 mL, or 15 mg/mL 17. 0.03 g/100 mL, or 0.3 mg/mL, or 300 mcg/mL

7-3. FINDING THE AMOUNT OF PURE DRUG IN A SOLUTION

Mr. Styrone has had an intravenous infusion of 100 mL of ticarcillin disodium solution. If the strength of the solution was 30 mg/mL, how much pure drug did Mr. Styrone receive? Whenever we know the strength of a solution and the volume administered, we can easily compute how much pure drug was administered.

Examples

1. Suppose that we have 100 mL of a solution with a strength of 30 mg/mL. Using the following table, we can easily compute the amount of drug in the solution.

Amount of Pure Drug		Amount of Solution
x mg	in	100 mL
30 mg	in	1 mL

By proportion, or formula, we find that there are 3000 mg (3 g) of pure drug in the solution.

2. If we need 75 mL of a solution with a strength of 0.5 mg/5 mL, we can easily find how much pure drug must be in the solution. The following table leads to a proportion or a formula.

Table:

Weight of Pure Drug		Total Volume
x mg	in	75 mL
0.5 mg	in	5 mL

Result (by proportion or formula): 7.5 mL

3. If 50 mL of a 10% v/v* solution are on hand, a fast method to compute the amount of pure drug is to take 10% of 50 mL, as the following computation demonstrates.

Table:

Amount of Pure Drug		Amount of Solution
x mL	in	50 mL
10 mL	in	100 mL

Since

$$\frac{x}{10} = \frac{50}{100}$$

$$x = \frac{50}{100} \times 10$$

$$= \frac{10}{100} \times 50$$

$$= 10\% \text{ of } 50$$

Result: 5 mL

4. If 4 mL of a 1:500 w/v† solution are available, you might simply use $\frac{1}{500} \times 4$ to find the amount of pure drug in the solution. The following computation shows why.

---

* *volume* (mL) of pure drug/total *volume* (mL) of solution.

† *weight* (g) of pure drug/total *volume* (mL) of solution.

Table:

Amount of Pure Drug		Amount of Solution
x g	in	4 mL
1 g	in	500 mL

Since

$$\frac{x}{1} = \frac{4}{500}$$

$$x = \frac{4}{500} \times 1$$

$$= \frac{1}{500} \times 4 = 0.008$$

Result: 0.008 g, or 8 mg

SAMPLE EXERCISES

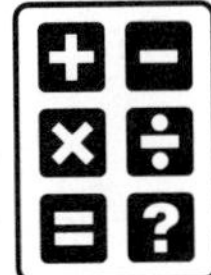

1. How much pure drug is in 15 mL of ticarcillin disodium solution with a strength of 10 mg/mL?

Exercises 2–4. The following chart gives information about weight per volume solutions (w/v). Complete the chart.

	Amount of Pure Drug (w)	Amount of Solution (v)	Strength
2.		100 mL	0.5 mg/5 mL
3.		50 mL	20%
4.		4 cc	1:300

ANSWERS

1. *Table:*

Weight (w)		Volume (v)
x mg	in	15 mL
10 mg	in	1 mL

Result: 150 mg

2. *Table:*

w		v
x mg	in	100 mL
0.5 mg	in	5 mL

Result: 10 mg

3. *Table:*

w		v
x g	in	50 mL
20 g	in	100 mL

Result: 10 g

4. *Table:*

w		v
x g	in	~~4 cc~~ 4 mL
1 g	in	300 mL

Result: $\frac{4}{300}$ g = 0.013 g, or 13 mg

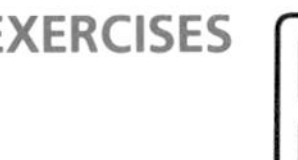

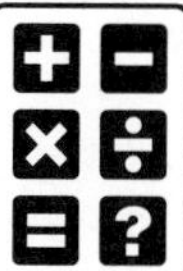

Exercises 1–8. The following chart gives information about certain solutions. Complete it by finding the amount of pure drug in each solution.

	Amount of Pure Drug	Amount of Solution	Strength
1.		200 mL	1 mg/mL
2.		100 mL	0.3 mg/5 mL
3.		20 mL	4 mg/mL
4.		30 mL	20% (w/v)
5.		120 mL	6:100 (w/v)
6.		30 g	5% (w/w)*
7.		45 g	20 mg/1 g
8.		3 fl oz	1:3 (v/v)

Exercises 9–12. How much pure drug is in 5 mL of a ticarcillin disodium solution that has the strength indicated?

9. 30 mg/mL
10. 0.1 g/mL
11. 45 mg/3 mL
12. 10 mg/0.5 mL
13. D10W, or D10%, is a 10% solution of dextrose in water. How much dextrose is in 200 mL of solution?
14. To treat an overdose of a medication, the doctor has given orders for administration of a 10% glucose solution. How much glucose should be in 1 L of the solution?
15. A saline solution called $\frac{1}{2}$ NS has a strength of 0.45%. How much sodium chloride is present in 1 L of $\frac{1}{2}$ NS?
16. Find the amount of pure drug in 3 L of neostigmine bromide solution, 1:1000 (w/v).

Exercises 17–20. Find the amount of pure drug in the following:

17. $\frac{1}{2}$ oz of amoxicillin trihydrate (Amoxil) suspension, 125 mg/5 mL
18. $\frac{1}{2}$ tsp of Amoxil suspension, 250 mg/5 mL
19. 2 g of fluocinonide (Lidex) cream, 0.05%
20. 1 gtt of timolol maleate (Timoptic), 0.5%
21. How much dextrose is needed to make 1 L of 5% dextrose solution?
22. How much sodium chloride is needed to make 500 mL of a 0.9% saline enema solution?

ANSWERS 1. 200 mg 3. 80 mg 5. 7.2 g 7. 900 mg 9. 150 mg 11. 75 mg 13. 20 g 15. 4.5 g 17. 375 mg 19. 1 mg 21. 50 g

7-4. FINDING THE AMOUNT OF SOLUTION TO ADMINISTER

Mrs. Enoryts is to receive a dose of 4 g of ticarcillin disodium in solution form. If the strength of the solution is 50 mg/mL, how much solution should she receive? Whenever you know the prescribed amount of pure drug and strength of solution, it is easy to compute how much solution to administer.

* *weight* (g) of pure drug/total *weight* (g) of solution.

Examples

1. To give a client 4 g of pure drug in a solution that is 50 mg/mL, you must compute the amount of solution to administer. The following table is the basis for the computation.

Table:

Amount of Solution		Amount of Pure Drug
x mL	contains	4000 mg ~~4 g~~
1 mL	contains	50 mg

Result: 80 mL

2. Suppose that we need 15 mg of pure drug in a solution with a strength of 0.5 mg/5 mL. Let us compute the required volume of the solution.

Table:

Volume of Solution		Weight of Pure Drug
x mL	contains	15 mg
5 mL	contains	0.5 mg

Result: 150 mL

3. If a 40% v/v solution contains 90 mL of a pure drug, we use the following table to compute the volume of the solution.

Table:

Volume of Solution		Amount of Pure Drug
x mL	contains	90 mL
100 mL	contains	40 mL

Result: 225 mL

4. If a 1:500 w/w solution contains 600 mg of pure drug, then there must be 300 g of solution. The following table is a basis for the computation.

Table:

Total Amount of Solution	Amount of Pure Drug
x g	0.6 g ~~600 mg~~
500 g	1 g

SAMPLE EXERCISES

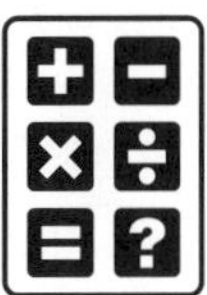

1. To administer a dose of 4 g of ticarcillin disodium, how much ticarcillin solution at a strength of 10 mg/mL do we need?

Exercises 2–4. The following chart gives information about weight per volume (w/v) solutions. Complete the chart by finding the volume of each solution.

	Volume of Solution (v)	Weight of Pure Drug (w)	Strength (w/v)
2.		2.5 mg	0.5 mg/5 mL
3.		18 g	20%
4.		400 mg	1:200

ANSWERS

1. *Table:*

v	w
x mL	~~4 g~~ 4000 mg
1 mL	10 mg

Result: 400 mL

2. *Table:*

v	w
x mL	2.5 mg
5 mL	0.5 mg

Result: 25 mL

3. *Table:*

v	w
x mL	18 g
100 mL	20 g

Result: 90 mL

4. *Table:*

v	w
x mL	~~400 mg~~ 0.4 g
200 mL	1 g

Result: 80 mL

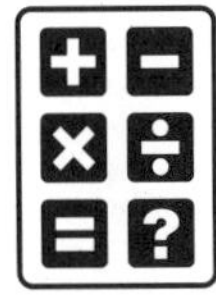

EXERCISES

Exercises 1–6. The following chart gives information about certain solutions. Complete the chart.

	Amount of Solution	Amount of Pure Drug	Strength
1.		5 mg	1 mg/mL
2.		600 μg	0.3 mg/5 mL
3.		10 mg	4 mg/mL
4.		24 g	20% (w/v)
5.		450 mg	6:100 (w/v)
6.		0.25 g	125 mg/5 mL

Exercises 7–10. How much solution is necessary for a 3.5-g dose of ticarcillin disodium from a solution that has the strength indicated?

7. 0.1 g/mL
8. 30 mg/mL
9. 45 mg/3 mL
10. 10 mg/0.5 mL

11. To be administered: naloxone 0.6 mg SC stat.
How supplied: in vials, 0.4 mg/mL.
(a) What is the route?
(b) What is the frequency?
(c) What is the amount in milliliters?

12. Ms. Sossue is receiving 4 mg of metaraminol bitartrate 1% IM. How many milliliters of solution should be administered?

13. Doctor's order: mannitol 12.5 g IV.
Available: 10% solution.
Find the number of milliliters to administer and the route.

14. Medication: labetalol hydrochloride solution, 200 mg:200 mL.
Dosage: repeated IV injections. Give 20 mg slowly over 2 min; repeat injections of 40 mg q10min until maximum dose of 300 mg is reached.
Find the number of milliliters for
(a) initial injection
(b) repeat injection

15. Doctor's order: clindamycin phosphate injection 300 mg IV q6h.
    Available: 1.2 g in 200 mL.
    (a) How is it administered?
    (b) How often?
    (c) How much?
16. As a test dose to assess tolerance to a thiopental drug, inject a small dose of 75 mg, using a 2.5% solution. How many milliliters is this?
17. If the drug order requires calcitonin 100 IU SC, and you have on hand a 2-mL vial of calcitonin containing 200 IU/mL, how much do you administer?
18. Doctor's order for pain following surgery: hydromorphone 4 mg SC q4h prn.
    Available: vial labeled 2 mg/1 mL.
    How much do you give?
19. Ampicillin 0.5 g PO q6h is ordered for Ms. Kinlob. An ampicillin oral solution is labeled 250 mg/5 mL. The nurse administers how much?
20. Doctor's order: amitriptyline 25 mg IM qid.
    Available: 10 mg/mL.
    How much should be injected?

ANSWERS 1. 5 mL 3. 2.5 mL 5. 7.5 mL 7. 35 mL 9. 233.3 mL 11. (a) subcutaneous (b) once (immediately) (c) 1.5 mL 13. 125 mL by intravenous administration 15. (a) intravenously (b) every 6 h (c) 50 mL 17. 0.5 mL subcutaneously 19. 10 mL every 6 h

---

7-5. EQUIPMENT FOR ADMINISTRATION OF SOLUTIONS

Medicine cups, droppers, and syringes are available for administration of liquid medications. We use droppers to administer a small amount of solution orally or into an eye or an ear. A syringe may be used either for an injection or, as in intravenous therapy, for adding one solution to another.

To administer the correct amount of solution, we need to read the scale on each piece of equipment very carefully. No matter what the scale, the principles are the same. The markings (calibrations) on each scale look like the markings on a ruler, but they represent volume of liquid rather than length.

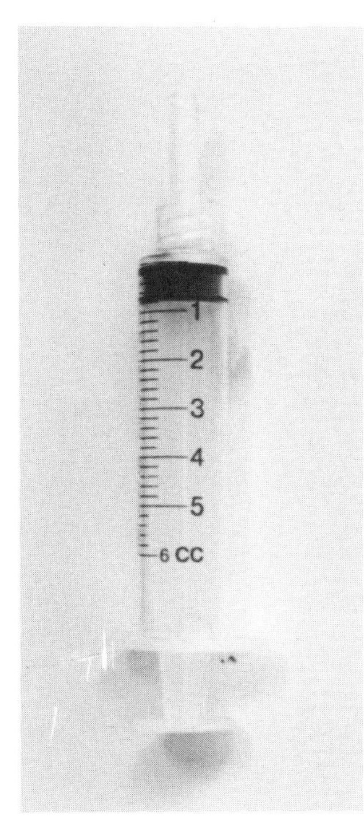

The Medicine Cup

A medicine cup is a small measuring cup. The one shown in Figure 7–3 has three scales, for (A) milliliters (cc), (B) tablespoons and teaspoons, and (C) ounces and grams. To check a measurement, hold the cup at eye level; the measurement should correspond to the marking at the base of the meniscus (crescent-shaped surface of liquid).

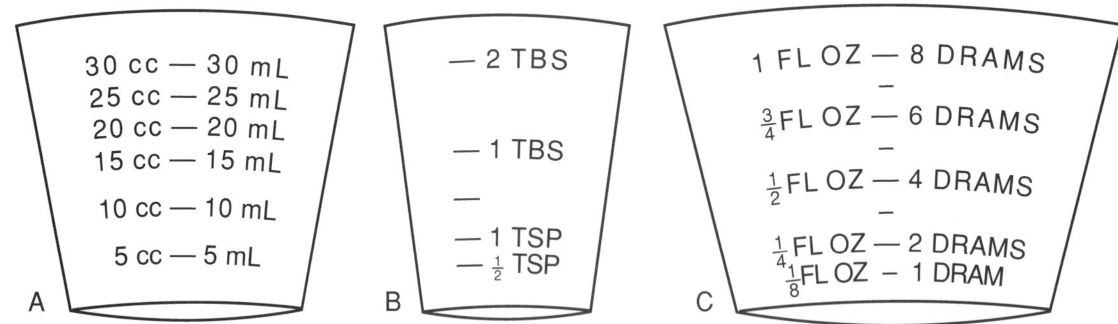

Figure 7–3 Three views of the same medicine cup.

The Dropper

To use a dropper, insert it into a liquid, squeeze the bulb, and draw up the quantity desired.

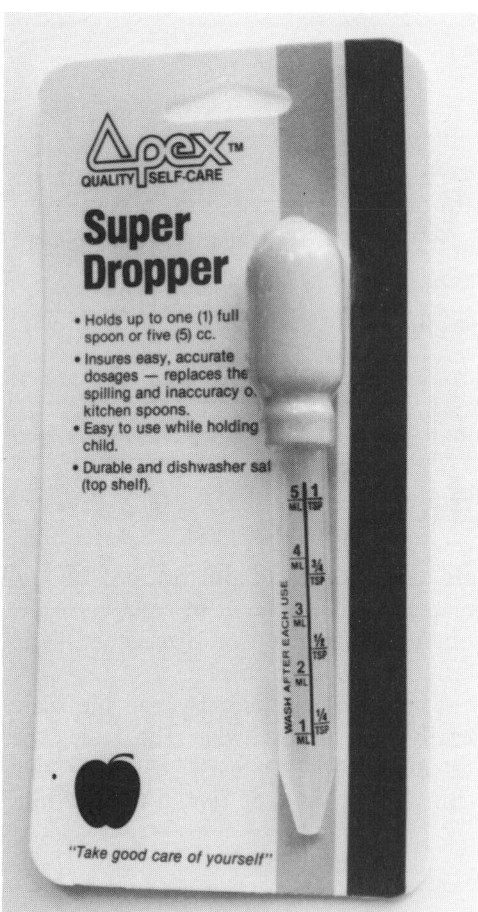

Classifying Syringes by Volume

A variety of syringes exist. We often choose a syringe by the maximum volume that it can measure. Therefore, the first thing to do with a syringe is to look at the largest number printed on the scale and the unit shown. One syringe can be mistaken for another; **careful attention is imperative.**

Examples

1. A 10-cc syringe (used for injecting one solution into another):

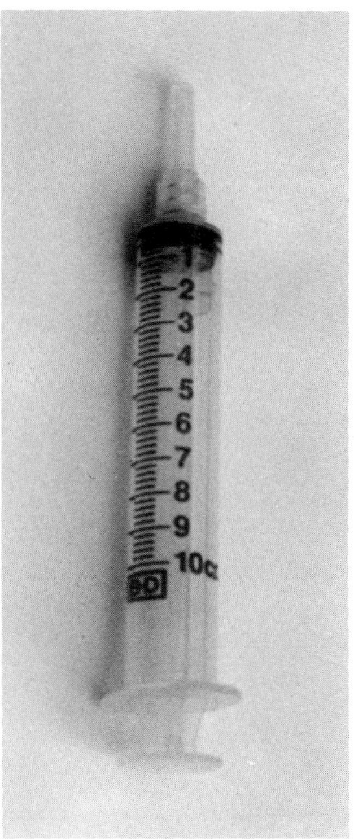

2. A 3-cc syringe (commonly used for IM and SC injections):

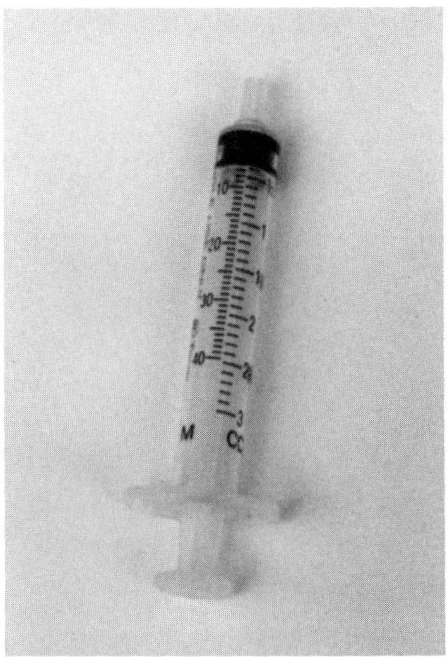

3. The 3-cc syringe also has a minim (M) scale, which shows markings up to 40 M.
4. The tuberculin syringe (Fig. 7–4), used for quantities less than 1 cc, has both a cubic centimeter (cc) scale (A) and a minim (M) scale (B), with markings up to 1 cc and 16 M.

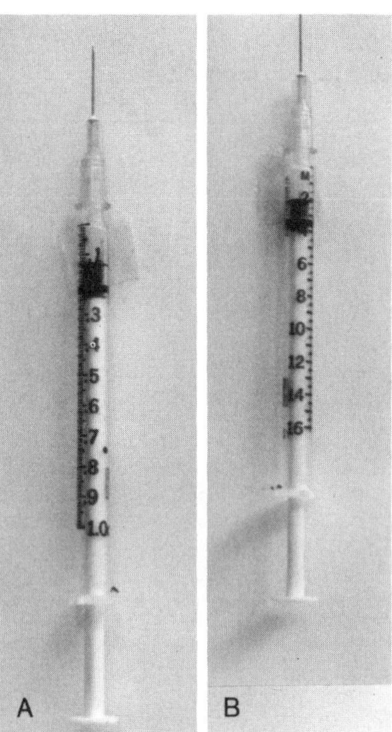

Figure 7–4 Two views of the same tuberculin syringe.

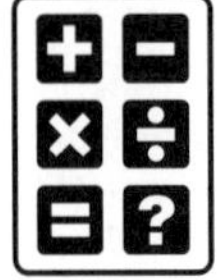

SAMPLE EXERCISES

Exercises 1 – 2. For each syringe shown, state the maximum volume it can measure.

1.

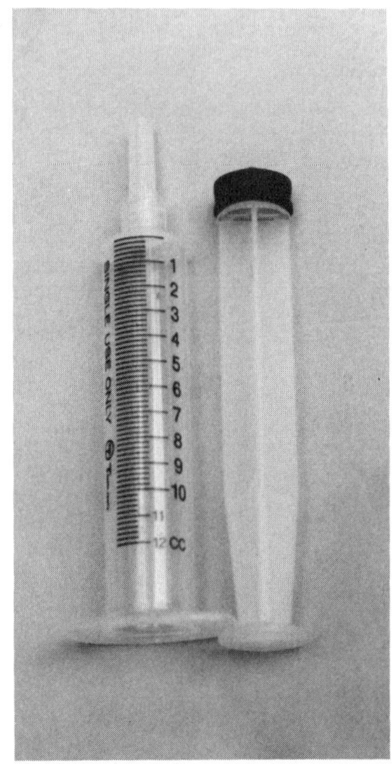

2.

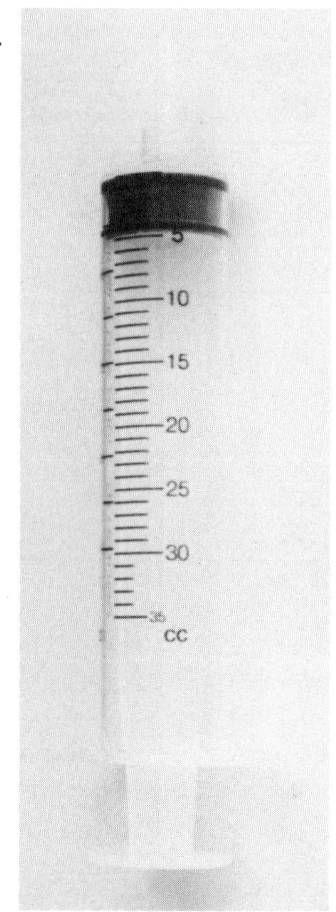

ANSWERS 1. 12 cc 2. 35 cc

Determining the Calibration of a Syringe

There are both long and short markings on a syringe, as on a ruler. Except for the first long mark (which represents 0), the long markings are usually labeled. Between the long markings are unlabeled short markings that create subdivisions. To determine the value of each subdivision (the calibration), find the difference between a pair of adjacent marked values and divide by the number of subdivisions (spaces) between the pair.

Examples

1. The 30-cc syringe is calibrated in 1-cc units.

$$\frac{25 - 20}{5} = 1$$

2. The 30-cc syringe has a second scale with a calibration of $\frac{1}{8}$ oz.

$$\frac{1 - \frac{3}{4}}{2} = \frac{\frac{1}{4}}{2} = \frac{1}{8}$$

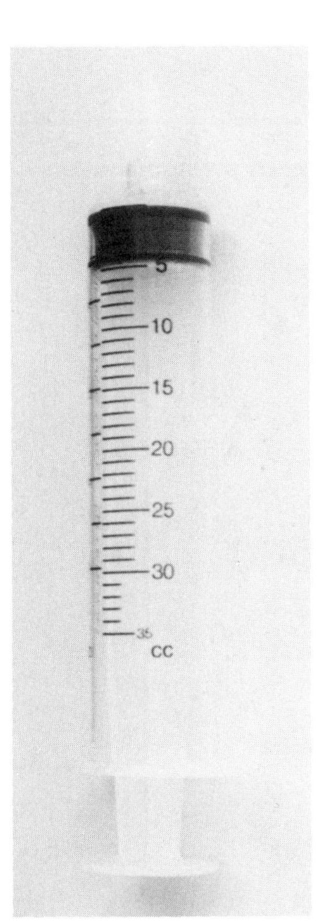

1.

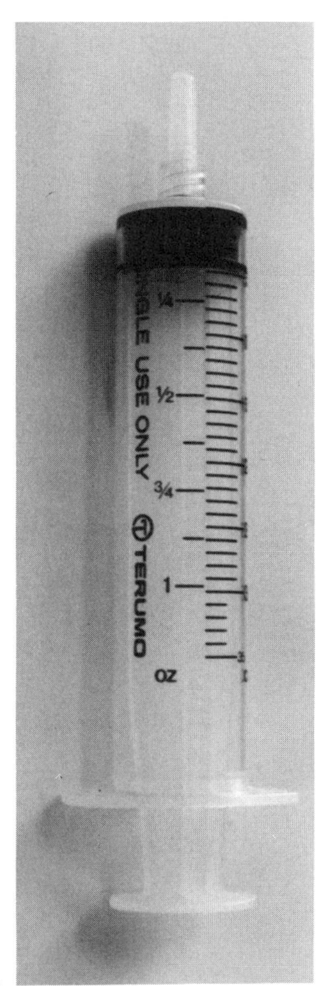

2.

3. The 10-cc syringe is calibrated in 0.2 cc.

$$\frac{9-8}{5} = 0.2$$

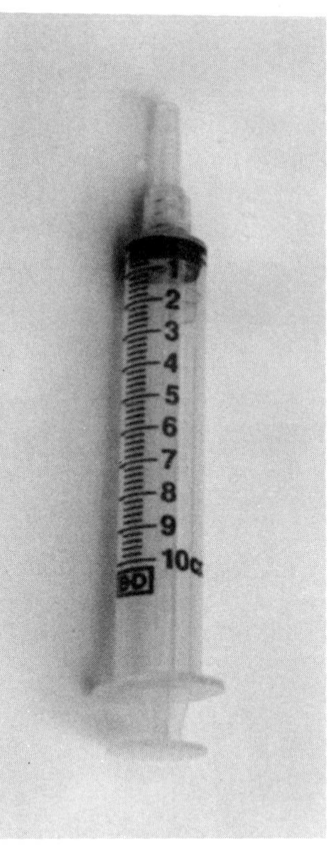

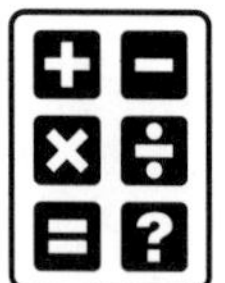

SAMPLE EXERCISES

Exercises 1–2. Determine the calibration of each syringe shown.

1.

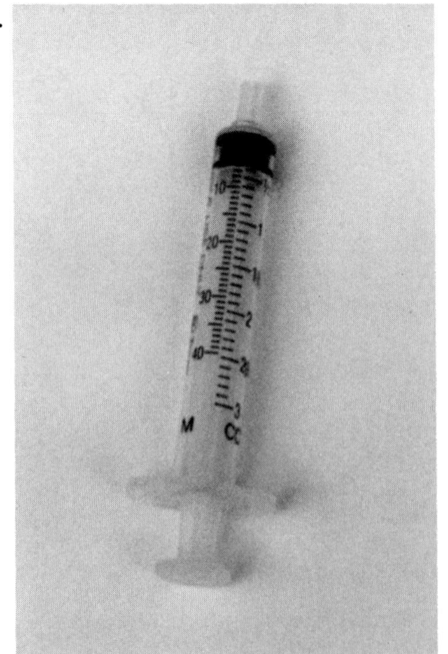

2.

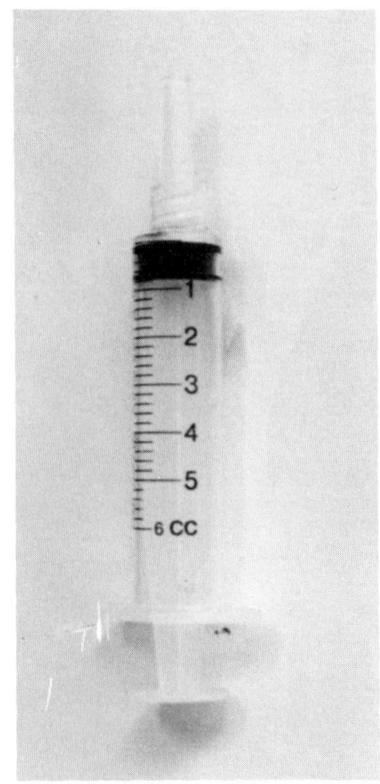

ANSWERS 1. 0.1 cc and 1 M 2. 0.2 cc

EXERCISES

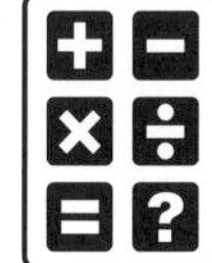

Exercises 1–2. From the scales of the medicine cup shown below, find:

1. The smallest volume (in cubic centimeters) that can be measured.
2. The largest volume (in ounces).

Exercises 3–6. On the medicine cup scales shown here, mark an arrow to indicate the given amount.

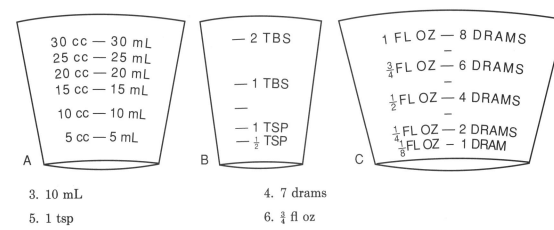

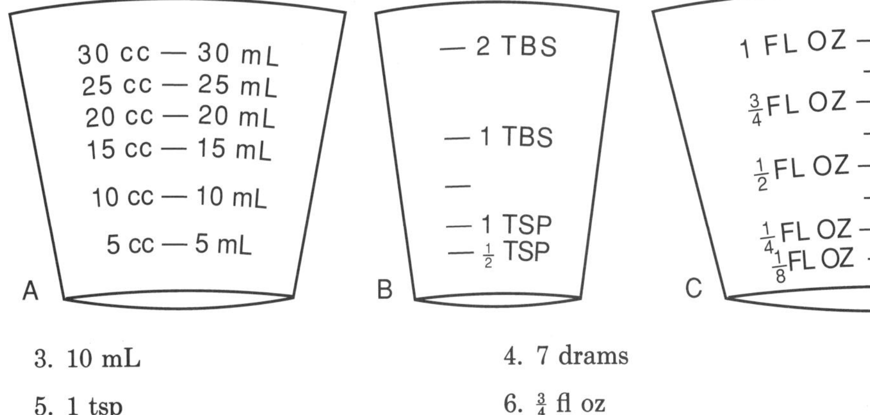

3. 10 mL
4. 7 drams
5. 1 tsp
6. $\frac{3}{4}$ fl oz

Exercises 7–11. Judging from the scale shown for each syringe below, state the maximum volume that the syringe can measure.

7.

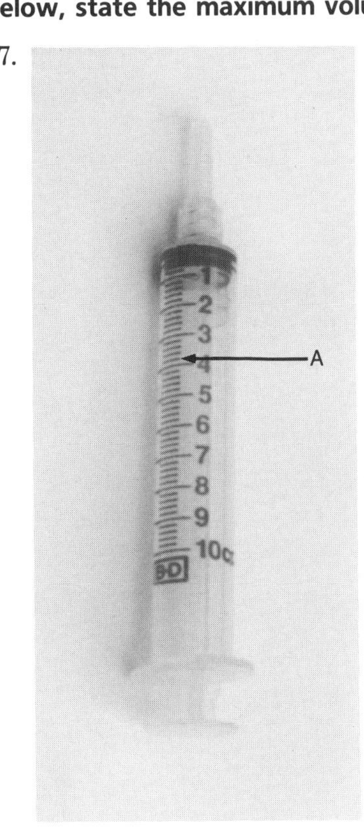

8.

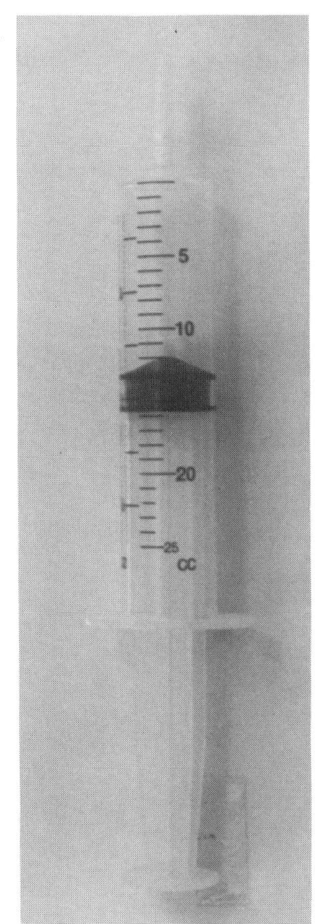

9.

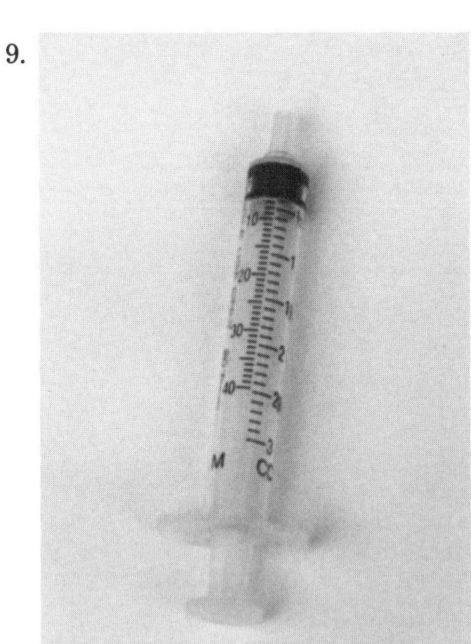

10.

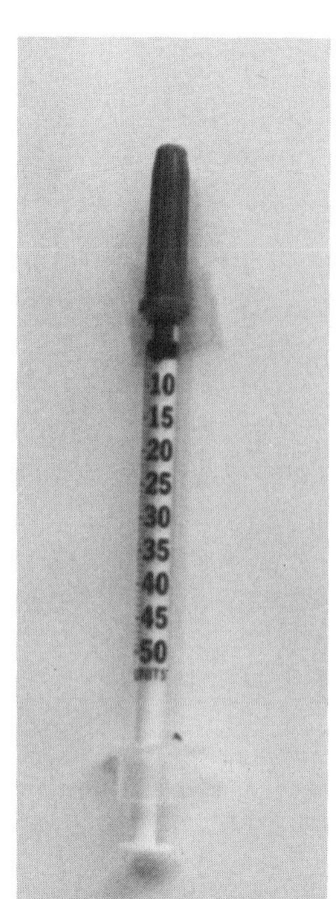

11.

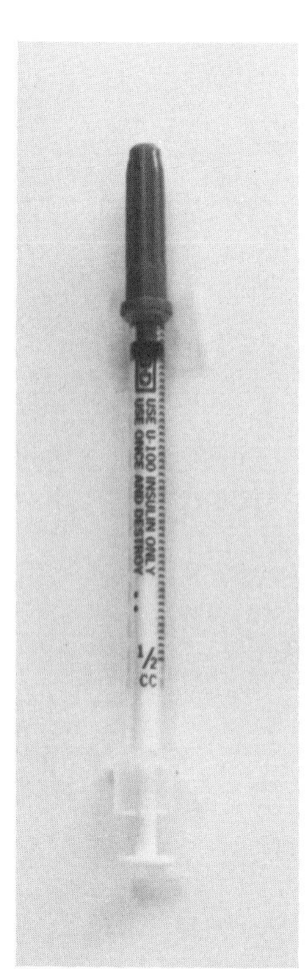

Exercises 12–16. Determine the calibration of each syringe shown.

12.

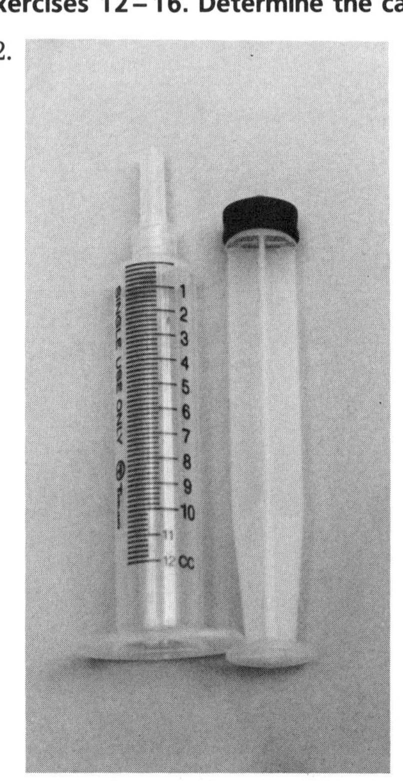

13.

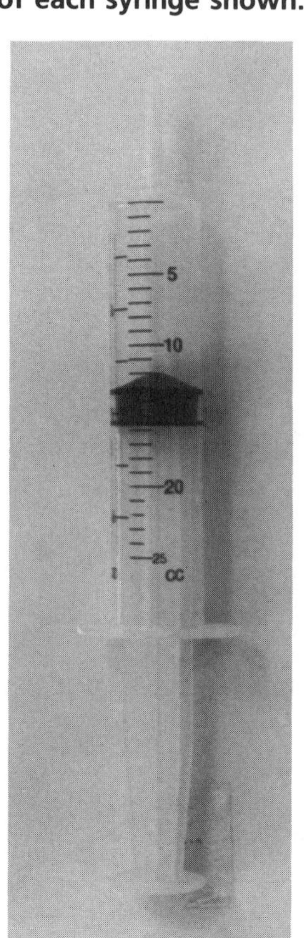

14.

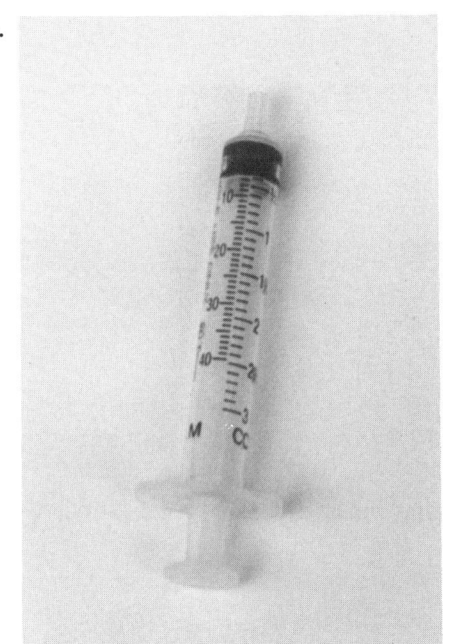

15.

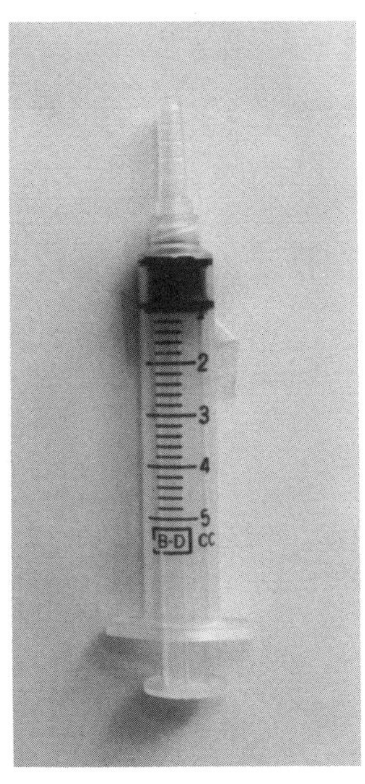

16.

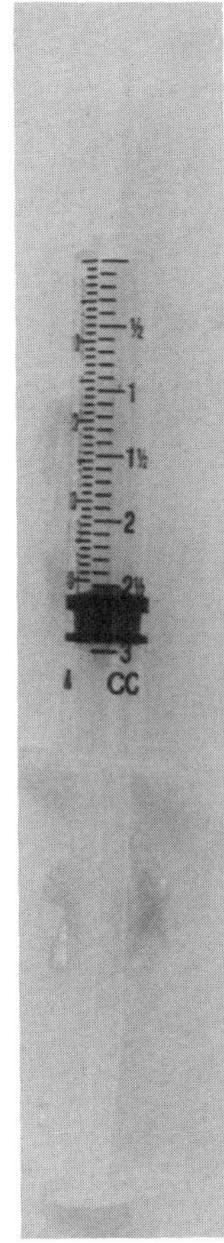

ANSWERS

1. 5 cc
3.

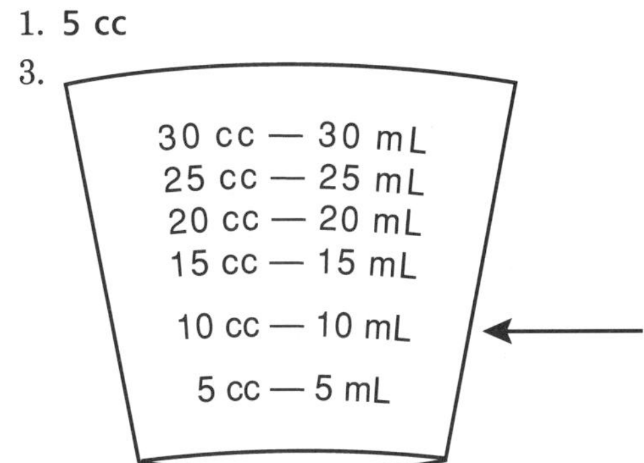

5.

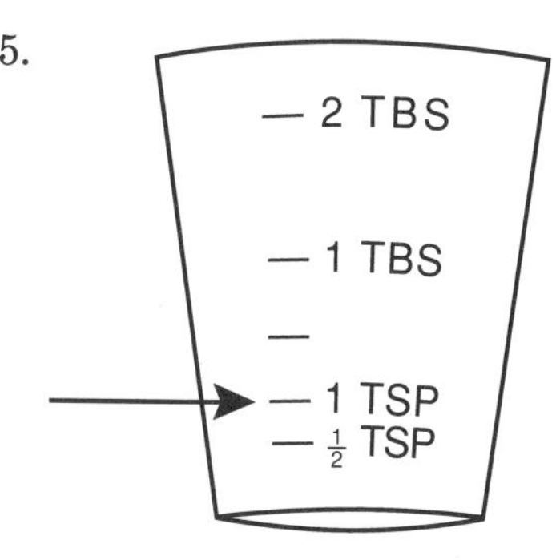

7. 6 cc
9. 3 cc
11. $\frac{1}{2}$ cc
13. 1 cc
15. 0.2 cc

7-6. READING A SYRINGE

HOW TO READ A MARKING

Find the closest smaller value.
Add the amount of the calibration for each marking.
Stop at the marking desired.

Examples

1. The 10-cc syringe below is calibrated in 0.2 cc.
   To find the volume indicated by the point marked A, we find the closest smaller value, 3 cc. We add 0.2 cc for each marking until we stop at A, or 3.8 cc (3.8 mL).
2. On the 3-cc syringe below, the point marked B represents 1.4 cc (1.4 mL).

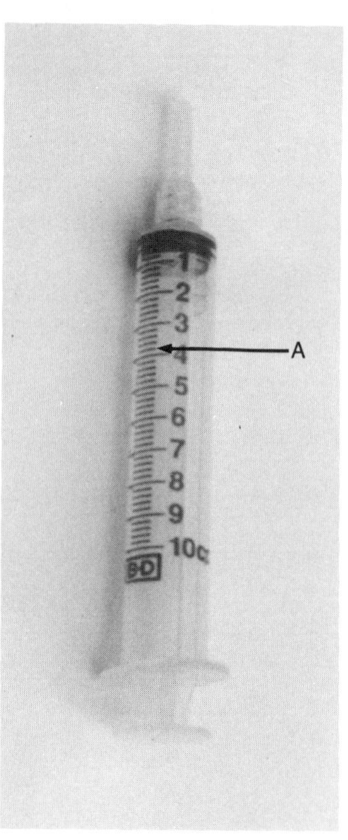

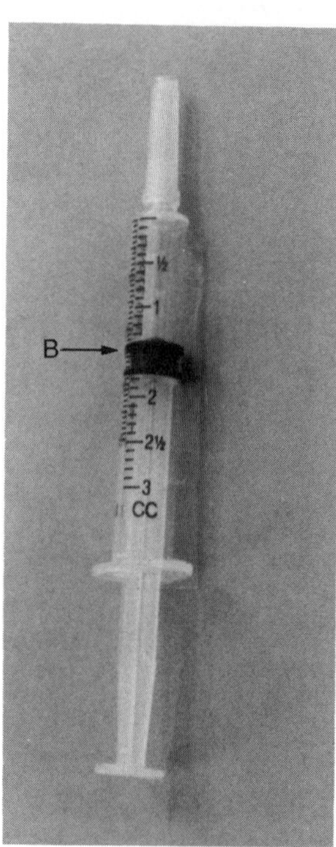

Exercises 1 – 2. Find the volume indicated by the arrows.

SAMPLE EXERCISES

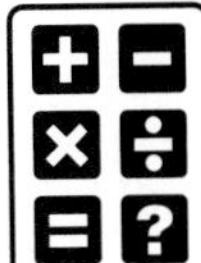

1.

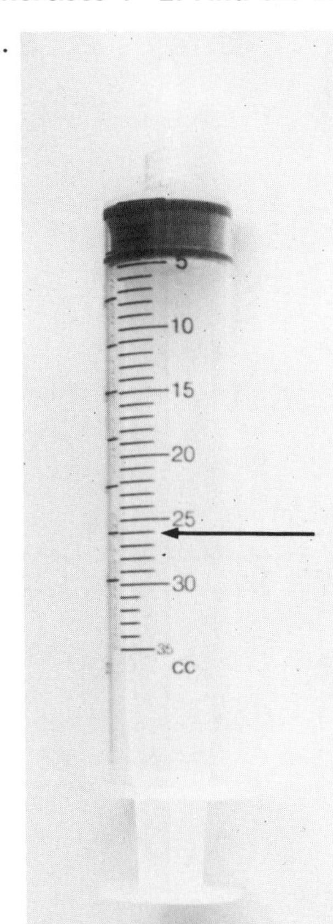

2.

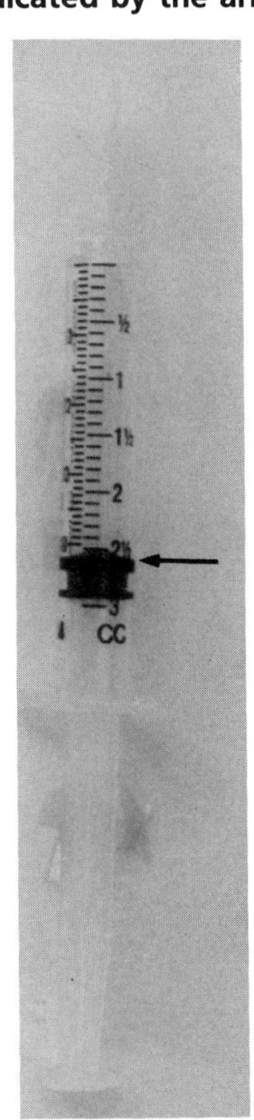

ANSWERS 1. 26 cc 2. 2.6 cc

HOW TO INTERPRET THE POSITION OF THE PLUNGER

Hold the syringe vertically, with the needle at the top.
Focus on the top ring of the plunger.
Read the marking at the level of the top ring.

Examples

1. On this 10-cc syringe, the volume is indicated by the position of the top ring of the plunger, that is, at 3.8 cc.

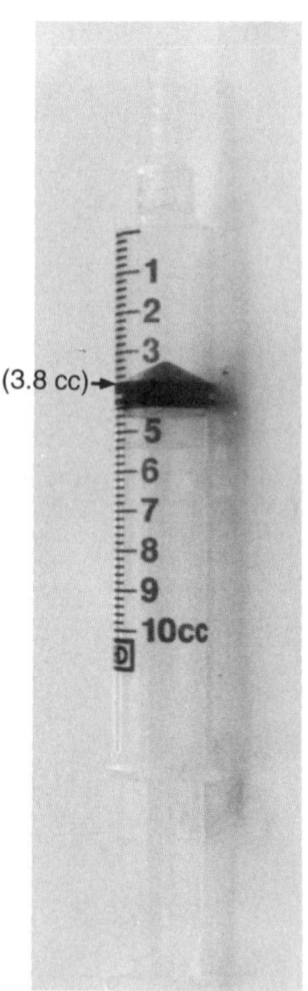

2. On this 3-cc syringe, the top ring indicates 1.4 cc.

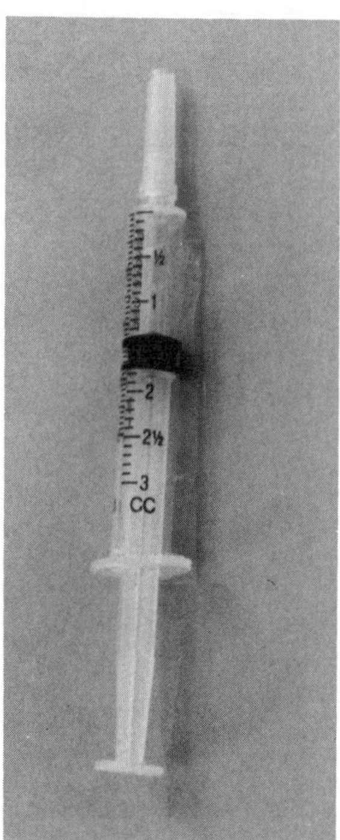

Exercises 1–2. Find the volume indicated by the position of the plunger.

SAMPLE EXERCISES

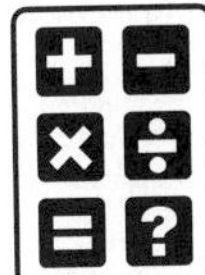

1.

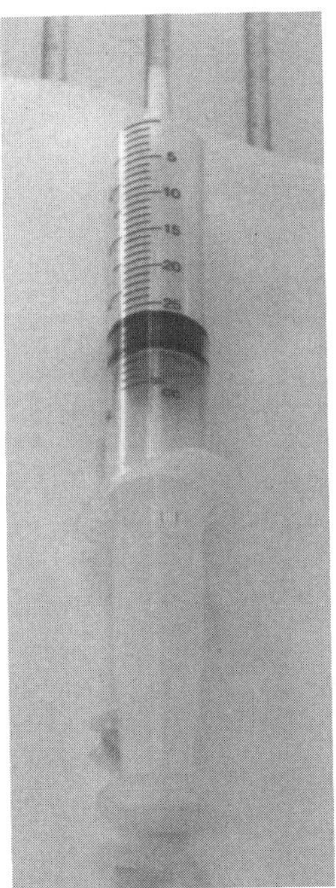

2.

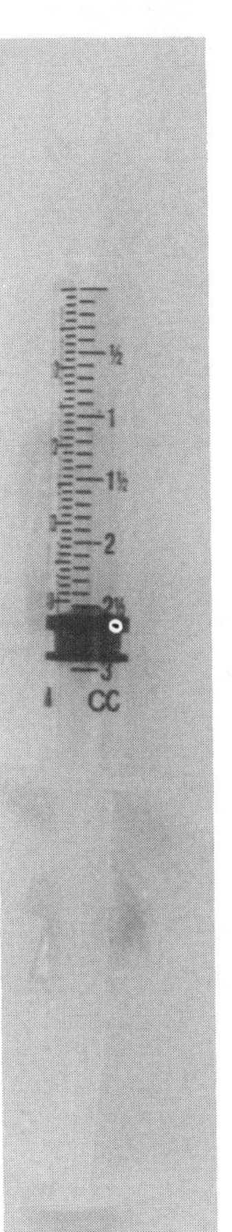

ANSWERS 1. 26 cc 2. 2.6 cc

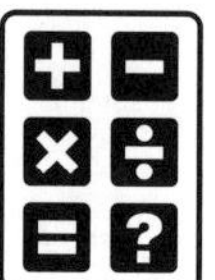

EXERCISES

Exercises 1 – 14. Find the volume indicated by each arrow.

1–5.

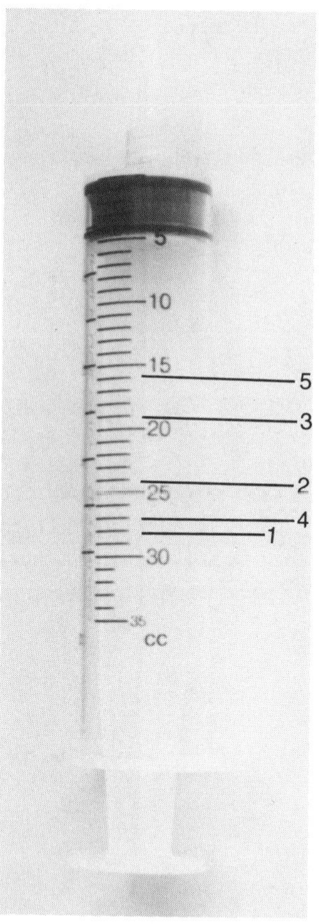

6–11.

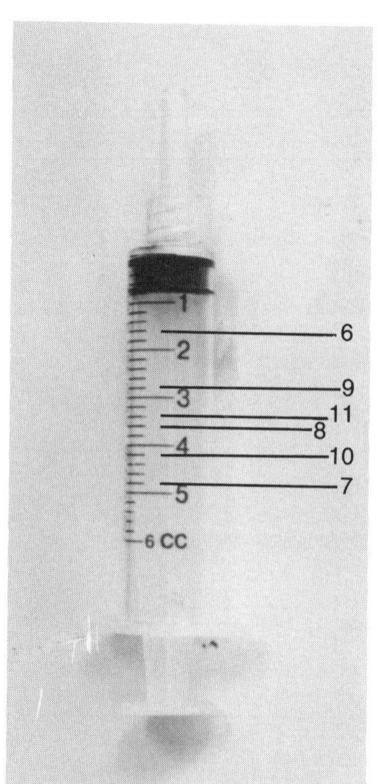

12.

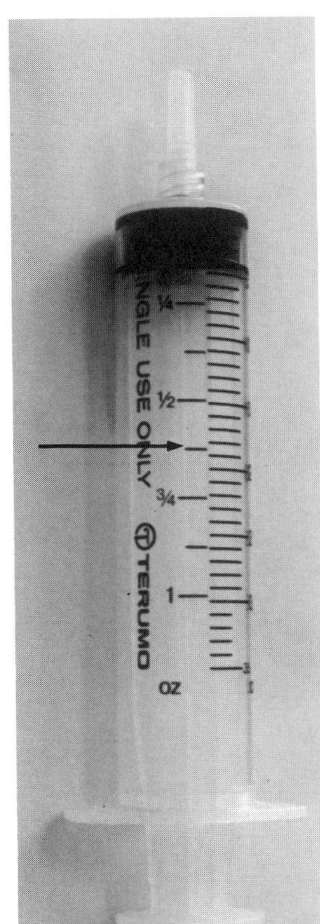

13.

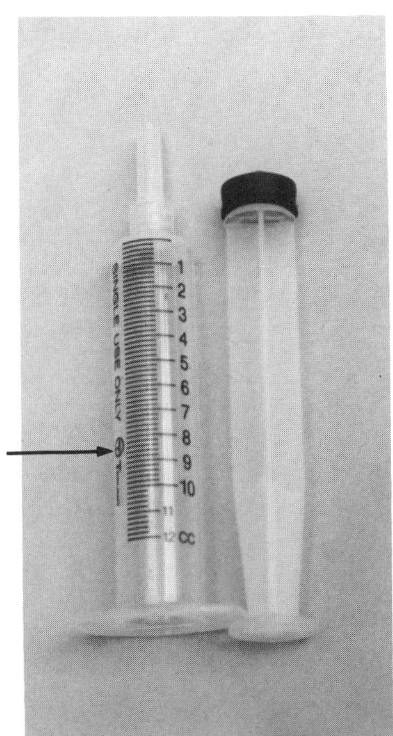

14.

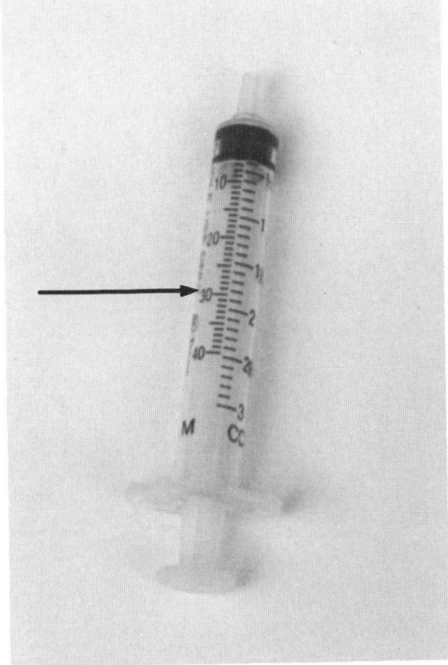

Exercises 15–20. Find the volume indicated by the plunger.

15.

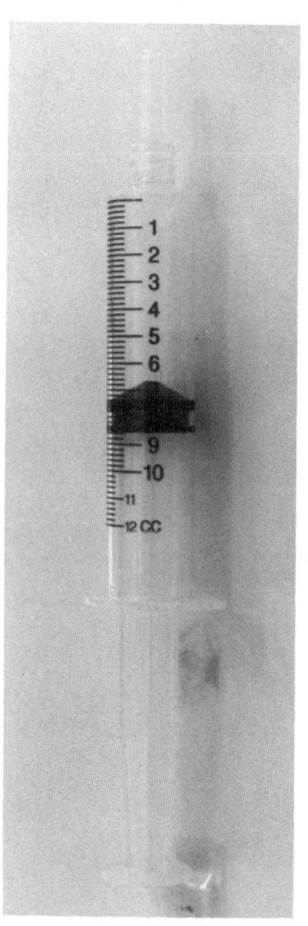

16.

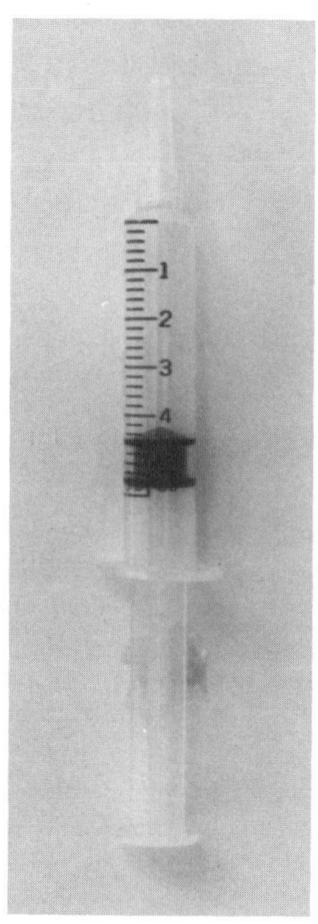

17.

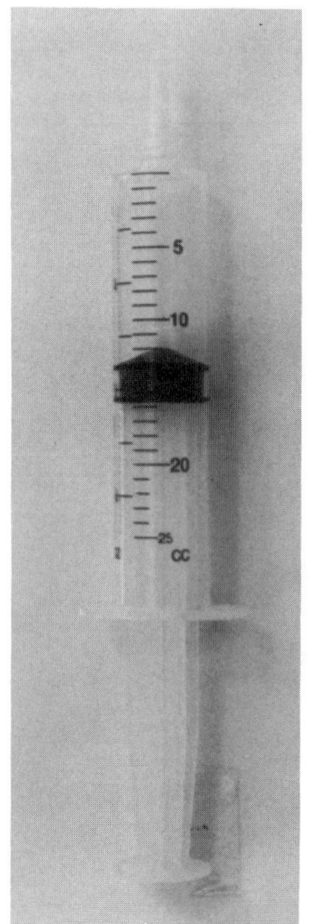

18.

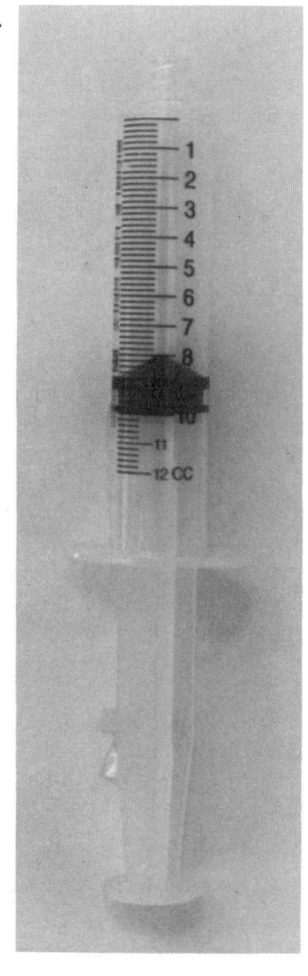

19.

20.

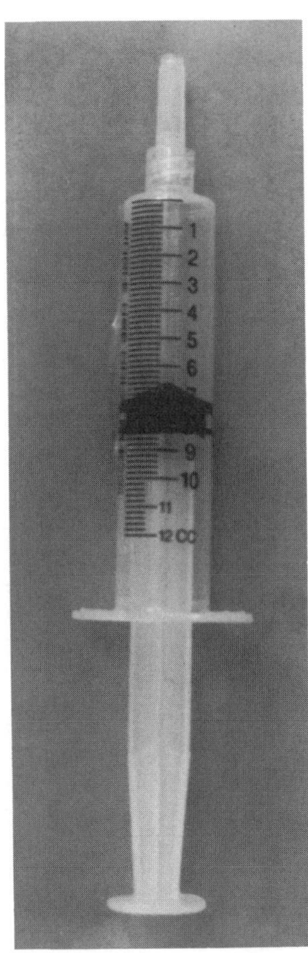

ANSWERS 1. 28 mL 3. 19 mL 5. 16 mL 7. 4.8 mL
9. 2.8 mL 11. 3.4 mL 13. 8.4 mL 15. 7.4 mL 17. 13 mL
19. 23 M

7-7. DRAWING A DESIRED VOLUME INTO A SYRINGE

To draw a desired amount into a syringe in preparation for an injection, the nurse must move the plunger so that the marking at the top ring of the plunger (nearest the needle) corresponds to the desired amount. The marking at the top ring of the plunger in the syringe shows the amount of liquid in the syringe.

HOW TO LOCATE A DESIRED MEASUREMENT ON A SYRINGE

Read from the smallest marked value to the greatest.
Find the approximate location between the two closest marked numbers.
Count markings to find the exact location and check.

When reading the scale on a syringe, always be aware of the direction from lesser to greater values.

Examples

1. To locate 7.2 cc on this 10-cc syringe (calibrated in 0.2 cc increments), look between 7 and 8, and find the first marking after 7, towards 8.

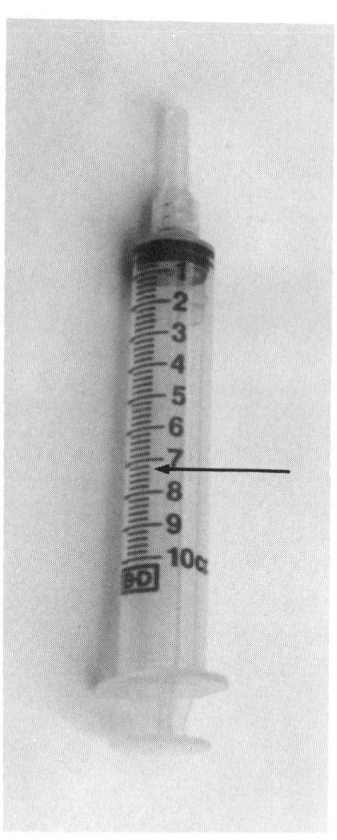

2. On the 3-cc syringe, find:
   (a) 1.4 cc, by looking between 1 and $1\frac{1}{2}$ on the cc scale;
   (b) 15 M, by locating the halfway point between 10 M and 20 M.

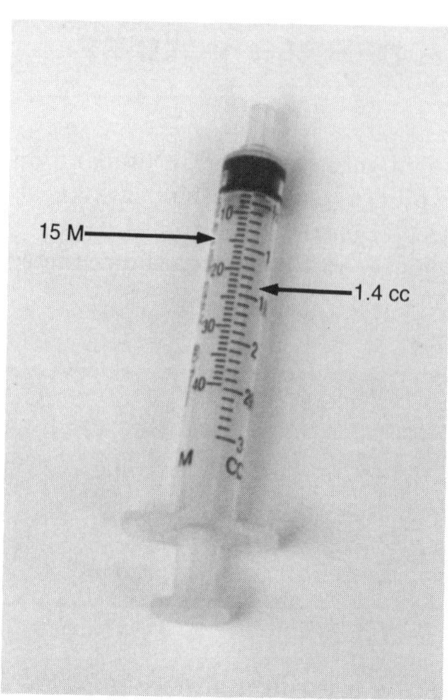

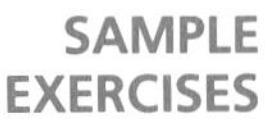

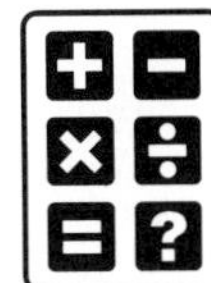

1. Find 0.8 mL on the 3-cc syringe.

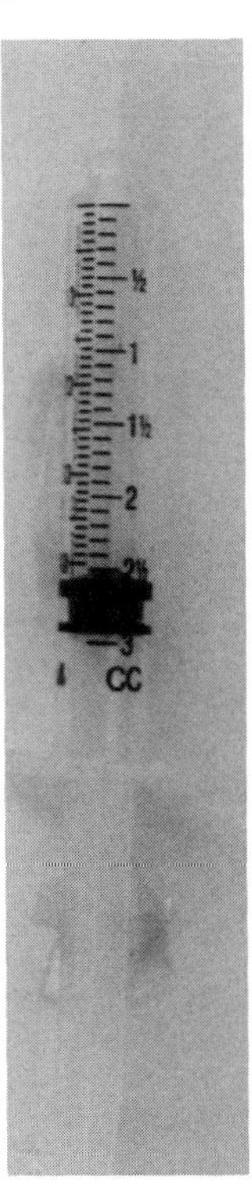

Exercises 2–3. For each dose, compute and mark (with an arrow) the desired volume on the 3-cc syringe. Label it with the computed volume.

Dose Required	Strength of Available Solution
2. dexpanthenol IM 500 mg	250 mg/mL
3. dicyclomine hydrochloride IM 5 mg	10 mg/mL

4. On the 30-cc syringe, locate 17 mL.

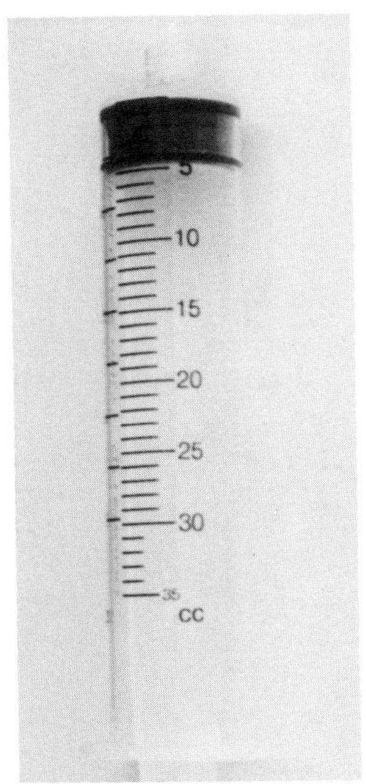

ANSWERS 1–3.

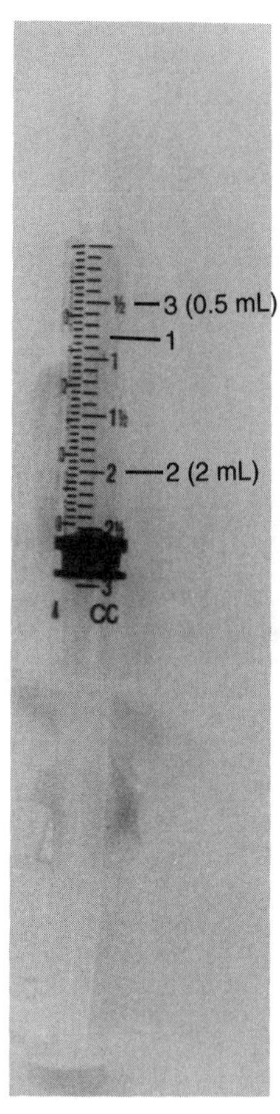

4.

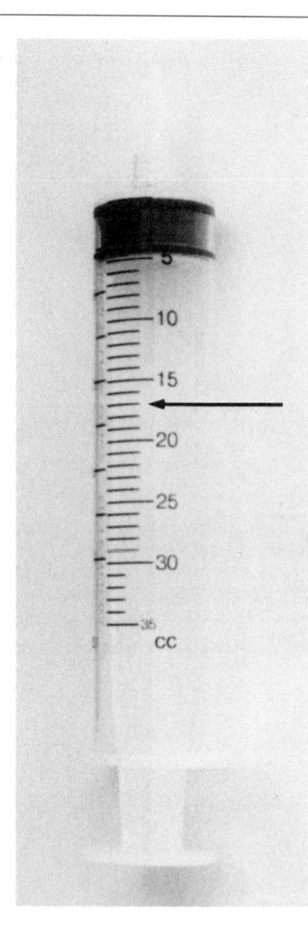

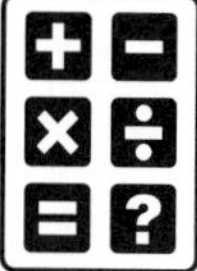

EXERCISES

Exercises 1–4. On the 10-cc syringe, locate the indicated measurement with an arrow. Label with the indicated volume.

1. 4 cc
2. 2.6 cc
3. 5.2 cc
4. 6.8 cc

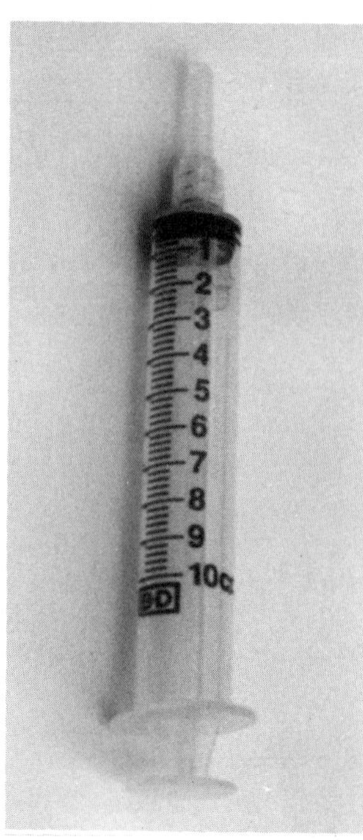

Exercises 5–12. On the 3-cc syringe, locate the indicated measurement. Label each arrow with the indicated volume.

5. 2 cc
6. 2.5 cc
7. 1.4 cc
8. 2.3 cc
9. 1.8 cc
10. 0.7 cc
11. 1.6 mL
12. 0.4 mL

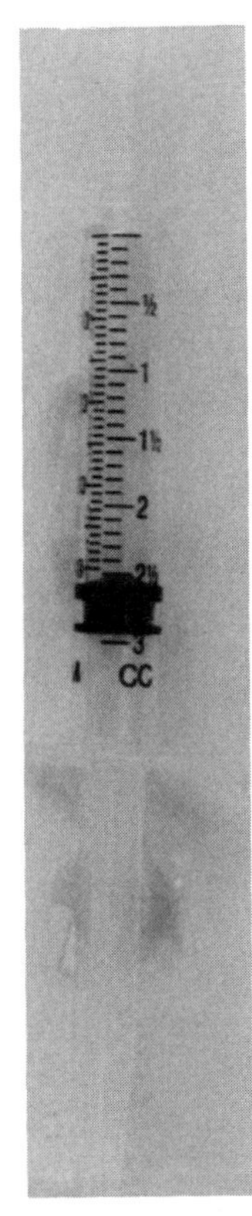

Exercises 13–14. On the 30-cc syringe, locate the indicated measurement and mark each arrow with the indicated volume.

13. 16 cc
14. 29 cc

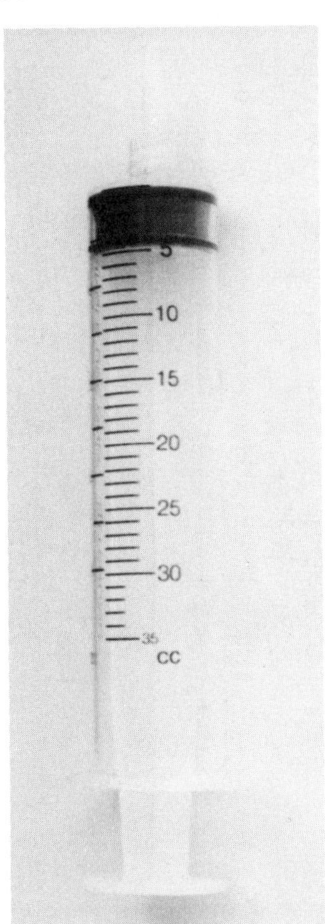

Exercises 15–22. For each dose, compute and mark the desired volume on the 3-cc syringe.

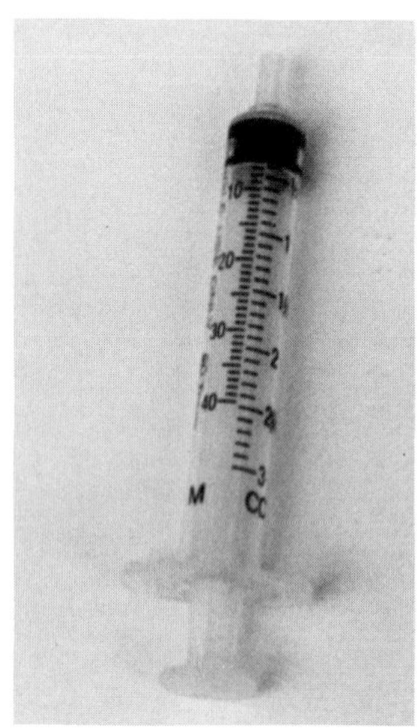

	Dose Required	Strength of Available Solution
15.	dicyclomine hydrochloride IM 15 mg	10 mg/mL
16.	glycopyrrolate IM 0.44 mg	0.2 mg/mL
17.	posterior pituitary hormone (Pituitrin) SC 15 U	20 U/mL
18.	belladonna (Bellafoline) SC 0.125 mg	0.5 mg/mL
19.	Bellafoline SC 0.25 mg	0.5 mg/mL
20.	Bellafoline SC 0.375 mg	0.5 mg/mL
21.	cyanocobalamin (vitamin B_{12}) IM 150 μg	120 μg/mL
22.	vitamin B_{12} IM 80 μg (Give answer in minims.)	120 μg/mL

ANSWERS

1–4.

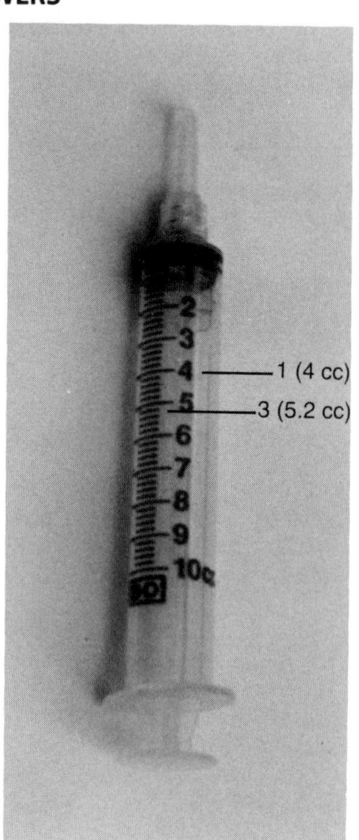

5–12.

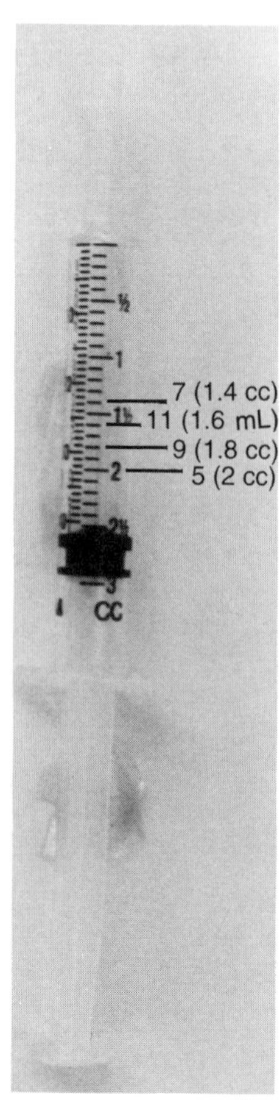

13, 14.

13 (16 cc)

15–22.

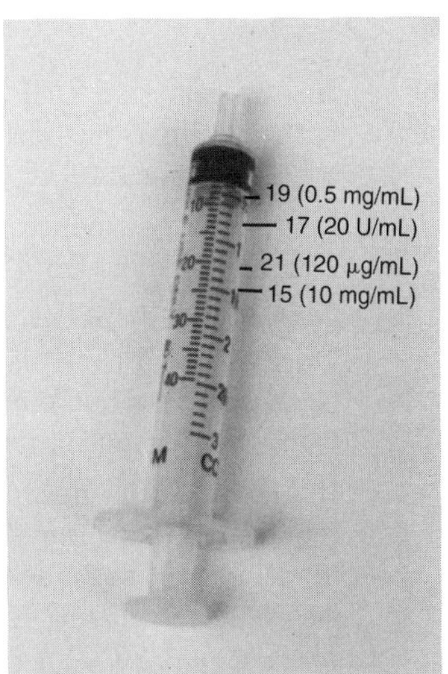

7-8. INSULIN SOLUTIONS

Insulin solutions are used to restore blood sugar levels to the normal range in diabetic clients. Today, insulin must be injected, although some researchers are optimistic that there will soon be an inhalable alternative. There are many types of insulins that are effective in the body for varying periods of time. Some clients require a combination of insulin types to regulate their blood sugar.

The commonly available strength of insulin solution is 100 U/mL, which is denoted as U-100; the solution is injected subcutaneously with a special insulin syringe. On rare occasions, a health care center (such as a nursing home) may face a very unusual emergency situation in which the mandated insulin syringe is not on hand; the nurse then uses a tuberculin syringe. In this case, it is necessary to calculate the number of milliliters corresponding to the number of insulin units prescribed. The label U-100 indicates 100 insulin units per milliliter.

U-100 = 100 insulin units per milliliter

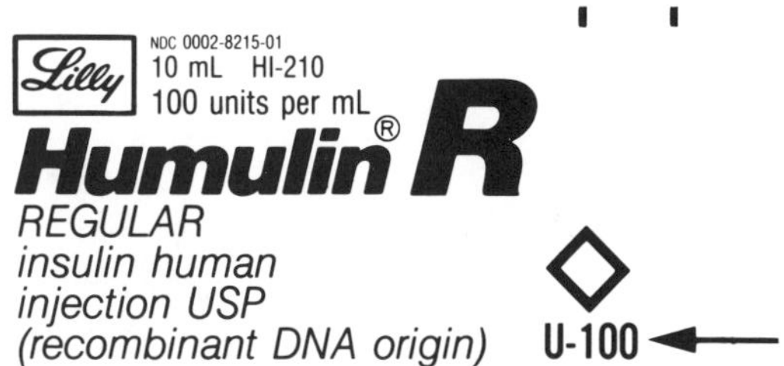

Lilly
NDC 0002-8215-01
10 mL HI-210
100 units per mL
Humulin® R
REGULAR
insulin human
injection USP
(recombinant DNA origin)
U-100

Examples

1. Insulin injection USP (regular pork insulin) is a solution prepared with insulin from pork pancreas. It is available in 10-mL vials with a strength of U-100.
2. Insulin zinc suspension USP (Lente) is a suspension prepared with zinc and insulin from beef pancreas and is available in a strength of U-100.
3. Human insulin (semisynthetic) injection (regular) is derived from pork pancreas but modified to be structurally identical to insulin from the human pancreas. It is available in U-100 form.
4. Individuals who need combinations of insulin vary greatly in their requirements. Some clients may use a commercially available combination of insulin solutions, such as Novolin 70/30. This preparation is a mixture of 70 U of NPH insulin (an intermediate-acting insulin) and 30 U of regular insulin (a short-acting insulin). In most cases, however, the client or the nurse has to mix two types of insulin together, using two separate insulin solutions.

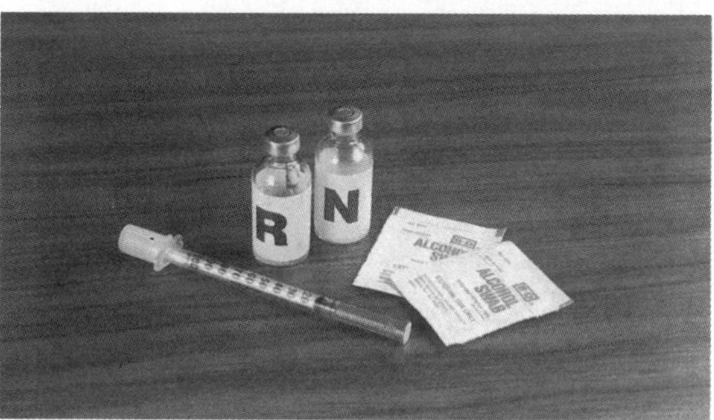

5. To calculate the volume (in cubic centimeters) of insulin suspension U-100 corresponding to a dose of 10 U, use a proportion or the formula $\frac{D}{H} \times Q$, based on the following table.

x cc	for	10 U
1 cc	for	100 U

Result: 0.1 cc

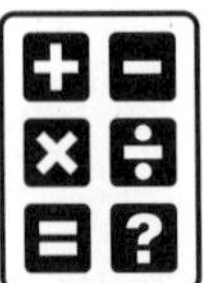

SAMPLE EXERCISES

1. Mr. Xan is having an injection of 0.5 mL of regular pork insulin. Using the strength U-100, determine how many units of insulin he is receiving.
2. Mrs. Yesper is to take 30 U of Lente. If the strength is U-100, state the corresponding number of milliliters in the dose.
3. The client must receive 28 U of NPH insulin and 6 U of regular insulin. A strict procedure is followed to mix the two insulins in one syringe. What is the total number of insulin units in the syringe?

ANSWERS

1. ***Table:***

x U	in	0.5 mL
100 U	in	1 mL

Result: 50 U

2. ***Table:***

x mL	for	30 U
1 mL	for	100 U

Result: 0.3 mL

3. **34 U**

The Insulin Syringe

Insulin syringes are used **only** for insulin injections. A typical U-100 syringe (shown below) has one scale calibrated for both cubic centimeters and insulin unit measurements, up to 1 cc and 100 U.

Examples

1.

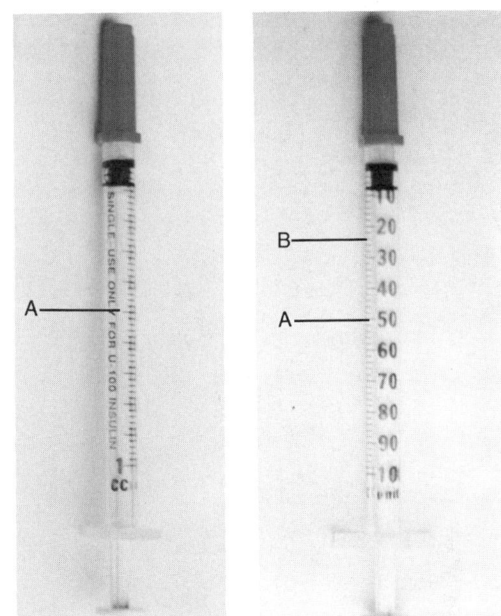

On this 1-cc (100-unit) insulin syringe, 10 U = 0.1 cc, and each small subdivision of the scale represents 2 U, or 0.02 cc.

(a) The arrows marked A measure 50 U (or 0.5 cc);

(b) To locate 24 U, or 0.24 mL, look between 20 and 30, and count markings in 2's from 20 to 30, until reaching 24 (the point marked B).

2.

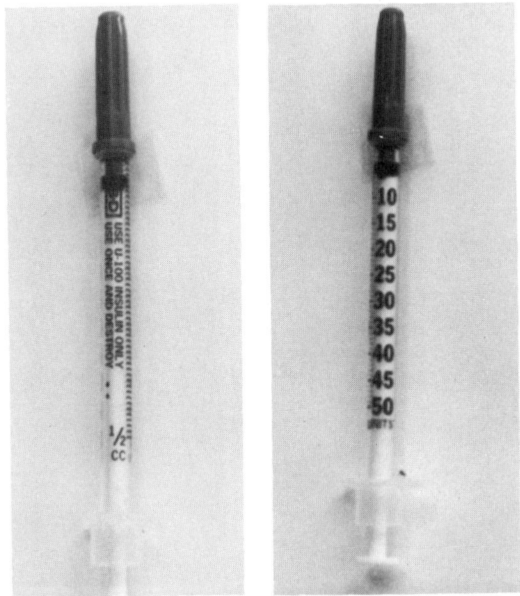

On this $\frac{1}{2}$-cc insulin syringe, 50 U = $\frac{1}{2}$ cc (0.5 cc); thus, 1 U = 0.01 cc. Each small subdivision of the scale represents 1 U, or 0.01 cc.

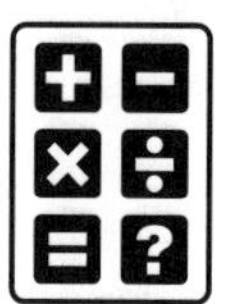

SAMPLE EXERCISES

Exercises 1 – 3.

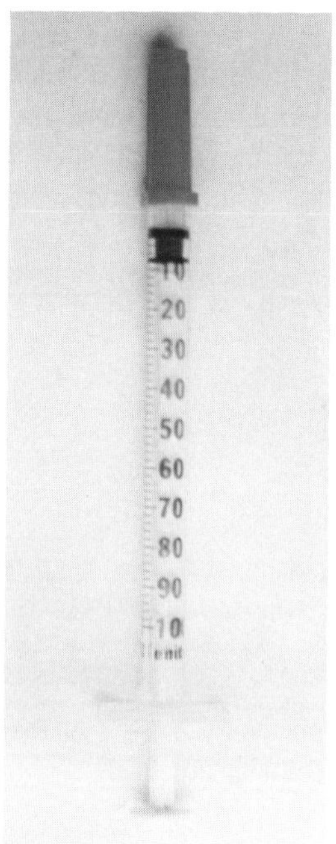

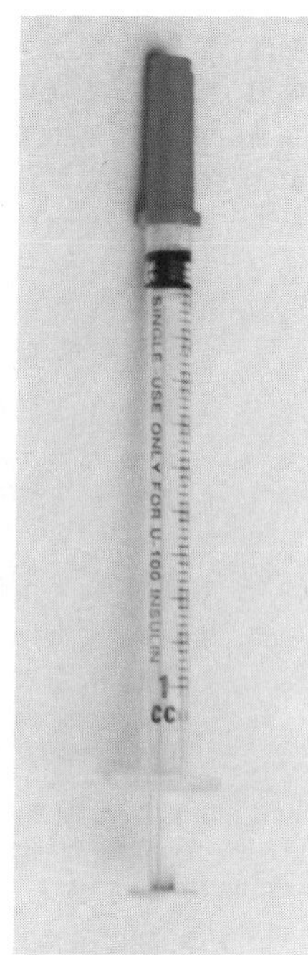

On this 1-cc, U-100 syringe:

1. Locate 64 U and place #1 next to your arrow.
2. Use an arrow to show 0.76 mL; label this arrow #2.
3. State the volume (in cubic centimeters) corresponding to 64 U.

ANSWERS

1–2.

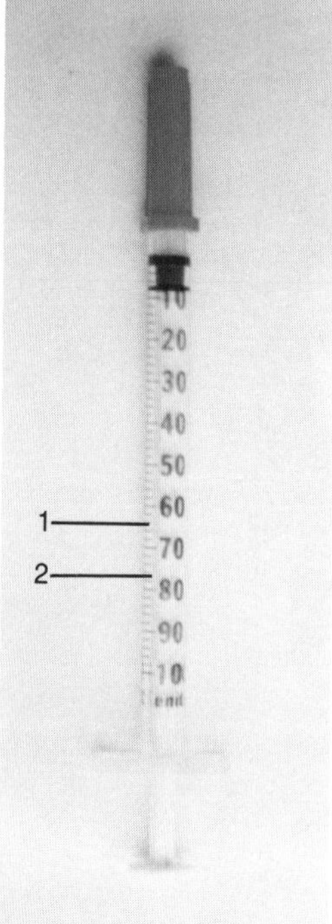

3. 0.64 cc

Exercises 1–8. Find the volume indicated by the plunger.

EXERCISES 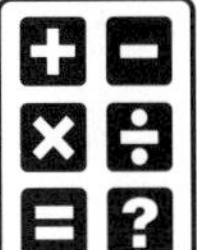

1. 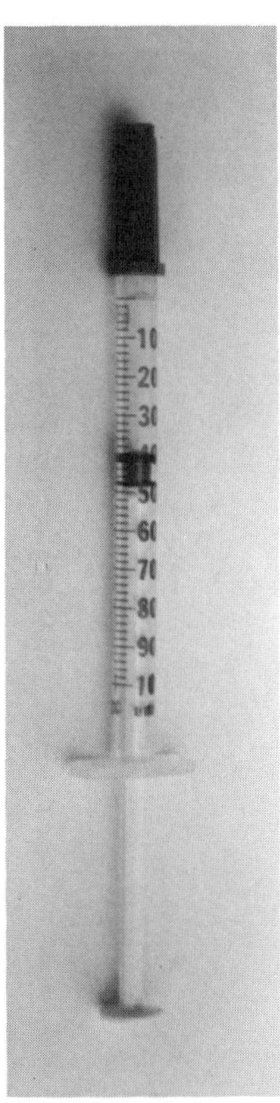

2. 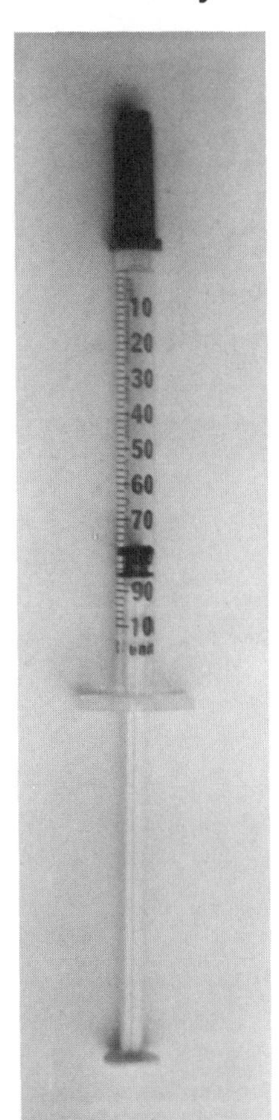

3. 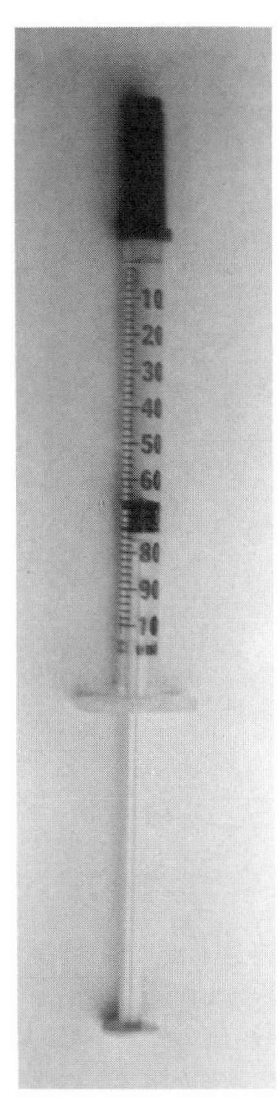

4. 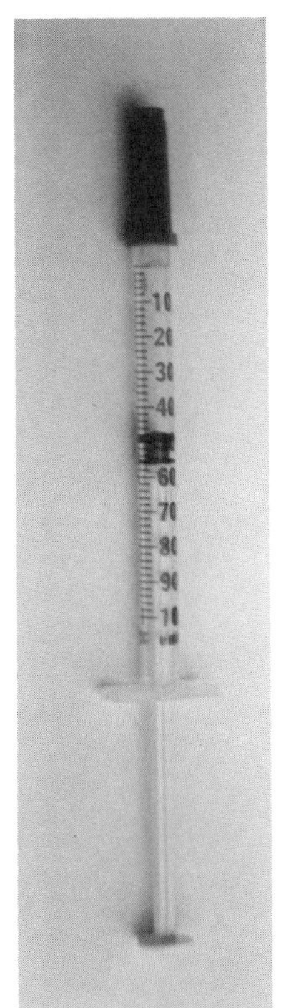

5. 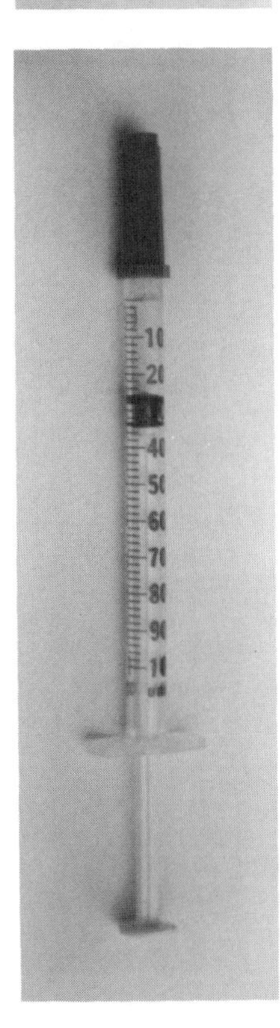

6. 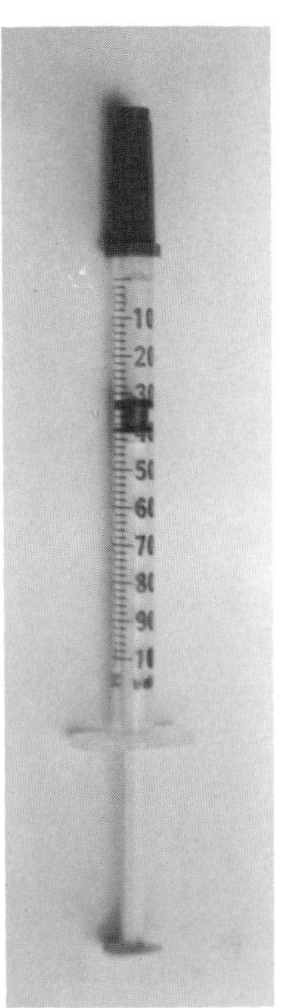

7.

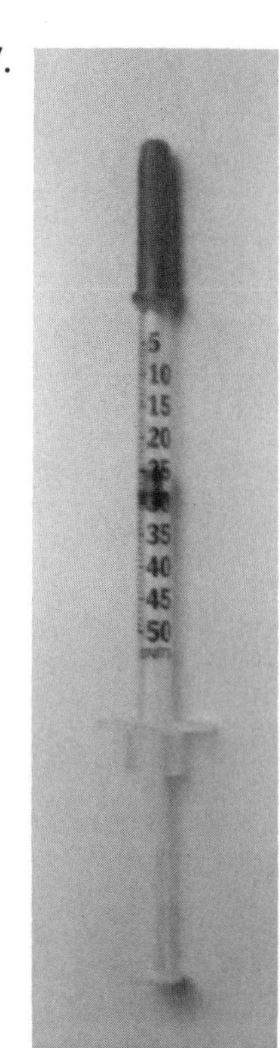

8.

Exercises 9–16. Mark each of the following doses on the accompanying syringe. Label each arrow with the indicated volume.

9. 50 U
10. 74 U
11. 58 U
12. 86 U
13. 42 U
14. 54 U
15. 63 U
16. 92 U

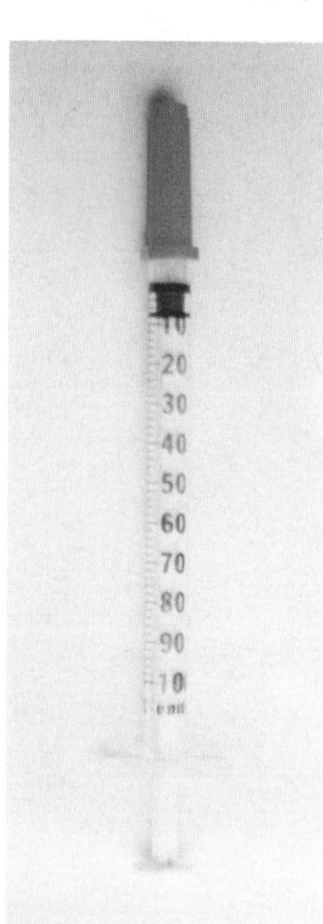

17. Doctor's order: Insulin suspension 30 U. Client has on hand: Insulin suspension U-100. How much (in cubic centimeters) should the patient be taking?
18. Some people need injections of U-500 insulin. What strength does the term U-500 imply?
19. U-100 insulin syringes come in various sizes including (a) $\frac{3}{10}$ cc, (b) $\frac{1}{2}$ cc, and (c) 1 cc. What is the maximum number of units of insulin that can be drawn from each of these syringes?

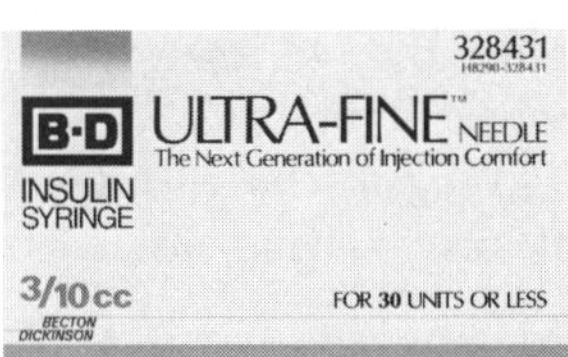

20. On the $\frac{1}{2}$-cc syringe for U-100 insulin, 25 U and 0.25 cc correspond. Why?

ANSWERS 1. 40 U 3. 66 U 5. 26 U 7. 25 U

9–15.

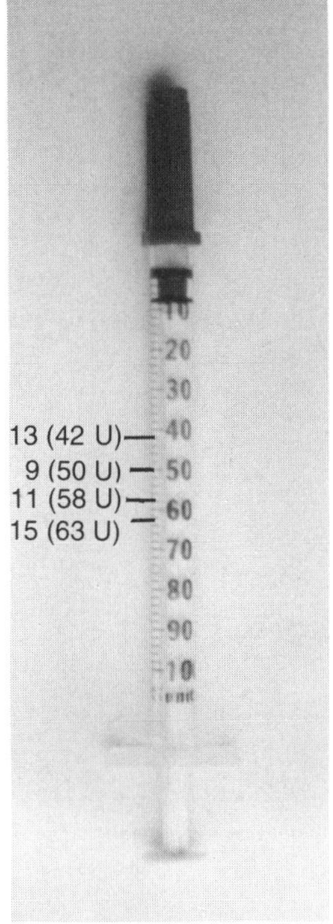

17. 0.3 cc 19. (a) 30 U (b) 50 U (c) 100 U

7-9. AVOIDING ERRORS: CHECKING THE STRENGTH OF THE SOLUTION

Because of the variety of syringes, it is possible to mistake one for another. Physicians and nurses have reported such medication errors as overdosage based on not reading the label or the scale on the syringe.

Errors may also occur when computing the amount of drug to add to a solution, the amount of solution to add to a drug, or the amount of solution to administer. To prevent errors, one may check by recalculating the strength of the resulting solution to see if it matches the original intentions.

Examples

1. Amount of solution desired: 10 mL
   Strength of solution desired: 1 g/5 mL
   Is the strength correct if, in 10 mL of the solution there are 2 g of drug?
   Yes, because 2 g/10 mL = 1 g/5 mL.
2. Amount of drug to be diluted: 40 mg
   Resulting strength desired: 1 mg/mL
   Is it correct to dilute 40 mg to the 40-mL level?
   Yes, because 40 mg/40 mL = 1 mg/mL.
3. Doctor's order: 25 g IV
   Available: 10% solution
   Is it correct to administer 2.5 mL of the solution?
   No, because 10% = 10 g/100 mL = 25 g/250 mL; thus, 250 mL must be administered.

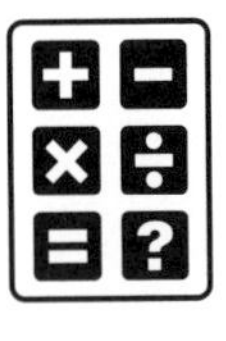

SAMPLE EXERCISES

1. Amount of solution desired: 350 mL
   Strength of solution desired: 1 g/5 mL
   Is it correct to have 70 mg of drug in 350 mL of solution?
2. Amount of drug to be diluted: 600 mg
   Resulting strength desired: 10 mg/mL
   Is it correct to add diluent to the 60-mL level?
3. Doctor's order: mannitol 20 g IV
   Available: 10% solution
   Is it correct to administer 200 mL?

ANSWERS 1. No, 70 mg/350 mL = 1 mg/5 mL, not 1 g/5 mL. 2. Yes, 600 mg/60 mL = 10 mg/mL 3. Yes, 20 g/200 mL = 10 g/100 mL = 10%

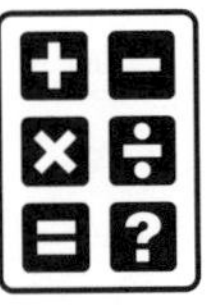

EXERCISES

1. Amount of drug to be diluted: 400 mg
   Resulting strength desired: 10 mg/mL
   Is it correct to add diluent to the 40-mL level?
2. Amount of drug to be diluted: 2.5 g
   Resulting strength desired: 10%
   Is it correct to add diluent to the 25-mL level?
3. Amount of drug to be diluted: 600 mg
   Resulting strength desired: 20 mg/mL
   Is it correct to add diluent to the 40-mL level?
4. Doctor's order: mannitol 15 g IV
   Available: 10% solution
   Is it correct to administer 150 mL?

5. Doctor's order: amitriptyline 20 mg IM qid
   Available: 10 mg/mL
   Is it correct to administer 2 mL?
6. Doctor's order: hydromorphone 5 mg SC q4h prn
   Available vial: 2 mg/mL
   Is it correct to administer 2.5 mL?
7. Doctor's order: bethanecol 2.5 mg SC q6h
   Label states: 5 mg/mL
   Is it correct to administer 2.5 mL?
8. Doctor's order: butorphanol tartrate 2.4 mg IM
   In stock: 2 mg/mL
   Is it correct to administer 1.2 mL?
9. Ordered: butorphanol tartrate 1.8 mg IV q4h prn
   Available: butorphanol tartrate 2 mg/mL
   Is it correct to administer 3.6 mL?
10. Amount of solution desired: 300 mL
    Strength of solution desired: 1:5
    Is it correct to have 60 mg of drug in 300 mL of solution?
11. Amount of drug to be diluted: 500 mg
    Resulting strength desired: 0.2%
    Is it correct to add diluent to the 200-mL level?
12. Amount of solution desired: 500 mL
    Strength of solution desired: 0.9%
    In 500 mL of solution, is it correct to have 4.5 g of drug?
13. Amount of solution desired: 800 mL
    Strength of solution desired: 5%
    Is it correct if the 800-mL solution contains 40 g of drug?
14. Amount of solution desired: 400 mL
    Strength of solution desired: 50 μg/mL
    Is it correct to have 20 mg of drug in 400 mL of solution?
15. Amount of solution desired: 30 minims
    Strength of solution desired: 1 grain/10 minims
    Is it correct to have 180 mg of drug in 30 minims?
16. Amount of drug to be diluted: 1 g
    Resulting strength desired: 0.4 g/cc
    Is it correct to add diluent to the 0.4-mL level?
17. Order: calcitonin 100 IU SC
    On hand: 2-mL vial of calcitonin 200 IU/mL
    Is it correct to administer 1 mL?
18. Doctor's order: clindamycin phosphate injection 360 mg IM
    Available: 1.2 g in 200 mL
    Is it correct to administer 0.3 mL?
19. Ampicillin 2 g q6h has been ordered.
    Available vial: 250 mg/mL
    Is it correct to administer 2.5 mL?
20. Ordered: atropine sulfate gr $\frac{1}{120}$ IM
    On hand: atropine sulfate injection USP 400 μg/mL
    Is it correct to administer 1.25 mL?

ANSWERS 1. Yes, 400 mg/40 mL = 10 mg/mL 3. No, 600 mg/40 mL = 15 mg/mL 5. Yes, 20 mg/2 mL = 10 mg/mL 7. No, 2.5 mg/2.5 mL = 1 mg/mL, not 5 mg/mL 9. No, 1.8 mg/3.6 mL = 0.5 mg/mL, not 2 mg/mL 11. No, 500 mg/200 mL = 250 mg/100 mL = 0.25 g/100 mL = 0.25%, not 0.2% 13. Yes, 40 g/800 mL = 5 g/100 mL = 5% 15. Yes, 180 mg/30 minims = 3 grains/30 minims = 1 grain/10 minims 17. No, 100 IU/mL is not = 200 IU/mL 19. No, 2 g/2.5 mL = 800 mg/mL

7-10. SUMMARY

1. A homogeneous mixture of at least one substance (the **solute**) dissolved in another substance (the **diluent**) is called a **solution.**

   Example

   A normal saline solution is a homogeneous mixture of salt (the solute) and water (the diluent).

2. STRENGTH OF SOLUTION

   Amount of solute/amount of solution. Because the solution is homogeneous, the strength is the same for any portion of the solution.

	Ratio Strength	Percent Strength
Solid in solid:	w/w	Number of grams in 100 g of solution
Solid in liquid:	w/v	Number of grams in 100 mL of solution
Liquid in liquid:	v/v	Number of milliliters in 100 mL of solution

   Whenever units are not specified, weight is understood to be measured in grams only, and volume is understood to be measured in milliliters only.

   Examples

   (a) A 2:5 w/v solution means 2 g of solid in a total of 5 mL of solution.
   (b) Strength of a magnesium sulfate w/v solution may be 5 g/10 mL = 50% or 1:2.

3. FINDING THE AMOUNT OF PURE DRUG IN A SOLUTION

   If we know the strength and volume of a therapeutic solution, we can compute the amount of pure drug in the solution.

   Example

   How much magnesium sulfate is in 20 mL of a 50% magnesium sulfate solution?

   Table: x g 20 mL
   50 g 100 mL

   Result (by proportion or formula): 10 g

   Shortcut: 50% of 20 = 0.5 × 20 = 10

4. FINDING THE AMOUNT OF SOLUTION TO ADMINISTER

If we know the prescribed amount of pure drug and the strength of the solution to be used, we can compute how much solution to administer.

Examples

(a) How much of a 50% magnesium sulfate solution should be administered for a dose of 15 g?

Table: x mL for 15 g
100 mL for 50 g

Result: 30 mL

(b) For a dose of 0.4 g, how much solution should we draw from a vial labeled 1 g/2.5 mL?

Table: x mL for 0.4 g
2.5 mL for 1 g

Result: 1 mL

5. TO LOCATE A DESIRED MEASUREMENT ON THE SYRINGE

The ring (nearest the needle end) of the plunger in the syringe shows the amount of liquid in the syringe.

(a) Read from the smallest marked value to the greatest.
(b) Find the approximate location between the two closest marked numbers.
(c) Count markings to find the exact location and check.

6. INSULIN SOLUTIONS

Insulin solutions are used to restore blood sugar levels to the normal range. The most common form of insulin solution is U-100 (100 insulin units per milliliter); this solution is injected subcutaneously with a special insulin syringe. On the scale of a typical U-100 syringe, there are both cubic centimeter and insulin unit calibrations. 10 U = 0.1 cc.

7. AVOIDING ERRORS: CHECKING THE STRENGTH OF THE SOLUTION

Two labels may name the same drug, but the strengths of the solutions may differ. Thus, it is important to check the details of the label. Sometimes you must do a calculation to check that the strength of a prepared solution is as desired.

Example

A powdered drug comes in a vial containing 2.4 g. To have a 40% solution, a diluent is injected into the vial. If the total volume in the vial is 6 mL after the diluent is injected, is the resulting strength correct?

Yes, because

$$\frac{2.4\text{ g}}{6\text{ mL}} = \frac{0.4\text{ g}}{1\text{ mL}} = \frac{40\text{ g}}{100\text{ mL}} = 40\%$$

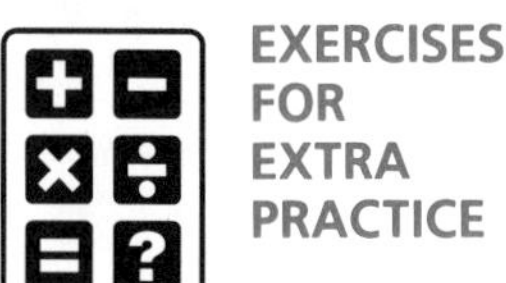

EXERCISES FOR EXTRA PRACTICE

1. If a solution is prepared by diluting 240 mg of pure drug to 30 mL with a compatible solution, what is the ratio strength of the result?
2. A 5% v/v solution means 5 mL of a liquid in sufficient solvent to make how much solution?
3. How much boric acid powder is contained in 40 mL of boric acid solution 1:500?
4. What is the weight of the solute in 500 mL of a 7.5% w/v solution?

Exercises 5–8. The following table gives information about required w/v solutions. Complete the table.

	Volume	Strength	Weight of Pure Drug
5.	30 mL		10 g
6.	20 mL	1:4	
7.		1 mg/5 mL	0.5 mg
8.		0.1%	1 g

Exercises 9–12. On the 10-cc syringe, locate the indicated measurement. Mark the appropriate volume next to each arrow.

9. 5.2 cc
10. 1.6 mL
11. 2.6 mL
12. 3.2 cc

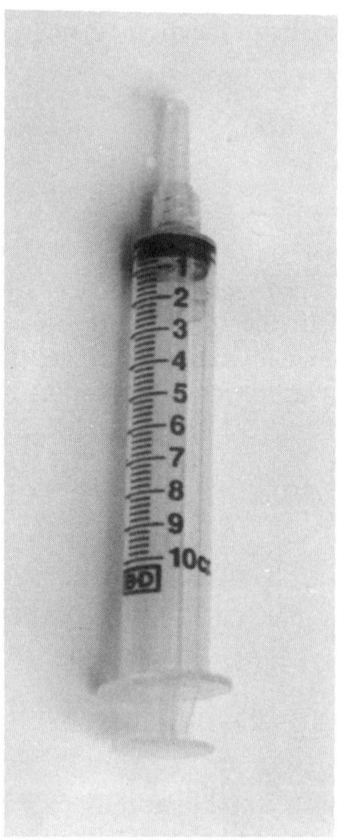

Exercises 13–16. On the 3-cc syringe, locate the indicated measurement. Mark the volume next to each arrow.

13. 2.2 cc
14. 1.3 mL
15. 20 M
16. 35 M

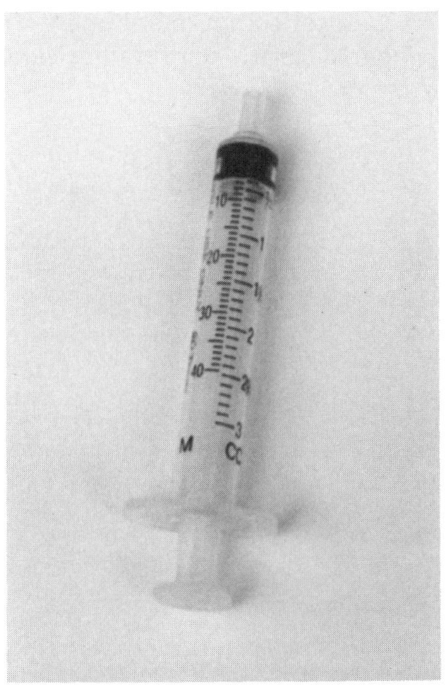

Exercises 17–20. On the 30-cc syringe, locate the indicated measurement. Mark the appropriate volume next to each arrow.

17. 28 cc

18. 18 mL

19. $\frac{1}{4}$ oz

20. $\frac{7}{8}$ oz

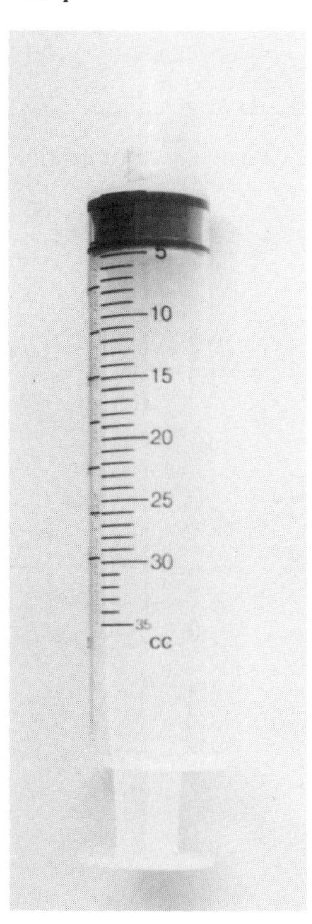

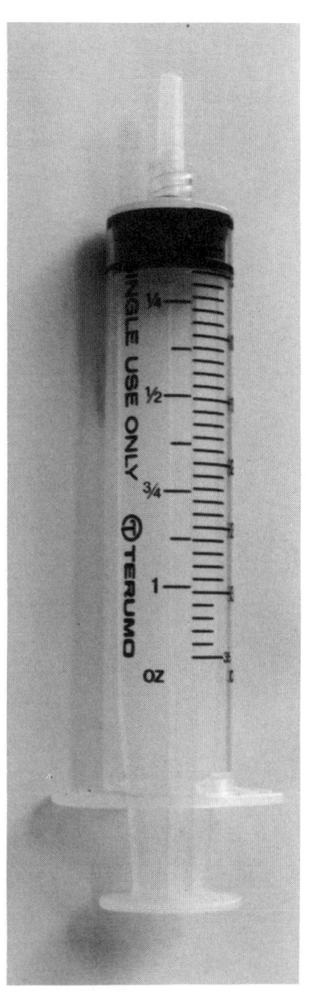

Exercises 21–24. For each dose, compute and mark the desired volume on the 3-cc syringe. Place the appropriate volume next to each arrow.

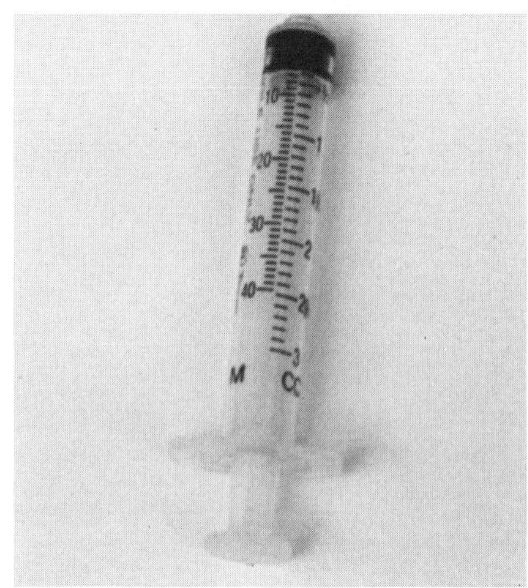

Dose Required	Strength of Available Solution
21. dexpanthenol IM 375 mg	250 mg/mL
22. glycopyrrolate (Robinul) IM 0.1 mg	0.2 mg/mL
23. magnesium sulfate IM 1 g	50%
24. belladonna (Bellafoline) SC 500 μg	0.5 mg/mL

Exercises 25–26. Check the following statements.

25. One liter of a 1:4 v/v glycerin solution contains 250 mL of glycerin.

26. To make 600 mL of a 0.9% w/v sodium chloride enema solution, the diluent must be combined with 5.4 g of sodium chloride.

ANSWERS 1. 8 mg/mL 3. 0.08 g, or 80 mg 5. $\frac{1}{3}$ 7. 2.5 mL

9, 11.

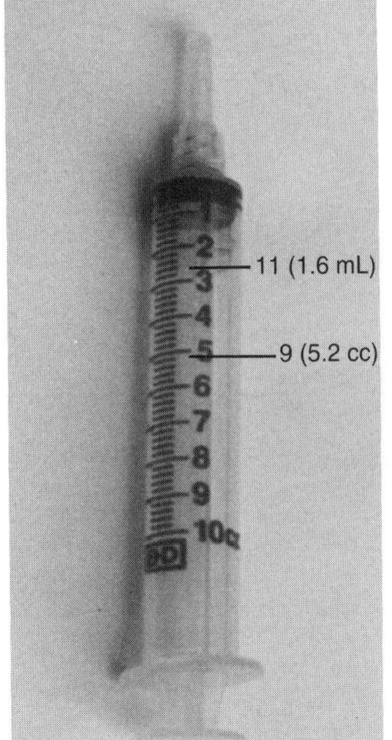

13–16.

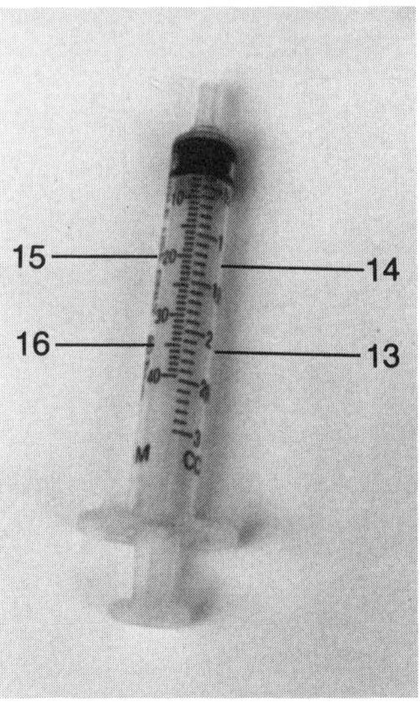

17, 19.

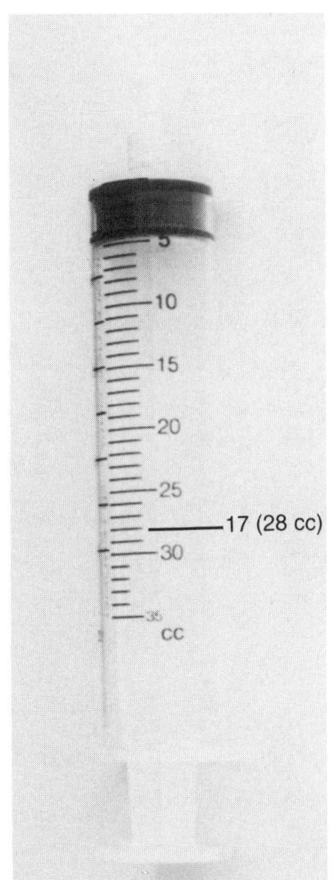

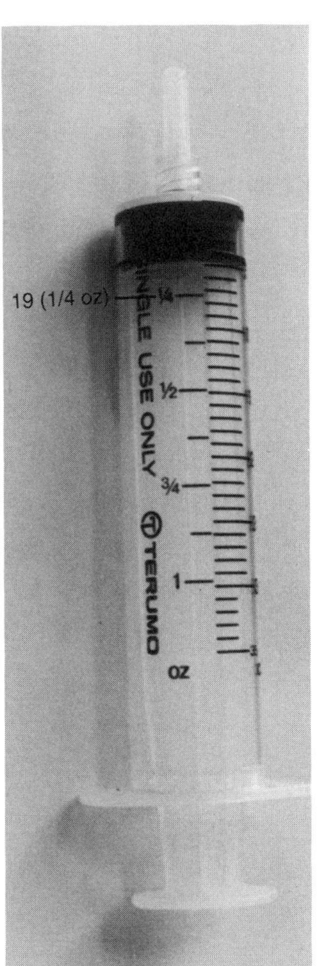

21–24.

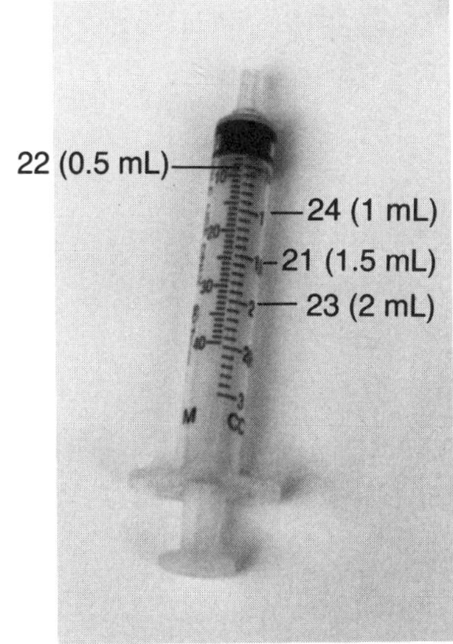

25. Check: $\dfrac{250\ \text{mL}}{1\ \text{L}} = \dfrac{250\ \text{mL}}{1000\ \text{mL}} = \dfrac{1}{4} = 1:4$

CHAPTER TEST

1. Express the strength of a solution that contains 2.8 mg in 4 mL. 1. ____________

2. How many grams of solute are in 550 mL of a 2.5% w/v solution? 2. ____________

3. How many milliliters of solute are in 1 L of a 9:10,000 v/v solution? 3. ____________

4. Doctor's order: gentamycin sulfate 100 mg q8h IM
   Available: gentamicin sulfate 60 mg/1.5 mL
   Explain how to carry out the doctor's order. 4. ____________

5. An insulin suspension is labeled U-100. What is the strength of the suspension? 5. ____________

6. Which is the weakest ferrous sulfate solution?
   (a) 75 mg/0.6 mL
   (b) 125 mg/mL
   (c) 220 mg/5 mL 6. ____________

7. Determine the calibration of the syringe shown below. 7. ____________

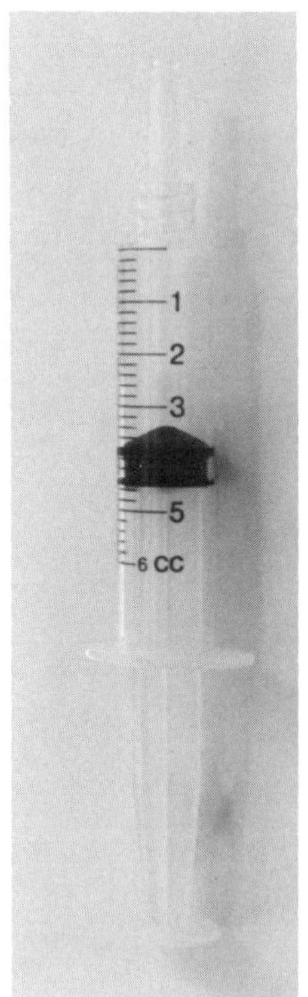

8. What volume is indicated by the position of the plunger in the syringe shown above? 8. ____________

9. On the same syringe, show 5.4 cc with an arrow.

10. Doctor's order: morphine sulfate 15 mg SC
    Available: morphine sulfate solution $\frac{1}{6}$ grain in 1 mL
    Mark the dose on the 3-cc syringe on the next page.

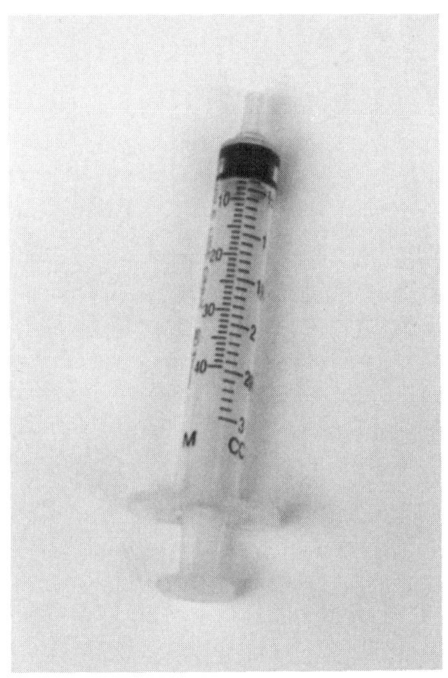

ANSWERS 1. 2.8 mg/4 mL, or 0.7 mg/mL, or 7 mg/10 mL 2. 13.75 g 3. 0.9 mL 4. Give an intramuscular injection of 2.5 mL every 8 h 5. 100 U/mL 6. (c) 7. 0.2 cc 8. 3.8 cc

9.

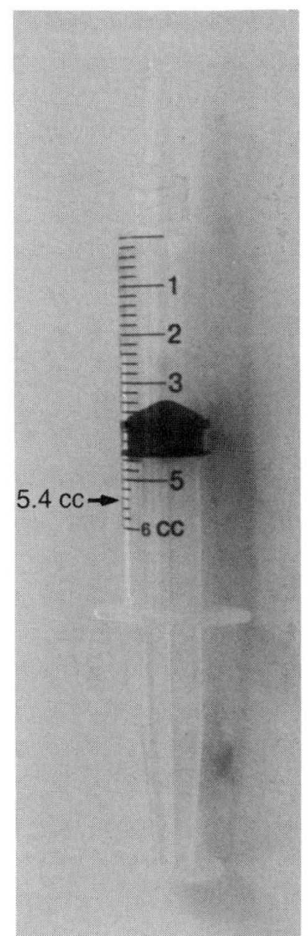

10.

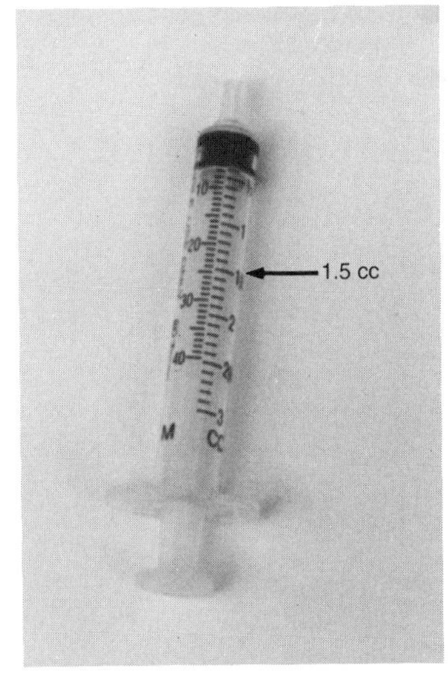

EIGHT

Intravenous Therapy

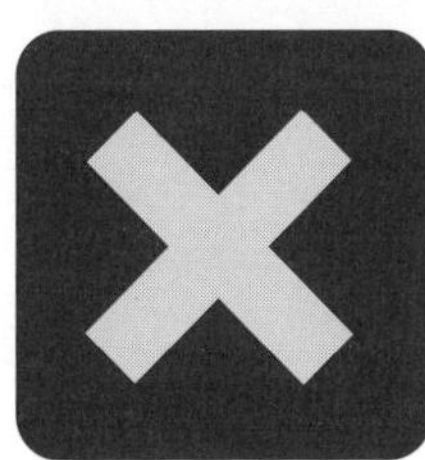

▶ OUTLINE

8-1. INTRODUCTION
8-2. DETERMINING DOSAGE
8-3. DETERMINING THE CALIBRATION ON AN IV SOLUTION BAG
8-4. FINDING THE IV DROP FACTOR
8-5. DETERMINING THE IV DRIP RATE
8-6. SHORTCUT FORMULA FOR DRIP RATE
8-7. IV THERAPY DELIVERY SYSTEMS
8-8. SPECIAL CALCULATIONS FOR IV DRUGS
8-9. AVOIDING ERRORS: ADHERING TO SAFE DRUG DOSAGE PARAMETERS
8-10. SUMMARY

▶ OBJECTIVES

After studying this chapter, you will be able to:

1. Identify abbreviations for common types of intravenous (IV) solutions.
2. Read the markings for calibration on an IV bag or bottle.
3. Differentiate between a macrodrip and a microdrip IV administration set.
4. Determine the drop factor for various types of IV administration sets.
5. Calculate IV flow rate and drip rate.
6. Describe the purpose of IV controllers and pumps.
7. Identify four systems for IV drug delivery.
8. Calculate the dosage of selected IV medications.
9. Calculate the flow rate and drip rate needed to deliver the prescribed dosage of IV medication.
10. Check drug dosages to avoid errors in medication administration.

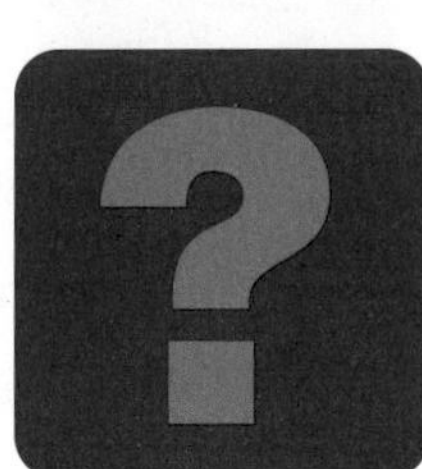

8-1. INTRODUCTION

What is intravenous therapy? Intravenous (IV) therapy is the method used to instill fluids or medications directly into the blood stream. The advantage of this medication administration method over subcutaneous or intramuscular injections is the *immediate* availability of the medication to the body.

In addition to medication administration, the intravenous route is used to meet nutritional requirements, replace electrolytes (chemicals such as sodium and potassium), or give blood and blood products. Whatever the need, the nurse is responsible for administering the IV therapy correctly.

Type of Calculations Necessary for IV Therapy

The intravenous administration of fluids often requires a calculation of the length of time that the infusion takes or the amount of fluid in milliliters that should be administered in 1 h. The nurse may also need to compute the amount of fluid per minute that is needed to deliver the total fluid volume prescribed by the physician. Determining the volume per minute allows the nurse actually to count the drops delivered by the IV system in 1 min.

Examples

1. The doctor orders 1000 mL of 5%D/$\frac{1}{2}$NS solution to be administered over 6 h. The nurse must calculate the number of milliliters the client should receive per hour.
2. An IV piggyback of vancomycin diluted in 100 mL of normal saline needs to infuse over a 60-min period. The nurse must calculate the solution rate in drops per minute.

Proficiency Gauge

You may already be experienced with intravenous therapy and know how to calculate dosages and rates. To determine whether you understand IV therapy sufficiently, complete the following exercises, checking your answers only after you have completed all the questions.

1. How many milliliters have infused from the 500 mL bag of IV solution shown on the next page? 1. ____________
2. The physician's order for IV fluids is: 1000 mL 5%D/RL to infuse over 6 h. How many milliliters should infuse each hour? 2. ____________
3. What is the usual drop factor for microdrip IV administration sets (IV tubing)? 3. ____________
4. An IV solution needs to infuse at 75 mL/h. If the drop factor of the IV tubing is 15 gtt = 1 mL, what should the drip rate of the IV fluid be? 4. ____________
5. The physician's order for IV fluids is: Give 1000 mL 5%D/0.2NS at 83 mL/h. How many

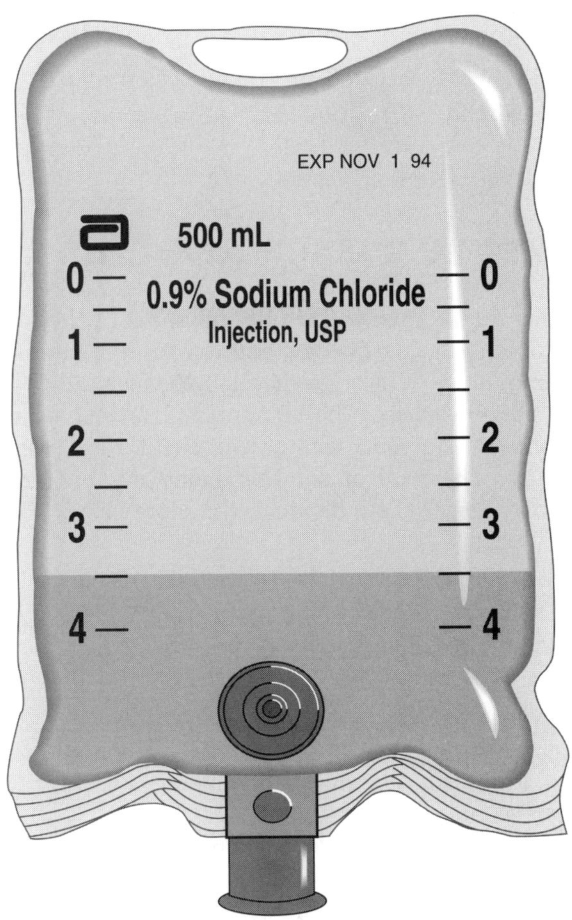

hours (approximately) does it take to complete the IV infusion? 5. ____________

6. Calculate the drip rate needed to provide the amount of IV fluid ordered in Exercise 5. The drop factor is 60 gtt = 1 mL. 6. ____________

7. The physician's order is: 1000 mL 5%D/$\frac{1}{2}$NS with 40 mEq KCl at 100 mL/h. How many milliequivalents of KCl (potassium) does the client receive each hour? 7. ____________

8. The physician's order is: Give continuous IV heparin infusion at 1500 U/h. The available solution from the pharmacy is 20,000 U in 1000 mL 5%D/W. What should the flow rate of the solution be to deliver the prescribed amount of heparin? 8. ____________

9. A client receives 60 mL/h of aminophylline 1 g diluted in 1000 mL normal saline. Calculate in milligrams the amount of drug the client is receiving per hour. 9. ____________

10. An IV solution is prepared with 400 mg of dopamine in 500 mL 5%D/W. The physician orders a dosage of 6 mcg/kg/min. Calculate the amount of drug in micrograms per minute and the drip rate for a client weighing 220 lb (DF: 1 mL = 60 gtt). 10. ____________

ANSWERS 1. 350 mL 2. 167 mL/h 3. 60 gtt = 1 mL 4. 19 gtt/min 5. 12 h 6. 83 gtt/min 7. 4 mEq/h 8. 75 mL/h 9. 60 mg 10. 600 mcg; 45 gtt/min

8-2. DETERMINING DOSAGE

Dosage instructions for IV therapy include the name of the solution or drug to administer and the quantity, frequency, and duration of administration.

The actual amount of fluid or medication that should be given to a client is determined by the physician. The amount and rate at which it is delivered depends on a number of factors, such as the client's age, weight, and general health condition and the type of solution being administered. As a general rule, the smaller or younger the individual, the more slowly the solution should be infused.

Common Types of Intravenous Solutions

Intravenous fluids most often come commercially prepared in heavy, transparent plastic bags. For solutions that may chemically react with the plastic material, glass bottles are used instead.

Intravenous bags come in various sizes depending on the amount of solution that they contain. The most common sizes are 50 mL, 100 mL, 150 mL, 250 mL, 500 mL, and 1000 mL. The larger bags are typically used to provide large volumes of fluid. The smaller bags are generally used to dilute IV medication.

The physician makes the decision about what type of solution or medication to give and how much. When prescribing IV fluids, the physician typically uses abbreviations to indicate the desired fluid for an individual client. Most of the solutions are either a combination of sugar (dextrose) and water, salt and water (saline), or electrolytes (body chemicals) in solution (such as Ringer's lactate). Some of the common prescribed intravenous fluids are shown below.

COMMONLY PRESCRIBED INTRAVENOUS FLUIDS

NS: Normal saline (label reads 0.9% sodium chloride)
RL: Ringer's lactate solution
5%D/W (also written D5W): 5% dextrose in water
5%D/$\frac{1}{4}$ NS (also written D5/ $\frac{1}{4}$ NS): 5% dextrose in $\frac{1}{4}$ strength normal saline (label reads 0.2% NS)
5%D/$\frac{1}{2}$ NS (also written D5/ $\frac{1}{2}$ NS): 5% dextrose in $\frac{1}{2}$ strength normal saline (label reads 0.45% NS)
5%D/RL (also written D5/RL): 5% dextrose in Ringer's lactate solution

Any combination and any strength of these basic solutions are available. The nurse is not required to prepare these solutions but must be aware that they are different. An example of a label found on an IV bag is shown here:

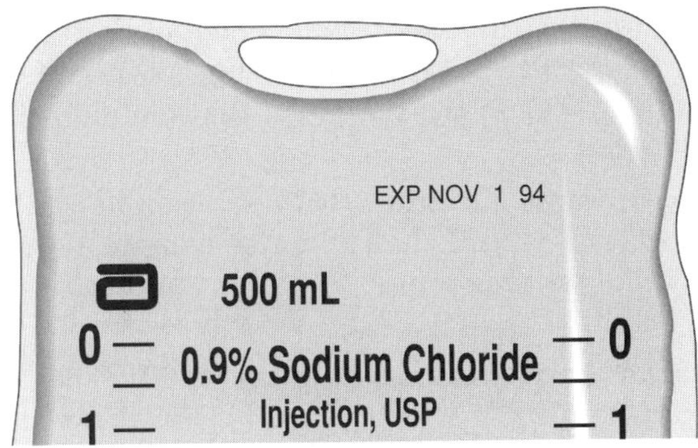

EXP NOV 1 94
500 mL
0.9% Sodium Chloride
Injection, USP

(Sodium Chloride = Normal Saline)

SAMPLE EXERCISES

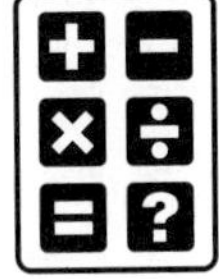

Exercises 1–3. Express the following abbreviations for intravenous fluids in words:

1. 10%D/W
2. 5%D/$\frac{1}{4}$NS
3. 5%D/RL
4. The physician orders an antibiotic to be given via the intravenous route. Which of the following size bags is the medication most likely to be mixed in: 1000-mL bag or a 100-mL bag?

ANSWERS 1. Ten percent dextrose in water 2. Five percent dextrose in quarter strength normal saline 3. Five percent dextrose in Ringer's lactate solution 4. 100-mL bag, because small bags are used for medication administration

Calculating the IV Flow Rate

Although the physician prescribes the actual amount of IV solution to give, the nurse calculates the hourly rate and marks the bag to indicate how much solution should be administered each hour. The hourly rate is also referred to as the **flow rate.** The process, or formula, for finding the amount of fluid to infuse in 1 h is:

AMOUNT OF SOLUTION INFUSED PER HOUR (FLOW RATE)

$$\text{Flow rate} = \frac{\text{Total amount of IV fluid}}{\text{Number of hours for infusion}}$$

Examples

1. The physician orders 1000 mL of 5%D/$\frac{1}{2}$NS to be infused in 10 h. The hourly rate needed for ensuring that the solution is administered in 10 h is 1000 mL/10 h = 100 mL/h.
2. The pharmacist recommends that 700 mg of acyclovir diluted in 150 mL of normal saline run in over 90 min (1.5 h). The hourly

rate needed for ensuring this recommendation is 150 mL/1.5 h = 100 mL/h. (*Note:* The dosage of the drug, 700 mg, is not used in the calculation. We use the *volume* of the solution to be infused to find the flow rate.)

3. The physician wants a continuous IV solution of 5%D/W to infuse at a rate of 125 mL/h. The nurse hangs a 1000-mL bag and calculates the total time that it takes for that bag to run in: $\frac{1000}{125} \times 1 \text{ h} = 8 \text{ h}$.
4. The physician orders 1000 mL to infuse in 6 h. The flow rate should be: 1000 mL/6 h = 166.66 mL/h. The answer is always rounded to the nearest whole number, or 167 mL/h.

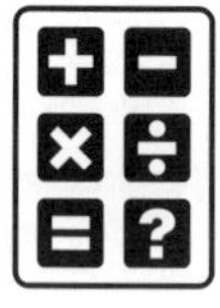

SAMPLE EXERCISES

1. The client should receive 500 mL of normal saline over 8 h. What should the hourly rate be?
2. The physician prescribes a liter of 5%D/RL to infuse in 5 h. What should the hourly rate of the infusion be?
3. The nurse wants to infuse 1 g of Rocephin in 50 mL of IV solution in 30 min (0.5 h). What is the hourly rate?

ANSWERS 1. 500 mL/8 h = 62.5, or 63 mL/h 2. 1000 mL/5 h = 200 mL/h 3. 50 mL/0.5 h = 100 mL/h (*Note:* Always convert minutes to hours when computing milliliters per hour.)

Determining Total Infusion Time and Volume

Even if the IV flow rate is prescribed by the physician, the nurse needs to compute the number of hours that a container of IV solution takes to infuse. Knowing the length of time for infusion helps the nurse carefully monitor the IV therapy. In some cases, the nurse also needs to compute how much fluid has infused over a specified period.

Examples

1. The order for IV therapy is 1000 mL to infuse at 150 mL/h. To find how long it takes for the solution to run in, we divide as shown in the table.

   Table: x h for 1000 mL
   1 h for 150 mL

   Result: $\frac{1000}{150} \times 1 \text{ h} = 6.7 \text{ h}$ (*Note:* Hours are rounded to the nearest tenth.)

2. The client's IV fluids are infusing at 100 mL/h. After 3 h, the nurse checks to determine how much fluid has infused. In this case, the table shows that we should multiply.

   Table: x mL in 3 h
   100 mL in 1 h

   Result: $\frac{3}{1} \times 100 \text{ mL} = 300 \text{ mL}$

SAMPLE EXERCISES

1. If 1000 mL of an IV solution infuses at 167 mL/h, how many hours does it take for the infusion to complete?
2. If an order is for 75 mL/h, how long does a 1000-mL bag last?
3. The client's intravenous fluids are infusing at a rate of 80 mL/h. After 4 h, how much fluid has run in?
4. The physician orders 1000 mL of IV fluid to infuse at 175 mL/h. How long does it take for the solution to run in?

ANSWERS

1. *Table:*
   x h for 1000 mL
   1 h for 167 mL
   Result: 6 h
2. *Table:*
   x h for 1000 mL
   1 h for 75 mL
   Result: 13.3 h
3. *Table:*
   x mL in 4 h
   80 mL in 1 h
   Result: 320 mL
4. *Table:*
   x h for 1000 mL
   1 h for 175 mL
   Result: 5.7 h

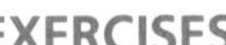

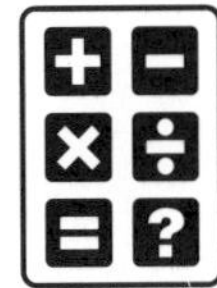

Exercises 1–3. Express the following abbreviations for intravenous fluids in words.

1. 0.9%NS
2. 50%D/W
3. 5%D/0.45 NS

Exercises 4–11. Calculate the flow rates for the following IV fluid orders.

4. 500 mL to infuse in 3 h
5. 250 mL to infuse in 4 h
6. 1000 mL to infuse in 12 h
7. 1000 mL to infuse in 5 h
8. 150 mL to infuse in 90 min
9. 50 mL to infuse in 45 min
10. 500 mL to infuse in 6 h
11. 1000 mL to infuse in 24 h

Exercises 12–20. Find the total infusion time for the following IV fluids.

12. 250 mL at 83 mL/h
13. 500 mL at 60 mL/h
14. 1000 mL at 40 mL/h
15. 1000 mL at 85 mL/h
16. 1000 mL at 120 mL/h
17. 1000 mL at 250 mL/h
18. 2000 mL at 125 mL/h
19. 3000 mL at 125 mL/h
20. 3000 mL at 150 mL/h

ANSWERS 1. Normal saline 3. Five percent dextrose in half strength normal saline 5. 63 mL/h 7. 200 mL/h 9. 67 mL/h 11. 42 mL/h 13. 8.3 h 15. 11.8 h 17. 4 h 19. 24 h

8-3. DETERMINING THE CALIBRATION ON AN IV SOLUTION BAG

The markings for calibration on an IV bag or bottle are not as precise as those on a syringe used for intramuscular or subcutaneous injection. Most bags have markings that indicate 50- and 100-mL increments of the solution as illustrated in Figure 8–1.

After calculating the amount of solution that should infuse in 1 h, the nurse may mark the bag before it is administered to show where the level of fluid should be at each hour. This practice varies, depending on the health care agency's policies. The purpose of marking the bag is to provide the nurse with a quick way of checking that the fluid is infusing on time as prescribed by the physician.

Many health care settings provide commercially prepared IV tapes that make this task a little easier. For settings where this tape is unavailable, regular white surgical tape can be used.

As shown in Figure 8–2, the commercially prepared tape has several preprinted time schedules that help with calculation of the IV rate. The time that the IV bag begins is written at the top next to "Starting time" and is again written at the "0" (zero) level at the top. Then the time is written in for each hour to indicate where the level of the fluid should be at each hour. The example in Figure 8–2 shows the bag labeled for infusion of 1000 mL over an 8-h period, or infusing at 125 mL/h. The start time is 8:30 AM and the "Discontinued time," or the time when the bag should be empty and ready to change, is 4:30 PM, 8 h later.

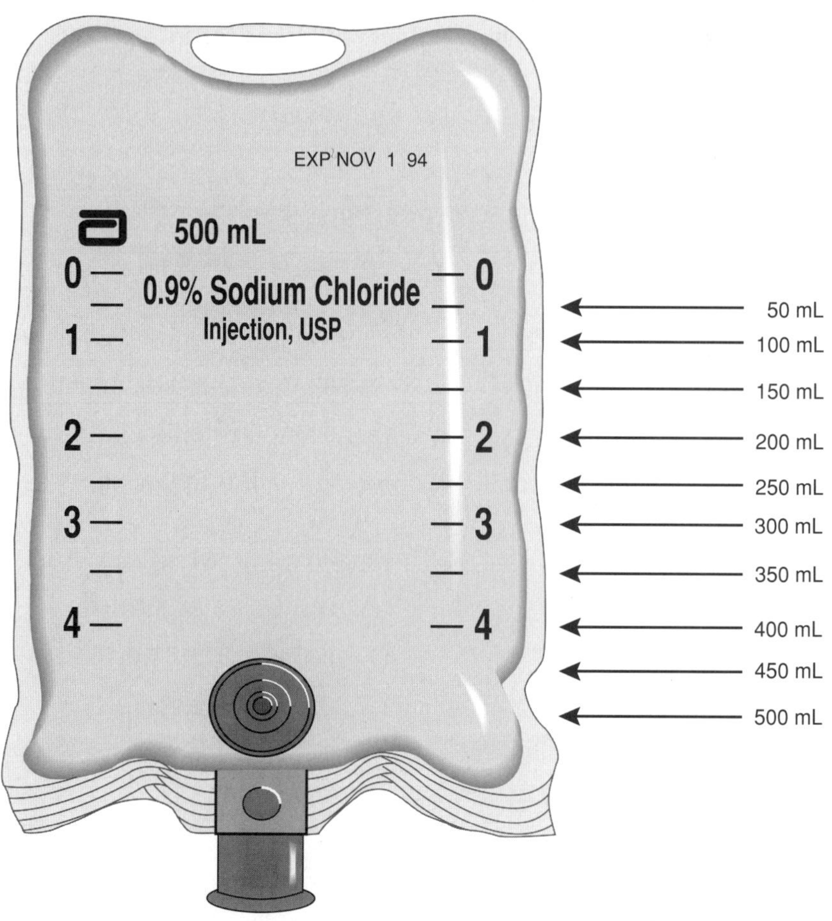

Figure 8–1 Intravenous bag calibrated in 50-mL increments.

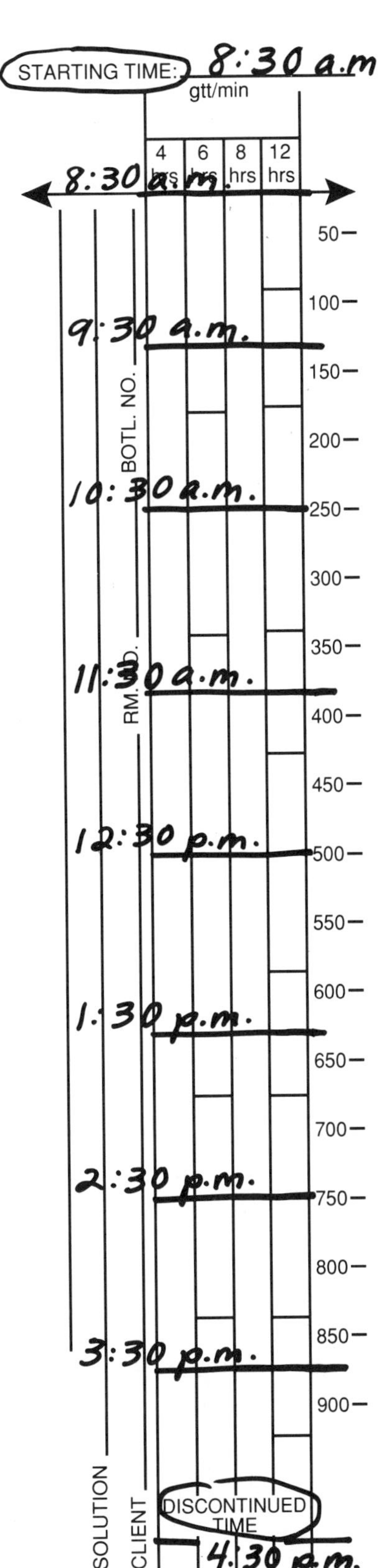

Figure 8–2 Commercially prepared tape for intravenous bags, showing preprinted times for easy calculation of infusion rate.

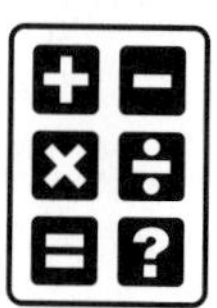

SAMPLE EXERCISES

1. On the tape provided here, label the 1000-mL IV bag to show a rate of 167 mL/h.

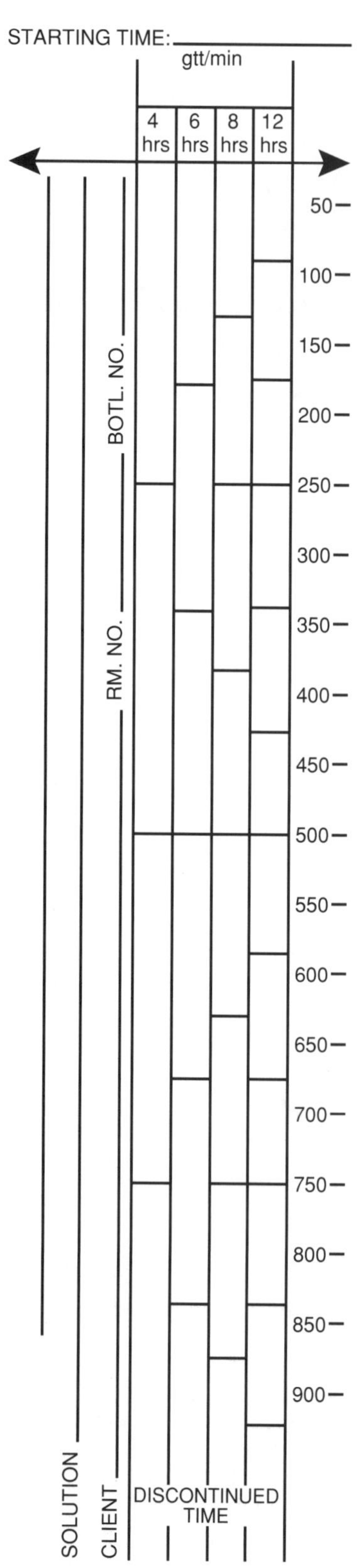

2. How many hours should the 1000 mL just shown take to complete?
3. On the tape provided here, label the 1000-mL bag to show that it runs in over 12 h.

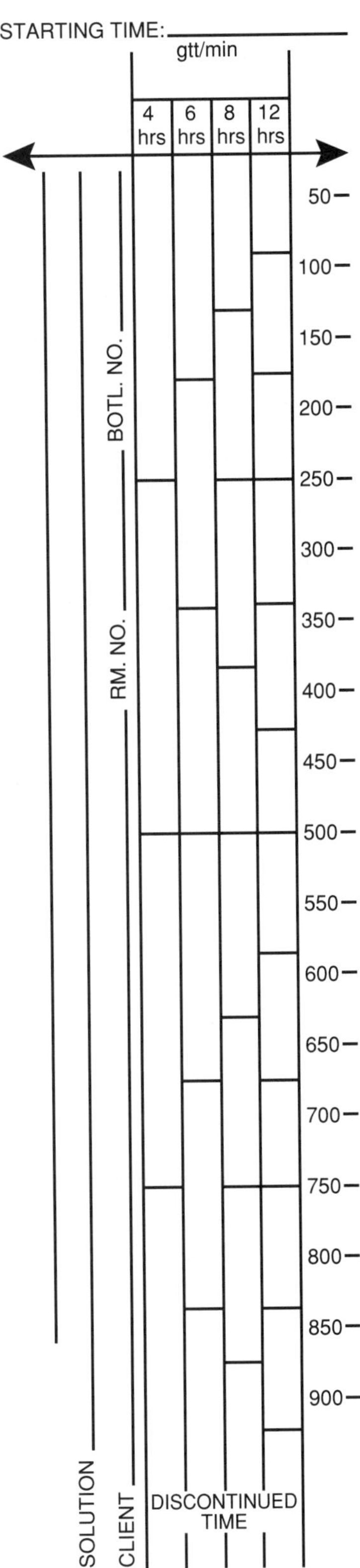

4. What is the hourly rate of the solution for the example in Exercise 3?

ANSWERS

1. STARTING TIME: ____________

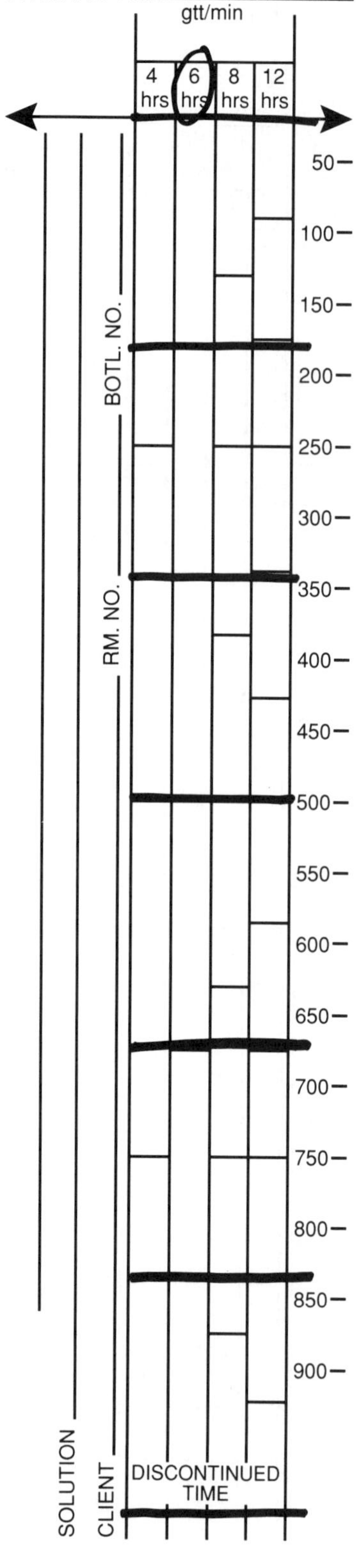

gtt/min

4 hrs	6 hrs	8 hrs	12 hrs

50— 100— 150— 200— 250— 300— 350— 400— 450— 500— 550— 600— 650— 700— 750— 800— 850— 900—

BOTL. NO. ______

RM. NO. ______

SOLUTION ______

CLIENT ______

DISCONTINUED TIME

2. 6 h

3. 

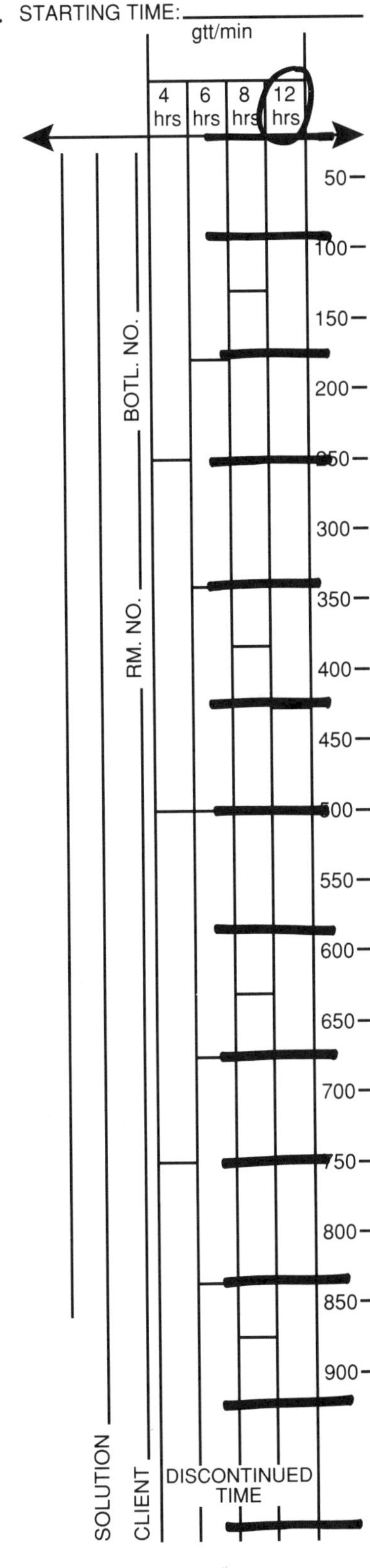

4. 83 mL/h

If the physician orders a rate that is not preprinted on the IV tape or if the commercial tape is not available, the nurse needs to calculate where the level of fluid should be at each hour. For example, if the order is for 75 mL/h, the nurse calculates that a 1000-mL bag lasts a little over 13 h (13.3 h). If the infusion was started at 12 noon, in 1 h, or at 1 PM, the level of the fluid should

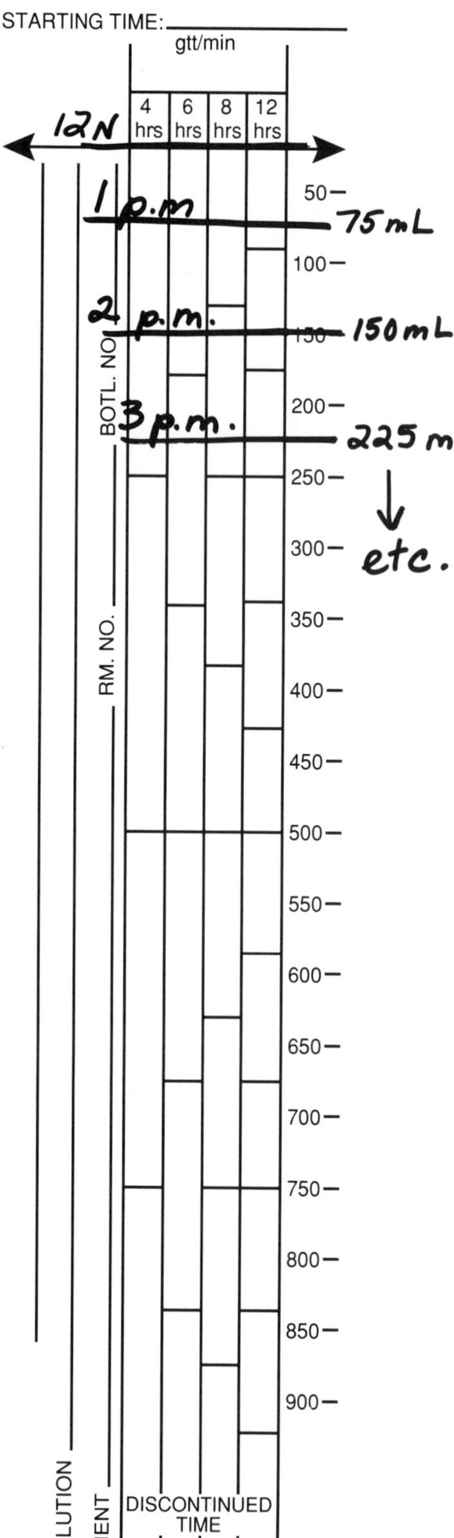

Figure 8–3 Markings on a commercially prepared intravenous tape, showing an infusion rate of 75 mL/h.

be at 75 mL/h, or halfway between the 50- and 100-mL markings on the bag as shown in Figure 8–3.

By 2 PM the level should be at 150 mL (75 mL + 75 mL). By 3 PM, another 75 mL should have infused, and the level should reflect 225 mL (150 mL + 75 mL) of fluid infused. The nurse continues marking the tape in this manner until all the fluid in the bag is accounted for.

Periodically the nurse needs to determine how much fluid has infused by a given time and how much is still left in the bag to be infused. Most often this calculation occurs at the end of the nurse's shift before leaving the work unit.

Examples

1. The client's intravenous fluids are infusing at a rate of 100 mL/h. A new 1000-mL bag was hung at 11:30 AM. At 2:30 PM, the nurse expects that 300 mL of the new bag has run in. The amount left in the bag should be 700 mL (1000 mL − 300 mL = 700 mL). These amounts are recorded on the appropriate fluid intake record (see Chapter 10).
2. The physician orders 1000 mL of 5%D/NS to run in over 8 h. The new bag was hung at 6 PM. At 10:30 PM, the nurse checked the bag to make sure that the correct amount of fluid was infusing. In 4.5 h about 560 mL had infused and there were 440 mL remaining in the bag. The nurse determined that the IV rate was correct and that the IV was "on time."

READING AN IV BAG

When reading the calibration on the IV bag, the nurse can observe the amount infused by gently grasping each side of the bag to level the fluid and estimating where the fluid level is. The amount infused is subtracted from the total amount that was in the bag when it was hung to determine the amount left in the bag.

SAMPLE EXERCISES

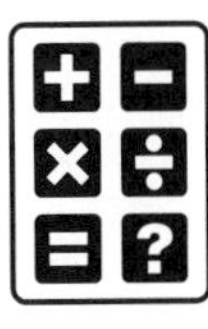

1. What is the amount left in a 500-mL bag of 5%D/W if 150 mL have infused?
2. At 6:30 AM, the nurse checks a client's IV bag and observes that 300 mL of fluid have infused since 3:30 AM. The physician's order states that the IV should infuse at 150 mL/h. Is the IV on time?
3. On the bag shown here, approximately what amount of fluid was infused by 4:00 PM? How much fluid is left in this 1000-mL bag?

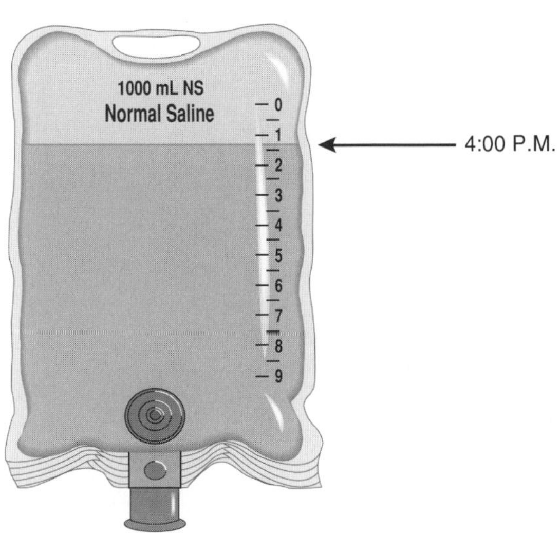

4. On the 250-mL bag shown here, how much fluid has been absorbed by the client? How much fluid is left in the bag?

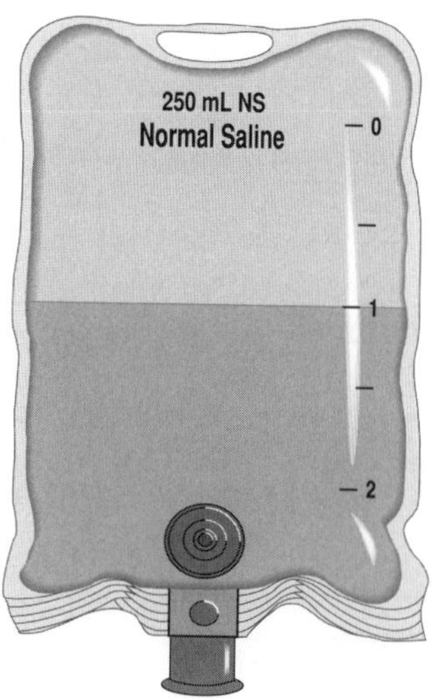

ANSWERS 1. 350 mL 2. The IV is *not* on time. 450 mL of solution should have been infused in 3 h. 3. 125 mL, 875 mL 4. 100 mL, 150 mL

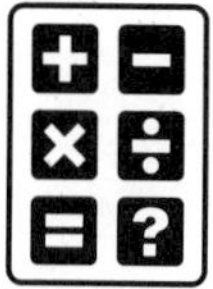

EXERCISES

Exercises 1–3. Determine the amount of fluid left in the IV solution bags shown here.

1.

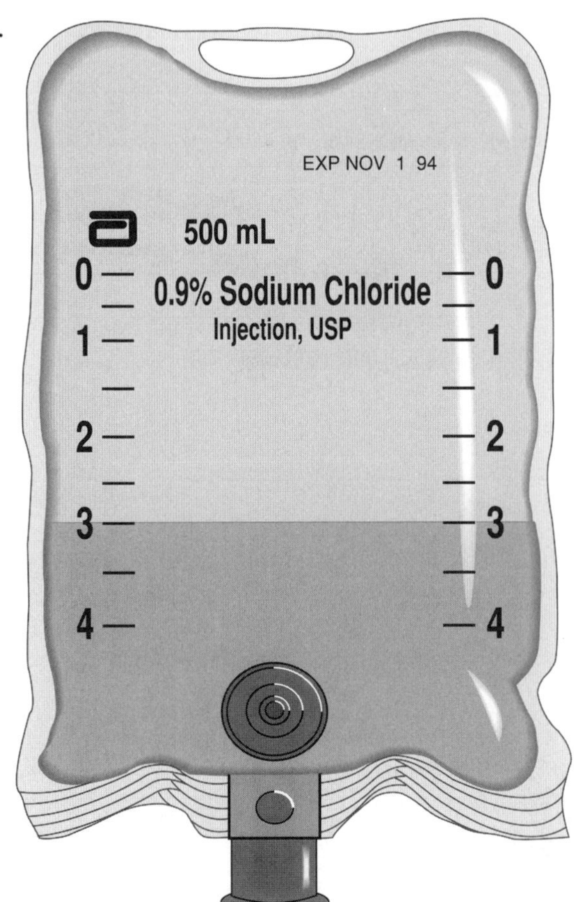

2.

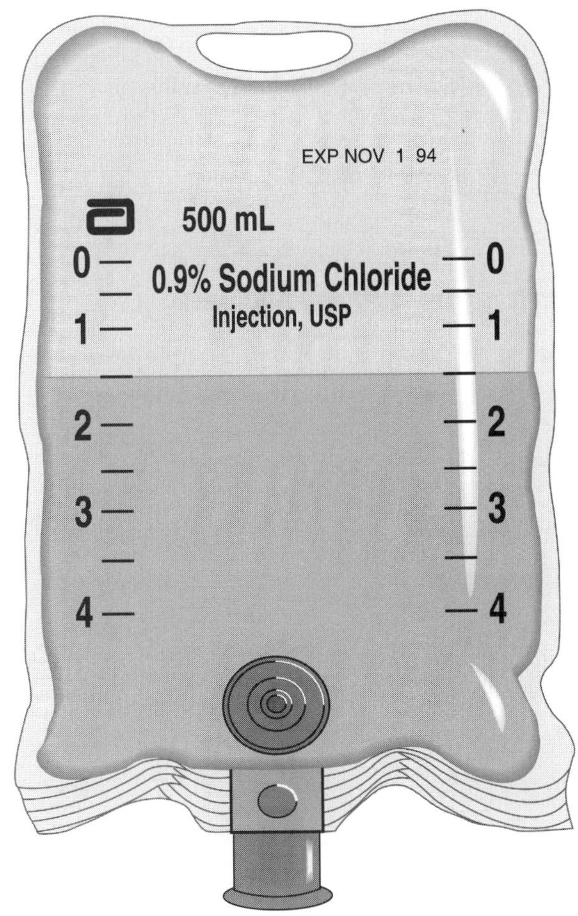
EXP NOV 1 94
500 mL
0.9% Sodium Chloride
Injection, USP
0
1
2
3
4
0
1
2
3
4

3.

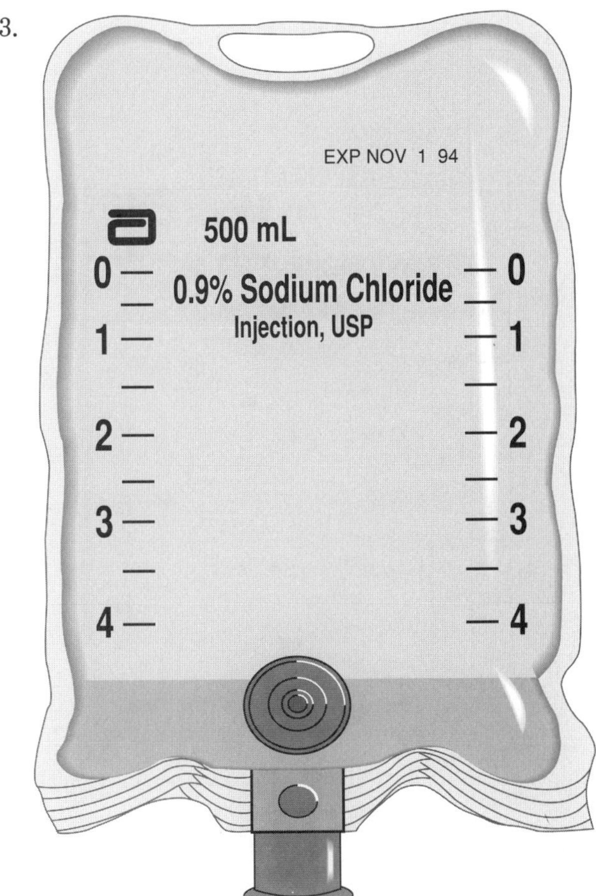
EXP NOV 1 94
500 mL
0.9% Sodium Chloride
Injection, USP
0
1
2
3
4
0
1
2
3
4

Exercises 4–6. Mark the tapes shown here to indicate delivery at the specified IV flow rates.

4. 200 mL/h STARTING TIME:____________

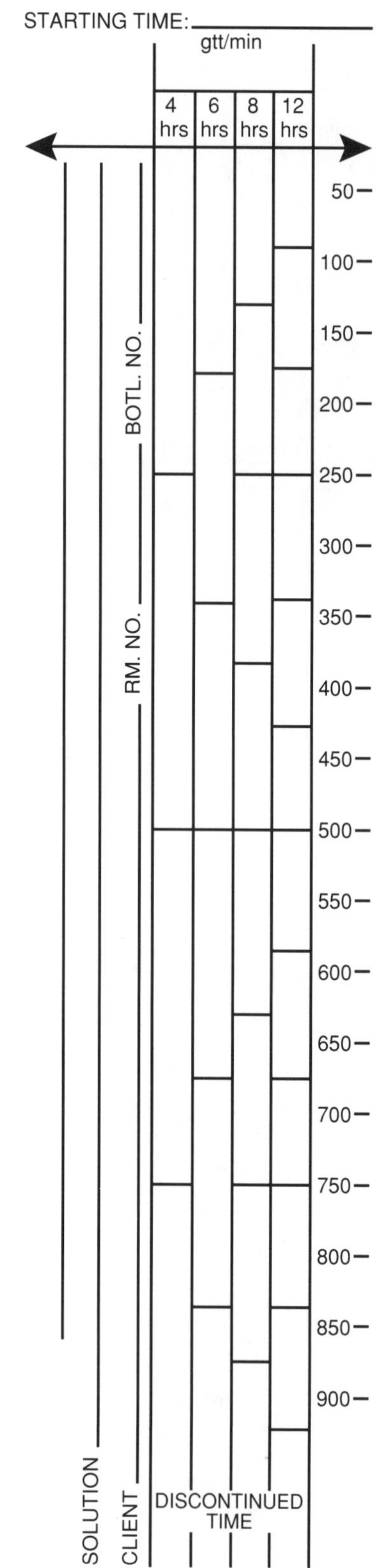

5. 75 mL/h

6. 120 mL/h

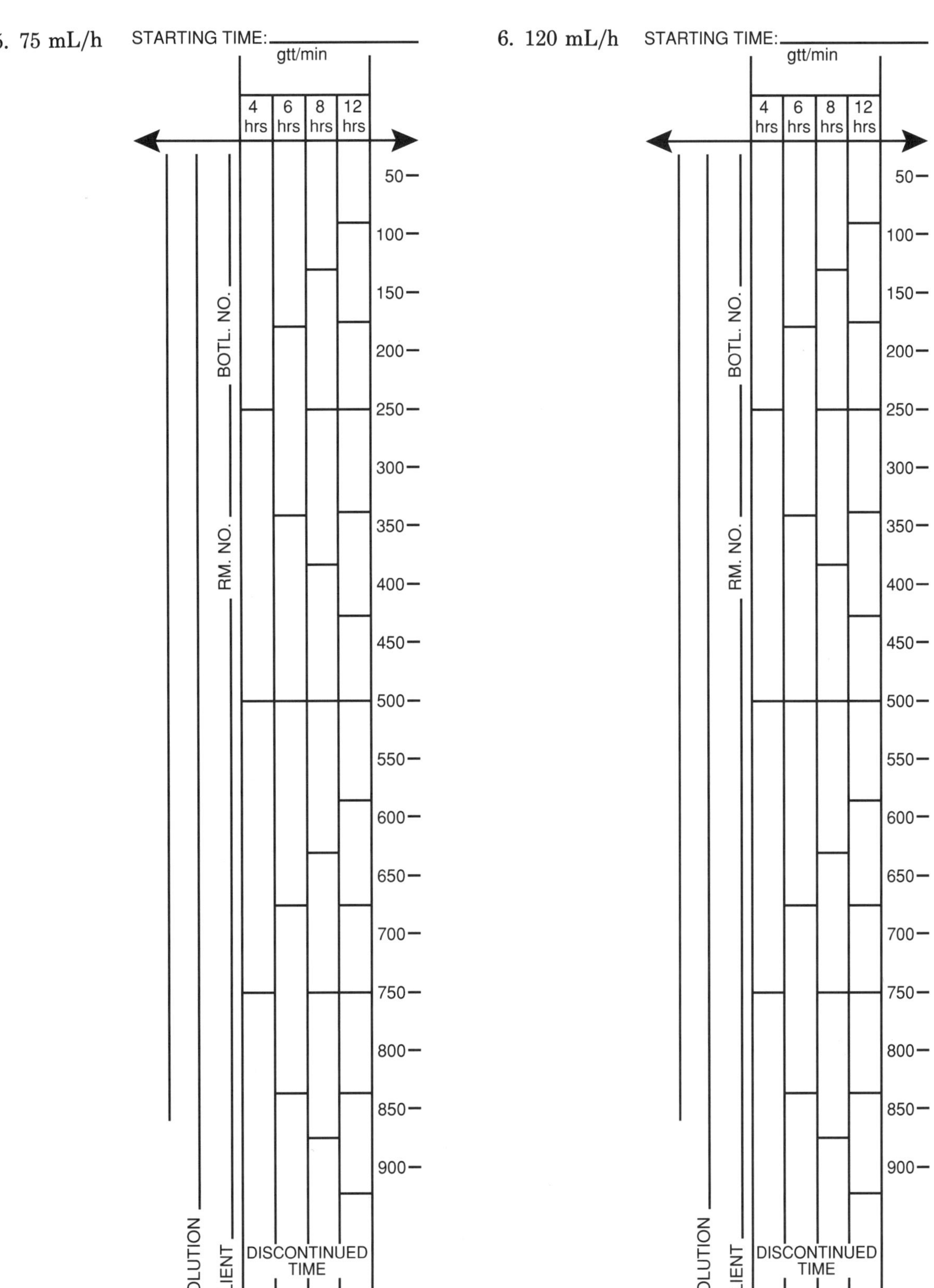

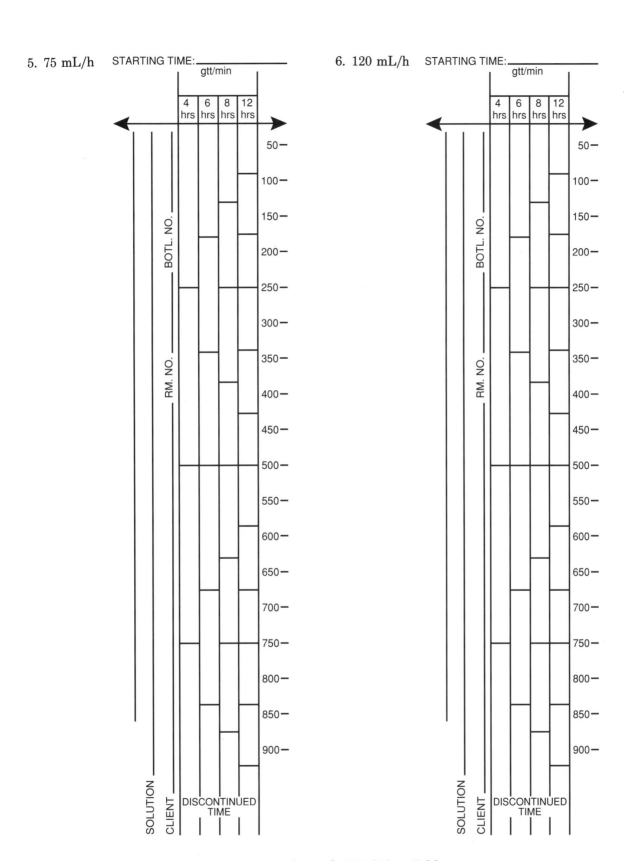

Exercises 7–9. The nurse hangs a 1000-mL bag of 5%D/NS at 7:30 AM. The flow rate is 50 mL/h. Answer the following questions about this situation.

7. If the fluid infuses on schedule, how many milliliters should have run in by 11:30 AM?

8. Mark the IV tape shown here to indicate where the level of the fluid should be at 11:30 AM.

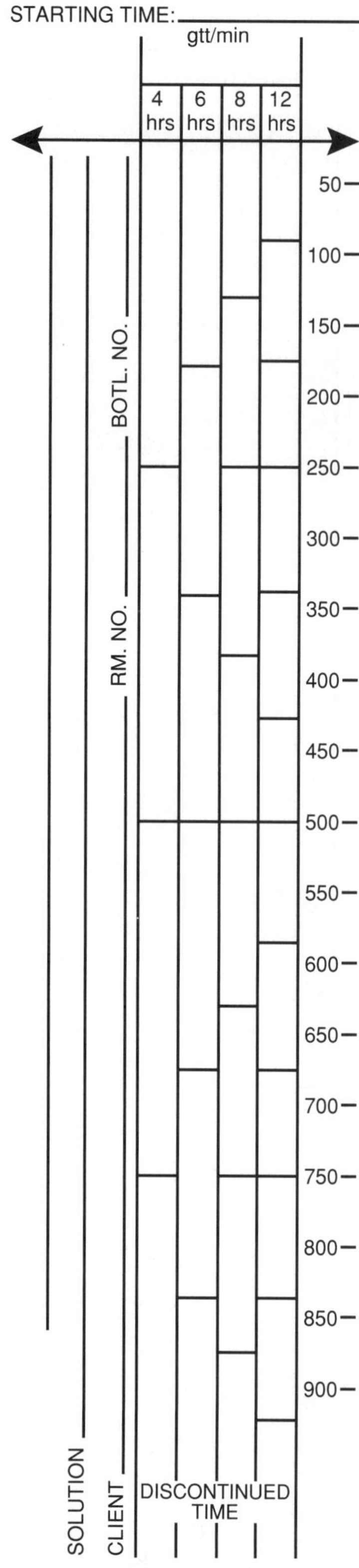

9. How many milliliters remain in the bag at 11:30 AM?

Exercises 10–12. The nurse hangs a 1000-mL bag of 5%D/RL at 9:00 AM. The flow rate is 75 mL/h. Answer the following questions about this situation.

10. If the fluid infuses on schedule, how many milliliters should have run in by 4:00 PM?

11. Mark the IV tape shown here to indicate where the level of the fluid should be at 4:00 PM.

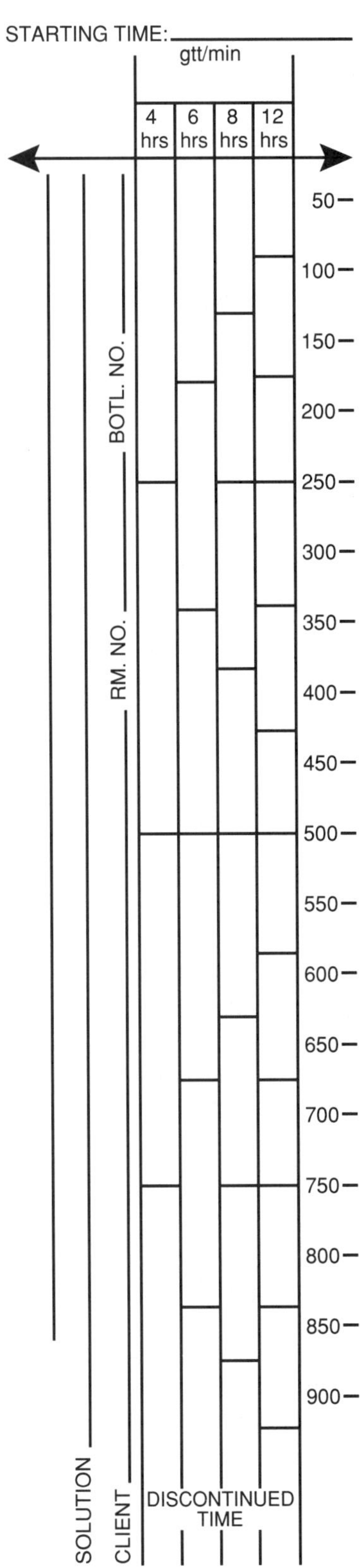

12. How many milliliters remain in the bag at 4:00 PM?

Exercises 13–20. Are the following IV fluids infusing on time?

13. 500 mL should infuse at 60 mL/h. The bag was started at 8:30 AM, and 325 mL have infused by 11:45 AM.

14. 1000 mL should infuse in 5 h. The bag was started at 10:15 PM, and 450 mL have infused by 2:30 AM.

15. 1000 mL should infuse at 150 mL/h. The bag was started at 12 noon, and there are 300 mL left in the bag at 6:00 PM.

16. 1000 mL should infuse at 125 mL/h. The bag was started at 4:20 AM, and there are 375 mL left in the bag at 9:20 AM.

17. 250 mL should infuse at 100 mL/h. The bag was started at 1:40 PM, and there are 150 mL left in the bag at 2:40 PM.

18. 500 mL should infuse at 80 mL/h. The bag was started at 12:30 AM, and 200 mL have infused by 2:00 AM.

19. 1000 mL should infuse at 40 mL/h. The bag was started at 6:45 PM, and 320 mL have infused by 2:45 AM.

20. 150 mL should infuse at 100 mL/h. The bag was started at 9:00 AM, and there are 75 mL left in the bag at 10:00 AM.

ANSWERS 1. 200 mL 3. 50 mL 5. See page 277 7. 200 mL 9. 800 mL 11. See page 277 13. No; 195 mL should have infused by 11:45 AM. 15. No; there should be 100 mL left in the bag at 6:00 PM. 17. Yes 19. Yes

---

8-4. DETERMINING THE IV DROP FACTOR

After calculating the amount of intravenous solution that should be infused per hour, the nurse needs to find the drip rate of the fluid (in drops per minute) to ensure that the prescribed amount is strictly followed. Intravenous solutions are administered with a special type of manufactured tubing (Fig. 8–4). The end with the drip chamber is attached to the IV bag. The other end is attached to a needle or catheter that is inserted into a vein. The entire IV set-up complete with bag, tubing (IV administration set), and venous access in the client is sometimes referred to as an **IV line.**

Determining Types of IV Tubing

There are two major types of IV tubing: a macrodrip and a microdrip. **Macrodrip** tubing delivers fairly large drops of solution and is usually reserved for administration of IV fluids in adults. These sets generally provide 10, 12, 15, or 20 drops (gtt) for each milliliter of solution. The differences in amounts of drops per milliliter depend on which manufacturer makes the tubing. The box that the tubing comes in states the number of drops per milliliter or **drop factor,** for that set, as shown on the label in Figure 8–5. The drop factor is also sometimes referred to as the **set calibration.** The nurse needs this information to calculate the drip rate of the IV solution.

5. STARTING TIME: ______

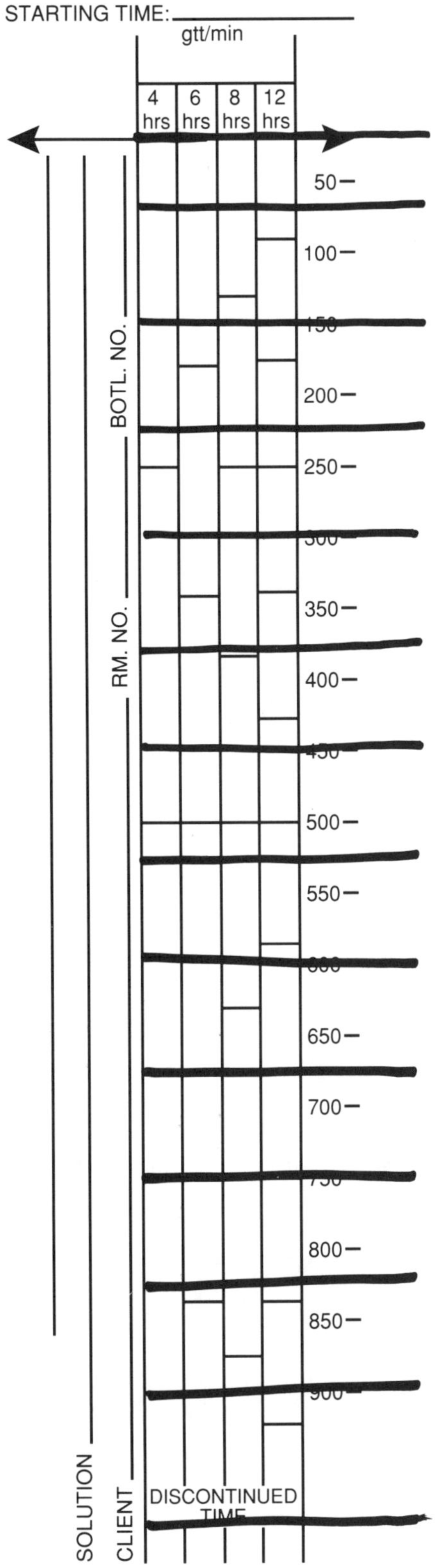

gtt/min

4 hrs	6 hrs	8 hrs	12 hrs

50 — 100 — 150 — 200 — 250 — 300 — 350 — 400 — 450 — 500 — 550 — 600 — 650 — 700 — 750 — 800 — 850 — 900 —

BOTL. NO. ______ RM. NO. ______

SOLUTION ______ CLIENT ______ DISCONTINUED TIME

11. STARTING TIME: ______

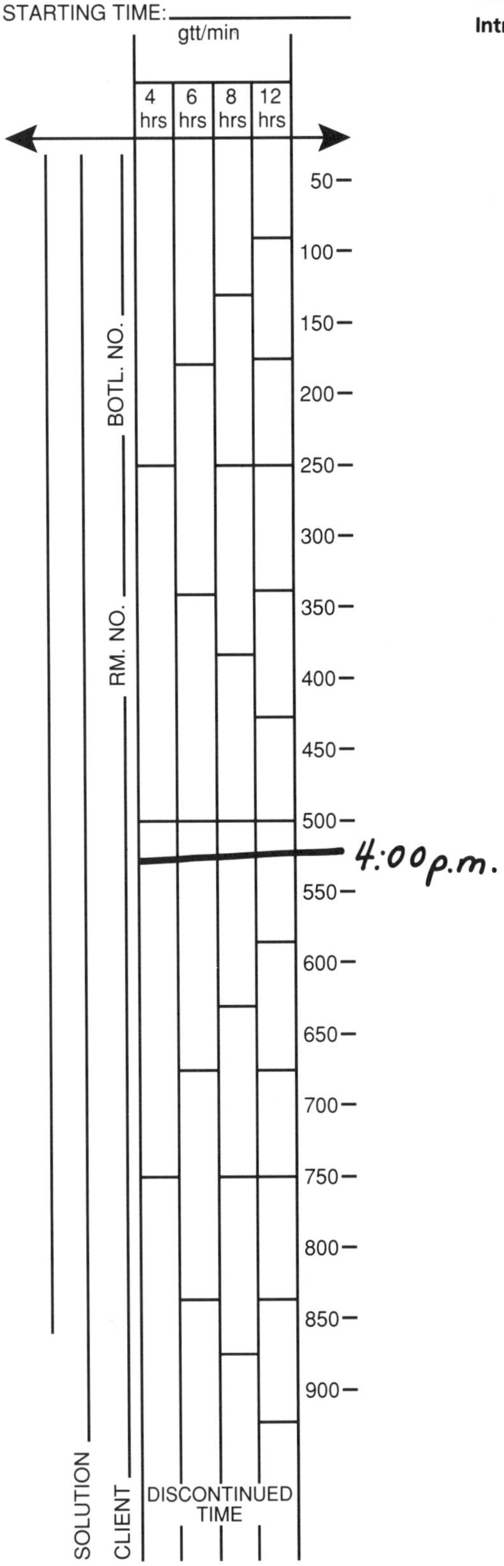

gtt/min

4 hrs	6 hrs	8 hrs	12 hrs

50 — 100 — 150 — 200 — 250 — 300 — 350 — 400 — 450 — 500 — 4:00 p.m. 550 — 600 — 650 — 700 — 750 — 800 — 850 — 900 —

BOTL. NO. ______ RM. NO. ______

SOLUTION ______ CLIENT ______ DISCONTINUED TIME

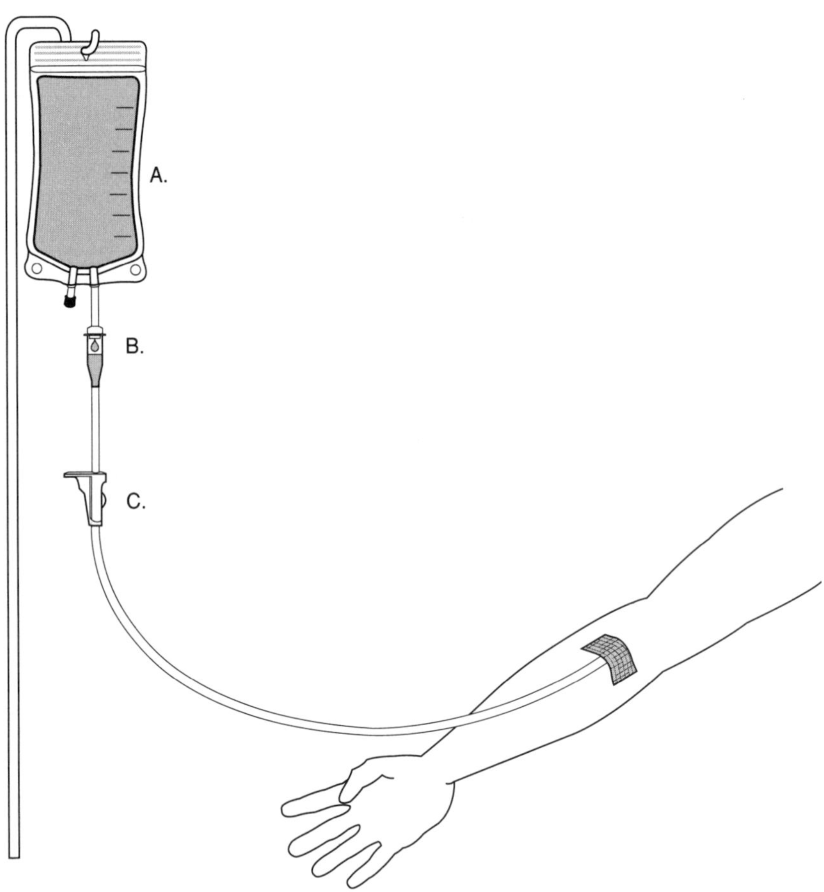

Figure 8–4 Manufactured intravenous solution bag and infusion set. (A) Intravenous solution bag. (B) Drip chamber. (C) Roller regulating clamp.

A **microdrip,** also called a **minidrip,** delivers very small drops. Most manufacturers provide microdrip tubing that delivers 60 gtt/mL. Again this information is provided on the tubing box label as shown in Figure 8–6. This type of tubing is used to deliver small amounts of fluid, usually less than 100 mL/h. Microdrip tubing is also commonly used for administering IV fluids to infants, children, and the elderly.

TYPES OF TUBING

Macrodrip tubing: 10, 12, 15, or 20 gtt/mL
Microdrip tubing: 60 gtt/mL, or 1 mL = 60 gtt

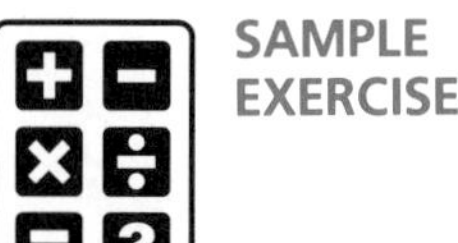

SAMPLE EXERCISES

1. The nurse prepares to start an IV solution for a 6-month-old baby. What type of tubing should be used: a macrodrip or a microdrip?
2. The nurse reads the following label on the IV tubing box:

   "Approximately 20 drops = 1 mL"

   What does this label mean? Is this macrodrip or microdrip tubing?
3. What is a drop factor?

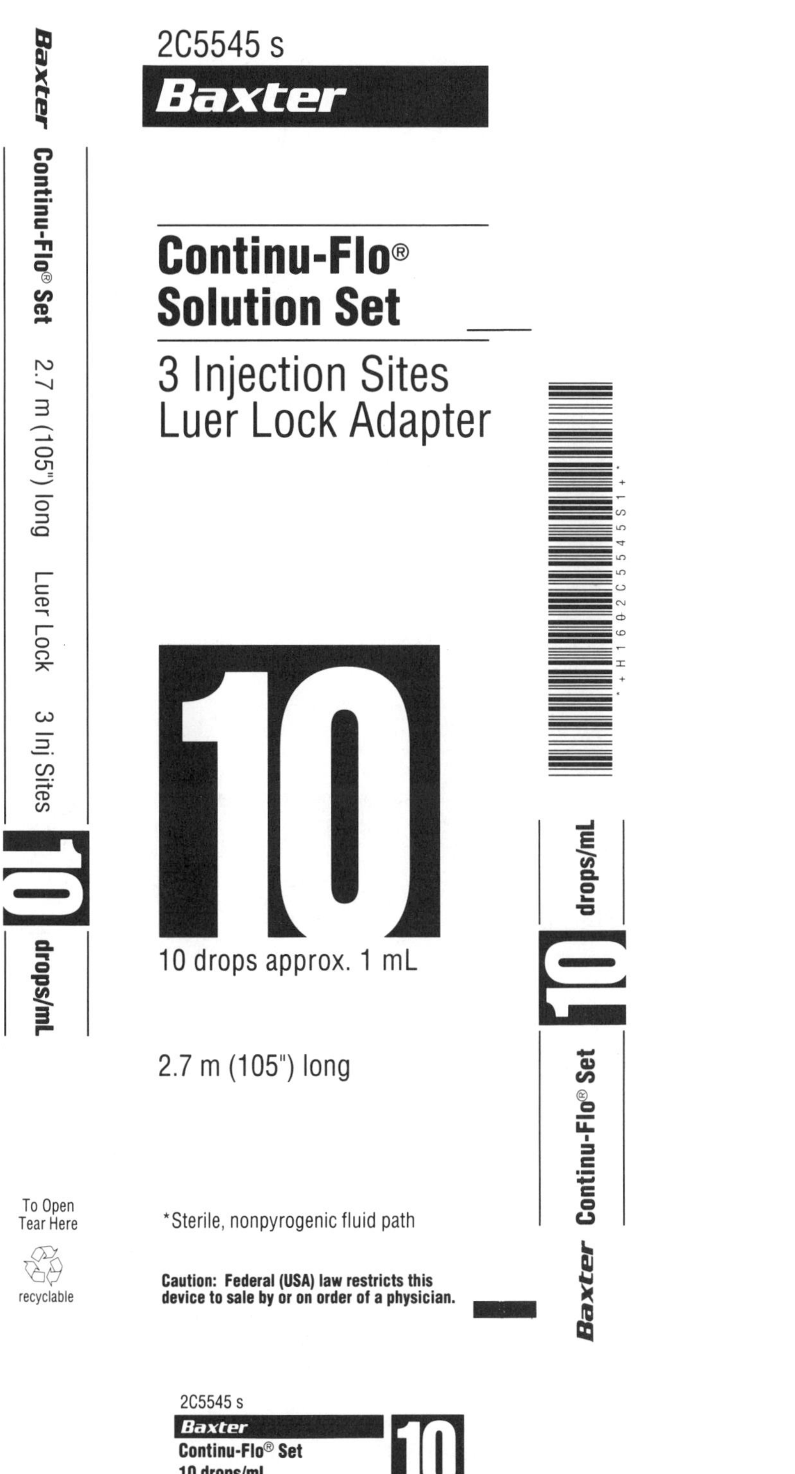

Figure 8–5 Baxter Continu-Flo primary intravenous set, showing drop factor of 10 drops per milliliter. (Courtesy of Baxter Healthcare Corporation, Deerfield, IL.)

ANSWERS 1. A microdrip to deliver a small amount 2. The tubing set delivers approximately 20 gtt for every milliliter of fluid; it is a macrodrip. 3. A drop factor is the number of drops in a milliliter of fluid that an IV tubing set delivers.

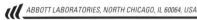

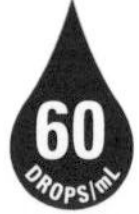

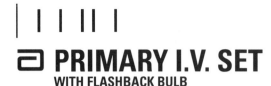

Figure 8–6 Label from an unvented primary IV set, a type of microdrip tubing. Note the drop factor of 60 gtt/mL. (Courtesy of Abbott Laboratories, Chicago, Illinois.)

Converting Milliliters to Drops

If a macrodrip tubing has a drop factor of 10, there are 10 gtt for every milliliter of IV solution. To find the number of drops in 4 mL, we multiply the number of milliliters by the drop factor.

Table: x gtt in 4 mL
10 gtt in 1 mL

Result: $\frac{4}{1} \times 10 \text{ gtt} = 40 \text{ gtt}$

> **CONVERTING MILLILITERS TO DROPS**
>
> To convert milliliters to drops, **multiply** the number of milliliters by the drop factor.

Examples

1. A nurse uses macrodrip tubing with a drop factor of 12 to administer an IV solution that infuses at 2 mL/min. We compute the number of drops in 2 mL by multiplying: $2 \times 12 \text{ gtt} = 24 \text{ gtt}$.

   Table: x gtt in 2 mL
   12 gtt in 1 mL

   Result: $\frac{2}{1} \times 12 \text{ gtt} = 24 \text{ gtt}$

2. Using a microdrip that has a drop factor of 60, the nurse administers an infusion of 0.8 mL/min. We compute the number of drops in 0.8 mL by multiplying: $0.8 \times 60 \text{ gtt} = 48$ drops.

   Table: x gtt in 0.8 mL
   60 gtt in 1.0 mL

   Result: $\frac{0.8}{1} \times 60 \text{ gtt} = 48 \text{ gtt}$

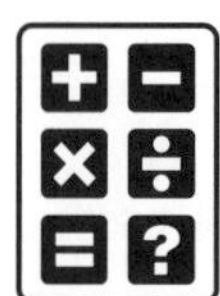

EXERCISES

Exercises 1–5. Convert milliliters into drops, using a drop factor of 15.

1. 3 mL
2. 2.6 mL
3. 1.8 mL
4. 0.9 mL
5. 1.2 mL

Exercises 6–10. Convert milliliters into drops, using a drop factor of 60.

6. 1.5 mL
7. 0.6 mL
8. 0.3 mL
9. 1.1 mL
10. 2.8 mL

ANSWERS 1. 45 gtt 3. 27 gtt 5. 18 gtt 7. 36 gtt 9. 66 gtt

8-5. DETERMINING THE IV DRIP RATE

After calculating the hourly IV rate and determining the drop factor as indicated on the IV tubing package, the nurse must calculate the IV **drip rate.** The drip rate is the number of drops per minute that the IV solution must run to deliver the prescribed volume per hour.

Some books present a formula for this calculation but do not fully explain how the answer is obtained. Two methods are presented in this chapter, so you can better understand the process.

The first step in calculating drip rate is to determine the **minute volume,** or amount of IV fluid that should infuse in 1 min. This is simply done by dividing hourly volume by 60.

MINUTE VOLUME

$$\text{Minute volume} = \frac{\text{Hourly volume of IV fluid}}{60 \text{ min}}$$

If the total amount of fluid should infuse in less than 1 h which is typical for drug administration, the process is very similar.

MINUTE VOLUME

$$\text{Minute volume} = \frac{\text{Amount of fluid to be infused (mL)}}{\text{Amount of time for infusion (min)}}$$

Examples

1. The physician orders an IV fluid to run at 80 mL/h. The amount of fluid that must be delivered in 1 min to provide the prescribed hourly rate is 80 mL/60 min = 1.3 mL/min (rounded to the nearest tenth).
2. The nurse receives an order to infuse 1000 mL of 5%D/W over 10 h. The hourly rate is 100 mL/h (1000/10). The minute volume is 100 mL/60 min = 1.7 mL/min.
3. The nurse wants to infuse clindamycin diluted in 50 mL of normal saline over 30 min. In this case, the rate is 50 mL/30 min. The minute volume is 50 mL/30 min = 1.7 mL/min.

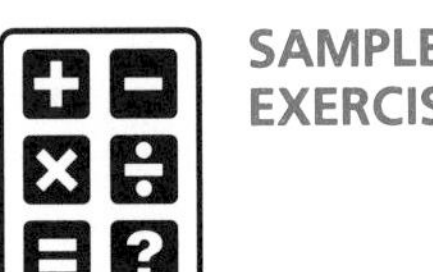

SAMPLE EXERCISES

1. If the nurse regulates the IV fluid to deliver 120 mL/h, what is the rate per minute (minute volume)?
2. The physician orders a liter of 5%D/$\frac{1}{4}$NS to infuse over 8 h. Find the rate per minute.
3. What is the rate per minute of an IV infusion of 250 mL that infuses in 120 min?

ANSWERS 1. 120 mL/60 min = 2 mL/min
2. 1000 mL/8 h = 125 mL/h = 125 mL/60 min = 2.1 mL/min
3. 250 mL/120 min = 2.1 mL/min

The minute volume indicates the number of milliliters that needs to be infused in 1 min. Since fractions of milliliters cannot be counted, for example, 2.1 mL/min, milliliters must be converted to drops to give the number of drops per minute that the fluid must run. If we know the drop factor (DF) of the tubing being used, we can easily compute the number of drops per minute (drip rate) by converting from milliliters to drops as shown previously.

Examples

1. The physician orders a continuous IV rate of 75 mL/h. If the drop factor of the tubing is 15 gtt/mL, the drip rate is calculated as:

   Step 1. Find the minute volume (rate per minute).

   $$\frac{75 \text{ mL}}{60 \text{ min}} = 1.3 \text{ mL/min}$$

   Step 2. Find the drip rate.

   1. 3 mL/min × 15 gtt/mL (drop factor) = 19.5, or 20 gtt/min

   (*Note:* Since half a drop cannot be counted, the answer is rounded to the nearest whole number.)

2. A client's IV solution should infuse at 50 mL/h. The microdrip tubing being used delivers 60 gtt/mL.

   Step 1. Find the minute volume.

   $$\frac{50 \text{ mL}}{60 \text{ min}} = 0.83 \text{ mL/min}$$

   Step 2. Find the drip rate.

   0.83 mL/min × 60 gtt/mL = 49.8, or 50 gtt/min

   (*Note:* When a microdrip IV tubing is used, the drip rate is always equal to the hourly rate. In this case, the hourly rate was 50, and the drip rate was also 50. As a shortcut, then, when using a microdrip, there is no need to calculate the drip rate if the hourly rate is known. The two numbers are always the same.)

3. The IV order reads: 1 L RL to infuse over 8 h. The drop factor is 20 gtt/mL.

   Step 1. Find the hourly IV rate.

   $$\frac{1000 \text{ mL}}{8 \text{ h}} = 125 \text{ mL/h}$$

Step 2. Find the minute volume.

$$\frac{125\text{ mL}}{60\text{ min}} = 2.1\text{ mL/min}$$

Step 3. Find the drip rate.

$$2.1\text{ mL/min} \times 20\text{ gtt/mL} = 42\text{ gtt/min}$$

SAMPLE EXERCISES

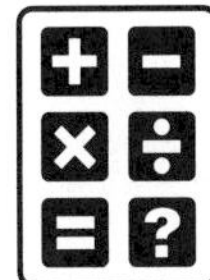

1. The physician orders a liter of 5%D/$\frac{1}{4}$NS to infuse over 12 h. The drop factor of the IV tubing that the nurse uses is 12 gtt/mL. What should the IV drip rate be?
2. The nurse regulates an IV to deliver 100 mL/h. What should the drip rate be to deliver this amount? (Drop factor = 15.)
3. An IV order reads: Give 500 mL of NS over 3 h. What should the drip rate be? (Drop factor = 10.)
4. The physician orders a medication to be mixed in 100 mL of 5%D/W. The nurse plans to run the IV over 90 min using a microdrip. What drip rate is needed to deliver this amount?
5. The physician prescribes an IV solution to run at 83 mL/h. If a microdrip is used, what should the drip rate be?

ANSWERS 1. 17 gtt/min 2. 25 gtt/min 3. 28 gtt/min 4. 67 gtt/min (*Note:* Remember that the drip rate is equal to the *hourly* IV rate.) 5. 83 gtt/min

---

EXERCISES

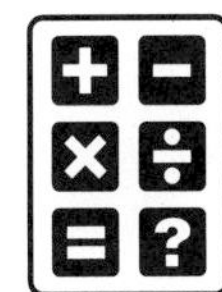

Exercises 1–10. Find the minute volume (rate per minute) for each of the IV exercises below.

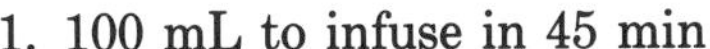

1. 100 mL to infuse in 45 min
2. 500 mL to infuse in 4 h
3. 50 mL to infuse in 30 min
4. 75 mL to infuse in 1 h
5. 1000 mL to infuse over 10 h
6. 250 mL to infuse in 4 h
7. 30 mL to infuse in 1 h
8. 500 mL to infuse in 8 h
9. 150 mL to infuse in 75 min
10. 1000 mL to infuse over 6 h

Exercises 11–20. Find the drip rate for each of the IV exercises below.

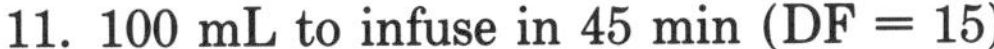

11. 100 mL to infuse in 45 min (DF = 15)
12. 500 mL to infuse in 4 h (DF = 20)
13. 50 mL to infuse in 30 min (DF = 10)
14. 75 mL to infuse in 1 h (DF = 60)
15. 1000 mL to infuse over 10 h (DF = 20)
16. 250 mL to infuse in 4 h (DF = 15)
17. 30 mL to infuse per hour (DF = 60)

18. 500 mL to infuse in 8 h (DF = 10)
19. 150 mL to infuse in 75 min (DF = 15)
20. 1000 mL to infuse over 6 h (DF = 10)

ANSWERS 1. 2.2 mL/min 3. 1.7 mL/min 5. 1.7 mL/min 7. 0.5 mL/min 9. 2.0 mL/min 11. 33 gtt/min 13. 17 gtt/min 15. 33 gtt/min 17. 30 gtt/min 19. 30 gtt/min

8-6. SHORTCUT FORMULA FOR DETERMINING IV DRIP RATE

A problem that many nurses encounter when using shortcut formulas is occasional confusion about what numbers to insert into which part of the formula. By learning the logic of the process explained in Section 8–5, the nurse can always compute the correct value. The following formula is a shortcut for computing IV drip rate.

SHORTCUT FOR COMPUTING DRIP RATE

$$\frac{\text{Amount of solution infused (mL)}}{\text{Amount of time for infusion (min)}} \times \text{Drop factor (gtt/mL)} = \text{Drip rate (gtt/min)}$$

Examples

1. Consider the example of administering 1000 mL over 8 h. The formula is easiest to use if the hourly rate (125 mL/h) is determined *before* using the formula. Then the numbers are inserted as follows:

$$\frac{125 \text{ mL}}{60 \text{ min}} \times 20 \text{ gtt/mL} = 42 \text{ gtt/min}$$

2. If a microdrip tubing is used in the above example,

$$\frac{125 \text{ mL}}{60 \text{ min}} \times 60 \text{ gtt/mL} = 125 \text{ gtt/min}$$

(*Note:* The 60's cancel. This is why the hourly rate is equal to the drip rate when microdrip tubing is used.)

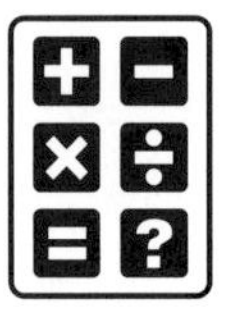

SAMPLE EXERCISES

1. The physician orders a continuous IV infusion of Ringer's lactate to run at 150 mL/h. What is the drip rate? (Drop factor = 10).
2. The nurse hangs a 150-mL bag to run in 75 min. What is the drip rate? (Drop factor = 15).

ANSWERS 1. 25 gtt/min 2. 30 gtt/min

Exercises 1–10. Find the drip rate for each of the IV exercises below, using the shortcut formula method.

EXERCISES

1. 100 mL to infuse in 45 min (DF = 10)
2. 500 mL to infuse in 4 h (DF = 15)
3. 50 mL to infuse in 30 min (DF = 60)
4. 75 mL to infuse in 1 h (DF = 20)
5. 250 mL to infuse in 4 h (DF = 20)
6. 40 mL to infuse per hour (DF = 60)
7. 500 mL to infuse in 8 h (DF = 15)
8. 150 mL to infuse in 75 min (DF = 60)
9. 1000 mL to infuse over 8 h (DF = 10)
10. 1000 mL to infuse over 10 h (DF = 15)

ANSWERS 1. 22 gtt/min 3. 100 gtt/min 5. 21 gtt/min 7. 16 gtt/min 9. 21 gtt/min

8-7. IV THERAPY DELIVERY SYSTEMS

The drip rate the nurse computes and regulates by the IV tubing clamp is subject to uncontrollable changes. If the client moves his or her arm where the IV is inserted or if the tubing becomes kinked, the drip rate may change. The result is an increase or a decrease in the hourly rate of the fluid, which could be harmful to the client's health. For example, if the client already has too much fluid in the body, a sudden increase in intravenous fluid could damage the heart or kidneys.

Electronic Control Systems

Several electronic control systems that mechanically regulate the IV fluid drip rate are commonly used. There are two general types of systems: controllers and pumps. **Controllers** allow the IV solution to infuse by gravity but keep the drip rate constant. The nurse sets the hourly rate (or minute volume depending on the type of machine) that follows the physician's order. Calculating the drip rate is not needed when a controller is used—the machine calculates and controls the drip rate. If the tubing becomes kinked or the bag is empty, an alarm on the controller signals the nurse that there is a problem.

Pumps are similar to controllers in that they deliver a constant flow determined by the setting on the machine (Fig. 8-7). Pumps mechanically force, or pump, the solution into the vein. The disadvantage of pumps is that many of them tend to continue pumping the fluid even if there is a tubing kink or the needle is not properly located in the vein (this problem is called an **infiltration**).

Special IV tubing that fits these machines must be used. The drop factor is not important since the machine is responsible for regulating the flow. The nurse may mark the bag with IV tape as discussed under Section 8-3, since the machine may experience mechanical failure. Marking the bag provides a

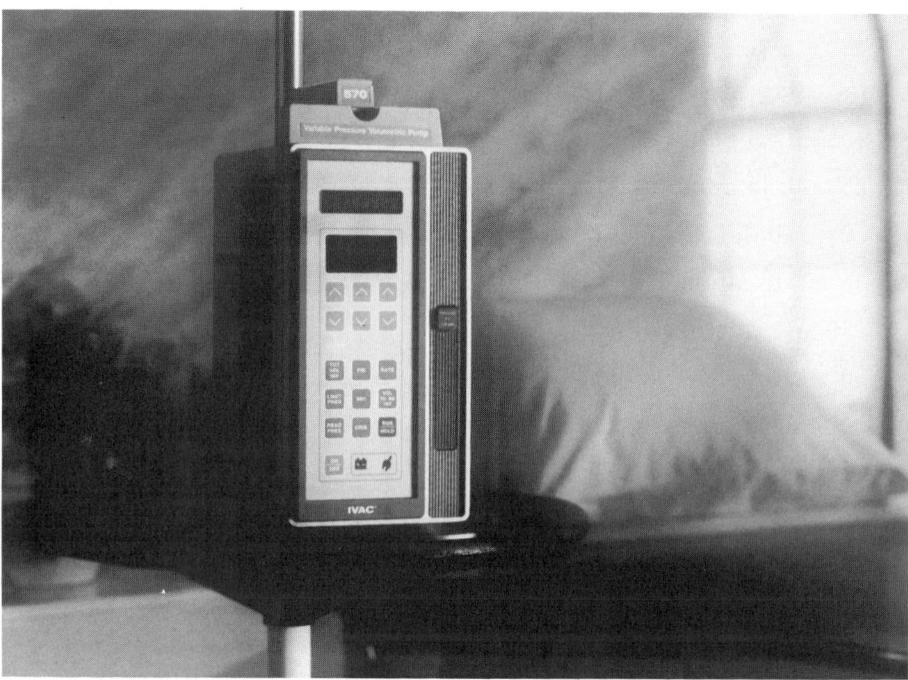

Figure 8–7 Example of an electronic pump used for regulating IV fluid flow rate.

quick check that the machine is functioning properly, but this practice depends on agency policy.

Intravenous Drug Delivery Systems

Intravenous drugs are commonly given in one of four ways: (1) intravenous push; (2) piggyback, using a secondary tubing system; (3) minibag via a heparin or saline lock (or lok), or (4) diluted in the primary IV solution. The **intravenous push (IVP)** method of drug delivery is reserved for medications that cannot be diluted or are needed in the body immediately. Examples are Lasix (furosemide) and Dilantin (phenytoin). These drugs are drawn up into a syringe in a manner similar to the procedure described in Chapter 7.

The second method of drug delivery, the **intravenous piggyback (IVPB)** system, is used much more commonly in general adult nursing practice. The health care agency pharmacy typically prepares the IV solution so that the medication is already mixed in a small bag of IV solution (usually 50- to 250-mL size) and properly labeled before the nurse is ready to administer it. In this method of intravenous drug delivery, a shorter IV tubing and small IV bag, or **minibag (IVMB)** is attached to the primary set for administration of the diluted drug as shown in Figure 8–8.

In the piggyback system, the medication can be mixed in a very small amount of solution, 50 mL for instance, but other more potent drugs or drugs of higher dosage may need to be mixed in amounts of up to 250 mL. The physician usually does not specify the hourly rate for administration of the medication. The nurse assesses the client and the nature of the medication to determine the rate of infusion. The pharmacist may recommend a safe flow rate, but this procedure is not universally practiced. Most 50-mL bags can be safely delivered over 30 min. If the nurse is unsure about a safe rate, the health care agency pharmacy can be contacted for more information.

The third system of IV drug delivery is similar to the piggyback method. In this system the minibag is administered directly into an intermittent infusion port—a heparin or saline lock. The **heparin** or **saline lock** is a plastic

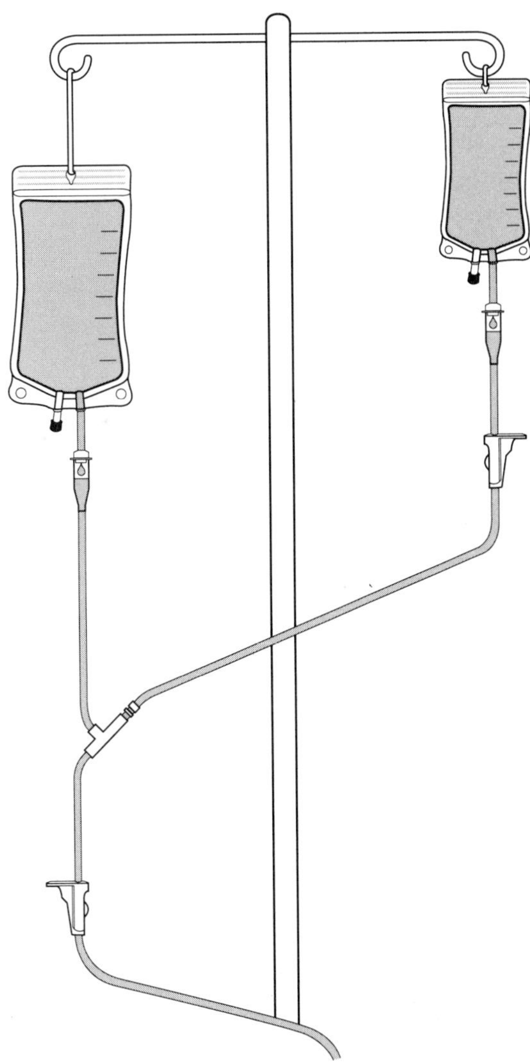

Figure 8–8 Intravenous piggyback (IVPB) system—an IV minibag (IVMB) connected to a primary IV line.

tube that is kept patent in the client's vein. For a heparin lock, a small amount of very diluted heparin, an anticoagulant, is instilled into the port. Saline is used for the saline lock.

The client with a heparin or saline lock does not receive a continuous IV infusion. Instead, the nurse connects the minibag containing the prescribed medication to the infusion port and disconnects it when the solution has infused. This procedure can occur once a day or many times a day, depending on the number of minibags prescribed. The heparin or saline lock is also used to instill IV push medications.

To prevent interaction with the prescribed medication, the nurse uses saline to flush the heparin out of the heparin lock.* Most health care settings use the SASH method for giving drugs via a *heparin* lock.

SASH METHOD

S: Saline flush* (step 1)
A: Add prescribed drug (step 2)
S: Saline flush (step 3)
H: Heparin flush (step 4)

---

* The amount of each flush is determined by specific health care agency policy.

The last system of IV drug delivery is the addition of medication into the large IV bags for continuous infusion or into small-calibrated cylindrical chambers, such as Buretrols, Volutrols, or Solusets, as illustrated and discussed in Chapter 9, Section 9–6. When these small cylinders are used, the nurse, rather than the pharmacist, usually adds the medication and labels the cylinder accordingly. These devices are used most often when giving drugs to infants and children.

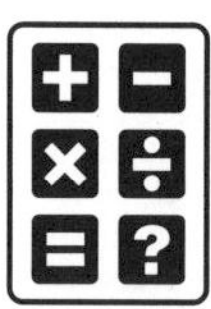

EXERCISES

1. Why are controllers or pumps used to deliver IV fluids?
2. Which method of IV drug delivery is used for drugs that cannot be diluted?
3. What is the name of a commonly used intermittent infusion port?
4. In the SASH technique for administering drugs through a heparin lock, what does the S stand for?
5. What is the name of a calibrated cylindrical chamber that can be used for IV drug delivery?

ANSWERS 1. To accurately regulate the IV flow rate 3. Heparin or saline lock 5. Buretrol, Volutrol, or Soluset

8-8. SPECIAL CALCULATIONS FOR IV DRUGS

Intravenous drugs that were once given only in critical care areas of a hospital are now commonly given in smaller doses on general hospital units. Many of these drugs are very potent and require careful monitoring by the nurse. A controller or pump is used to ensure that the rate of drug delivery is accurate, but the physician, nurse, and pharmacist play a major role in assuring safe drug administration.

The physician or pharmacist usually prescribes the concentration or dosage of the drug to be delivered (in mg/hr or mcg/kg/min), but may not specify the rate of IV administration (in mL/hr or gtt/min). Therefore, at times the nurse is responsible for calculating the dosage of the drug and the flow rate necessary to deliver the dosage.

For every drug, the nurse must know the characteristics of the drug, the therapeutic and safe dosage for the drug, the health care agency policies about IV drug delivery, and the condition of the client before making a determination about flow rate.

Although the pharmacist typically prepares IV medications and makes recommendations for IV administration, the nurse must know the parameters for safe drug delivery. In some cases, the drug dosage range is prescribed on the basis of the client's body weight. In other cases, drug dosage is prescribed on the basis of the concentration of the drug delivered over a specified period. In most cases, microdrip tubing is used because the amount of drug ordered is very small.

Examples

1. The physician orders 1000 mL of IV solution with 40 mEq KCl (potassium chloride) added to run over 8 h. The nurse calculates the dosage of drug delivered each hour.

Step 1. Find the milliequivalents per hour.

$$\frac{40 \text{ mEq}}{8 \text{ h}} = 5 \text{ mEq/h}$$

In this example, only one step is required to find the answer.

2. Mr. Amos has a new IV order: 1000 mL D5/NS with 30 mEq KCl. There are 400 mL left in his current IV bag. The nurse calculates the amount of KCl that should be added to the current partial bag. The KCl is 20 mEq/10 mL.

Step 1. Use ratio and proportion to find how much KCl in milliequivalents should be added.

$$\frac{1000 \text{ mL}}{400 \text{ mL}} = \frac{30 \text{ mEq}}{x \text{ mEq}}$$

$$1000x = 12000$$

$$x = 12$$

Result: 12 mEq should be added.

Step 2. Determine the number of milliliters of KCl solution to add using ratio and proportion.

$$\frac{10 \text{ mL}}{x \text{ mL}} = \frac{20 \text{ mEq}}{12 \text{ mEq}}$$

$$20x = 120$$

$$x = 6$$

Result: 6 mL should be added.

3. The physician orders an infusion of 400 mg of lidocaine in 250 mL 5%D/W to run at 50 mL/h. The nurse calculates the dosage in milligrams per hour and milligrams per minute.

Step 1. Use ratio and proportion to find dosage per hour.

$$\frac{250 \text{ mL}}{50 \text{ mL}} = \frac{400 \text{ mg}}{x \text{ mg}}$$

$$250x = 20{,}000$$

$$x = 80$$

Rate of dosage = 80 mg/h.

Step 2. Calculate milligrams per minute.

$$\frac{80 \text{ mg}}{60 \text{ min}} = 1.3 \text{ mg/min}$$

4. The physician orders dopamine to infuse at 20 mL/h. The solution comes from the pharmacy as 400 mg of dopamine diluted in 500 mL 5%D/W. The nurse calculates the amount of drug being delivered per hour (in milligrams per hour and in micrograms per minute).

Step 1. Use ratio and proportion to find dosage per hour.

$$\frac{500 \text{ mL}}{20 \text{ mL}} = \frac{400 \text{ mg}}{x \text{ mg}}$$

$$500x = 8000$$

$$x = 16$$

Rate of dosage = 16 mg/h.

Step 2. Calculate the rate in milligrams per minute.

$$\frac{16 \text{ mg}}{60 \text{ min}} = 0.267 \text{ mg/min}$$

Step 3. Convert milligrams per minute to micrograms per minute.

$$0.267 \text{ mg/min} \times 1000 \text{ mcg/mg} = 267 \text{ mcg/min}$$

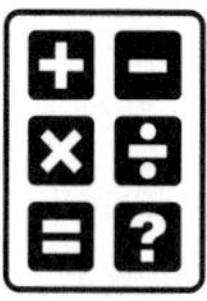

SAMPLE EXERCISES

1. The physician orders a liter of 5%D/RL with 40 mEq of potassium to infuse at 100 mL/h. Find the amount of potassium the client receives each hour.
2. The physician orders a continuous infusion of dopamine at 25 mL/h. The medication comes as 400 mg of dopamine in 500 mL 5%D/W. Calculate the delivery rate of the drug in mg/h and mcg/min.
3. The physician orders a continuous infusion of heparin to run at 25 mL/h. The solution available is 1000 mL containing 40,000 U of heparin. Calculate the dosage of heparin that the client receives per hour.
4. The physician orders a continuous infusion of aminophylline to run in at 80 mL/h. One gram of the drug comes diluted in 1000 mL of 5%D/NS. Calculate the hourly rate of the drug infusion.

ANSWERS 1. 4 mEq 2. 20 mg/h; 333 mcg/min 3. 1000 U 4. 80 mg/h

At times the nurse must calculate the flow rate when the drug dosage is ordered by the physician.

Examples

1. The physician orders a continuous infusion of heparin at 1100 U/h. The solution comes as 20,000 U of heparin diluted in 1000 mL 5%D/NS. The nurse determines the IV flow rate needed to deliver the prescribed amount of medication.

   Step 1. Use ratio and proportion to determine the flow rate.

$$\frac{1000 \text{ mL}}{x \text{ mL}} = \frac{20{,}000 \text{ U}}{1100 \text{ U}}$$

$$20{,}000x = 1{,}100{,}000$$

$$x = 55$$

Result: 55 mL/h.

2. The nurse uses an electronic IV pump to infuse the heparin solution in Example 1. The setting on the pump requires drops per minute. The nurse calculates the rate and sets the machine accordingly, using tubing with a drop factor of 60.

   Step 1. Use the shortcut formula for calculating IV drip rate.

$$\frac{55 \text{ mL}}{60 \text{ min}} \times 60 \text{ gtt/mL} = 55 \text{ gtt/min}$$

(*Remember:* The 60's cancel so the flow rate and the drip rate are the same number.)

3. A client is receiving a continuous morphine sulfate infusion at 6 mg/h. The solution comes as 125 mg of morphine in 250 mL of 5%D/W. The nurse calculates the flow rate needed to deliver the prescribed amount of medication.

   Step 1. Use ratio and proportion to determine flow rate.

$$\frac{250 \text{ mL}}{x \text{ mL}} = \frac{125 \text{ mg}}{6 \text{ mg}}$$

$$125x = 1500$$

$$x = 12$$

Result: 12 mL/h.

4. The physician orders IV amrinone to infuse at 3 mcg/kg/min for Mrs. Johnson (weight = 140 lb). 250 mg of amrinone is diluted in 250 mL of normal saline. The nurse calculates the drip rate. (*Note:* In this case, the drug dosage is ordered per minute rather than per hour. In addition, the order is based on body weight.)

   Step 1. Convert body weight from pounds to kilograms (2.2 lb = 1 kg).

$$\frac{140}{2.2} = 63.6$$

   Step 2. Determine the ordered drug dosage per minute.

$$63.6 \times 3 \text{ mcg} = 190.8 \text{ mcg}$$

   Step 3. Use ratio and proportion to determine the number of milliliters per minute.

$$\frac{250 \text{ mL}}{x \text{ mL}} = \frac{250{,}000 \text{ mcg}}{190.8 \text{ mcg}}$$

$$250{,}000x = 47{,}700$$

$$x = 0.2$$

Result: 0.2 mL/min

   Step 4. Calculate the drip rate in drops per minute (DF = 60).

$$0.2 \times 60 \text{ gtt} = 12 \text{ gtt}$$

Result: 30 gtt/min

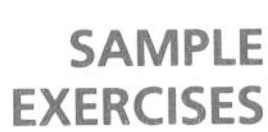

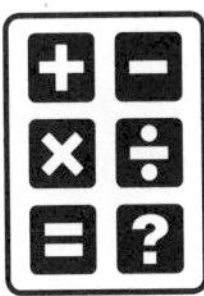

1. The order for a client is 10 mg/h of continuous morphine sulfate infusion. The solution is prepared as 125 mg morphine in 250 mL 5%D/W. Calculate the flow rate needed to deliver the correct drug dosage.

2. The physician orders lidocaine at 125 mg/h. The solution available is 500 mg lidocaine in 250 mL normal saline. Calculate the flow rate needed to deliver the prescribed dosage.

3. The nurse uses an electronic pump for the lidocaine infusion in Exercise 2. The pump setting is in drops per minute. If a microdrip tubing is used, find the drip rate that is needed to deliver the correct drug dosage.

ANSWERS 1. 20 mL/h 2. 63 mL/h 3. 63 gtt/min

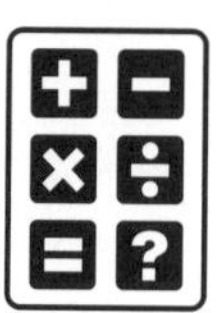

EXERCISES

Exercises 1–5. Calculate the drug dosage per hour for each of the IV potassium (K^+) exercises below. The solution is prepared as 40 mEq of potassium in 1000 mL of 5%D/½NS.

1. 1000 mL to infuse in 6 h
2. 1000 mL to infuse in 20 h
3. Continuous IV rate of 150 mL/h
4. Continuous IV rate of 75 mL/h
5. Continuous IV rate of 83 mL/h

Exercises 6–10. Calculate the drug dosage per hour for each of the IV aminophylline exercises below. The solution is prepared as 1 g aminophylline in 1000 mL 5%D/W.

6. 24 mL/h
7. 30 mL/h
8. 45 mL/h
9. 50 mL/h
10. 65 mL/h

Exercises 11–13. Calculate the drug dosage per hour for each of the IV dopamine exercises below. The solution is prepared as 200 mg dopamine in 250 mL 5%D/W.

11. 18 mL/h
12. 24 mL/h
13. 27 mL/h

Exercises 14–16. Convert the answers to the preceding exercises (11–13) to drug dosages in micrograms per minute.

17. The physician orders IV Isuprel to run at 4 mcg/min. The available solution is 1 mg Isuprel in 250 mL 5%D/NS. Calculate the flow rate in mL/h needed to deliver the prescribed drug dosage.
18. The physician orders a dopamine infusion of 400 mg in 250 mL 5%D/W at 6 mcg/kg/min. The client weighs 165 lb. Calculate the IV drip rate. (DF = 60.)

Exercises 19–20. Calculate the flow rate in milliliters per hour needed to deliver the correct drug dosages of heparin below. The available solution is 25,000 U of heparin in 500 mL 5%D/W.

19. 1300 U/h
20. 1800 U/h

ANSWERS 1. 6.7 mEq 3. 6 mEq 5. 3.3 mEq 7. 30 mg 9. 50 mg 11. 14.4 mg 13. 21.6 mg 15. 320 mcg/min 17. 60 mL/h 19. 26 mL/h

---

8-9. AVOIDING ERRORS: ADHERING TO SAFE DRUG DOSAGE PARAMETERS

Even though the physician orders IV drugs and the pharmacist checks and prepares them, the nurse is responsible for checking the dosage to ensure that the order is within the safe dosage range and that the pharmacist has prepared the proper strength of the IV solution. Recommendations about safe drug dosage are found in either the hospital policy manual or in drug reference books that should be available for the nurse to use. The nurse usually learns from experience the safe parameters for commonly used medications.

If the nurse discovers a potential problem with a dosage that is prescribed by the physician, he or she notifies the physician about the discrepancy. The pharmacist for the health care facility may be contacted as well. The nurse follows the protocol established by the individual work setting for notification of errors or potential problems with drug dosing.

Examples

1. The physician orders 40 mEq of potassium to be added to 500 mL 5%D/W and orders a flow rate of 125 mL/h. Using the calculation method described in Section 8–8, the nurse calculates an hourly potassium dosage rate of 10 mEq/h. The hospital policy for general medical-surgical units is a rate of no more than 5 mEq/h. Therefore, the nurse notifies the physician before giving the medication.
2. A client is receiving 1200 U/h heparin by continuous IV infusion. The recommended daily dosage is 20,000–40,000 U in 24 h. To compute the total number of units that the client is receiving, we multiply: 1200 U × 24 = 28,800 U in 24 h. This dosage is within the safe parameters for this drug.
3. The physician orders dopamine to infuse at 20 mL/h. The solution from the pharmacy is 400 mg of dopamine in 500 mL 5%D/W. The nurse calculates the dosage per minute as 267 mcg. The recommended dosage is 2–5 mcg/kg/min. The client weighs 154 lb (70 kg). To find micrograms per kilogram of body weight, we divide; $\frac{267}{70}$ = 3.8 mcg, which is within the safe dosage range.

SAMPLE EXERCISES

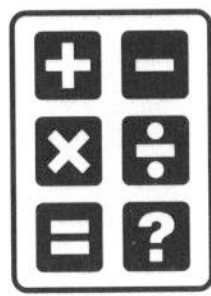

1. The physician orders a continuous heparin drip of 2100 U/h. The safe dosage range is 20,000–40,000 U in 24 h. Is this order within safe drug dosage parameters?
2. The physician orders lidocaine IV at 50 mL/h. The medication comes as 500 mg in 250 mL of solution. The recommended dose is 1–4 mg/min. Is the dose ordered within safe parameters?
3. A client is receiving Dobutrex at 100 mL/h. The IV is prepared with 250 mg in 1 L of 5%D/W. The recommended dose is 2.5–10 μg/kg/min. The client weighs 178 lb. Is the drug dosage ordered within safe parameters?

ANSWERS 1. No; infusion provides 50,400 U in 24 h. 2. Yes 3. Yes

EXERCISES

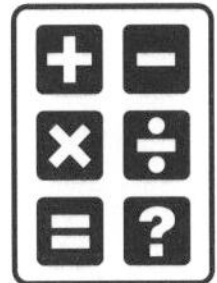

Exercises 1–5. For each of the IV heparin orders below, determine whether the dosage is within safe parameters if the recommended dosage range is 20,000–40,000 U/24 h. The solution has 30,000 U of heparin in 1000 mL 5%D/W.

1. 1000 U/h
2. 1500 U/h
3. 1800 U/h
4. 26 mL/h
5. 36 mL/h

Exercises 6–10. For each of the IV potassium orders below, determine whether the dosage is within safe parameters if the recommended dosage according to hospital policy is no more than 5 mEq/h. The solution has 30 mEq of potassium in 1000 mL of 5%D/NS.

6. 80 mL/h
7. 100 mL/h
8. 125 mL/h
9. 167 mL/h
10. 200 mL/h

Exercises 11–15. For each of the IV Dobutrex orders below, determine whether the dosage is within safe parameters if the recommended dosage is 2.5–10 mcg/kg/min. The solution available is 250 mg of Dobutrex in 1 L 5%D/W. In each example, the client weighs 132 lb.

11. 20 mg/h
12. 30 mg/h
13. 333 mcg/min
14. 630 μg/min
15. 80 mL/h

ANSWERS 1. Yes 3. No; 43,200 U/24 h 5. Yes 7. Yes 9. Yes 11. Yes 13. Yes 15. Yes

---

8-10. SUMMARY

1. WHAT IS INTRAVENOUS (IV) THERAPY?

Intravenous therapy is the method used to instill fluids or medications directly into the blood stream. The rate of fluid and drug administration often has to be determined by the nurse.

2. DETERMINING DOSAGE

Intravenous fluids come prepared in bags or, less often, in bottles. The large bags containing 500 or 1000 mL of fluid are generally used to administer fluids and certain chemicals that are lost from the body during illness. Smaller bags between 50 and 250 mL are usually used for medication administration. Many types of fluids are available, but most contain dextrose (sugar), saline (salt water), and/or chemicals, such as Ringer's lactate.

The number of milliliters administered in 1 h is called the **flow rate.** Flow rate is calculated by dividing the total amount of fluid to be infused by the number of hours allowed for the infusion. In some cases, we know the flow rate but need to compute the number of hours that the infusion lasts. To find this value, we divide the amount of solution by the flow rate.

3. DETERMINING THE CALIBRATION ON AN IV SOLUTION BAG

After finding the flow rate, the nurse marks the bag to show where the level of fluid will be for each hour that the solution is infusing. This helps determine whether the infusion is running on time, how much of the solution has infused over a specified period, and how much solution remains in the bag.

4. DETERMINING THE IV DROP FACTOR

Before the IV fluid can be regulated, we need to find the **drop factor,** or **set calibration,** of the tubing. Macrodrip tubing provides large drops of fluid, with 10, 12, 15, or 20 gtt approximately equivalent to 1 mL. Microdrip tubings provide smaller drops at 60 gtt/mL. Milliliters can be converted to drops by multiplying the number of milliliters by the drop factor. For example, assume a drop factor (DF) of 20 gtt/mL. Then in 2.4 mL, there are 48 gtt.

5. DETERMINING THE IV DRIP RATE

The **drip rate** is the number of drops per minute at which the IV solution must run to deliver the prescribed volume of fluid. The first step in finding the drip rate is to determine the minute volume by dividing the hourly volume by 60. Then we multiply the minute volume by the drop factor to find the drip rate. For example, an IV of 100 mL/h delivers a minute volume of 1.7 ($\frac{100}{60} = 1.7$). If the drop factor is 10, 1.7×10 yields 17 gtt/min as the drip rate.

6. SHORTCUT FORMULA FOR DETERMINING IV DRIP RATE

The shortcut formula is:

$$\frac{\text{Amount of solution infused}}{\text{Amount of time for infusion}} \times \text{Drop factor} = \text{Drip rate}$$

For example,

$$\frac{100 \text{ mL}}{60 \text{ min}} \times 10 \text{ gtt/mL} = 17 \text{ gtt/min}$$

7. IV THERAPY DELIVERY SYSTEMS

There are several methods for administering IV fluids and drugs. The safest is to connect the IV to an electronic control device, such as a controller or pump. These systems control the IV rate and signal the nurse when there are problems with IV fluid delivery.

Several systems are available to deliver IV medication. The most common method on general hospital units or in other health care settings is mixing the drug in a continuous IV infusion or administering the drug intermittently via a minibag.

8. SPECIAL CALCULATIONS FOR IV DRUGS

The physician may order IV drugs in a variety of ways. The nurse calculates the dosage of the drug first, then finds the flow rate that delivers the prescribed dosage. The calculation required is similar to that for determining the dosage of any medication. Most IV drugs are administered in milligrams per minute or micrograms per minute.

9. AVOIDING ERRORS: ADHERING TO SAFE DRUG DOSAGE PARAMETERS

The nurse checks the dosage prescribed and the solution prepared to ensure that the dose is safe for the client. The nurse compares the order with the recommendations for dosage ranges. Some recommendations require knowledge of the client's weight in kilograms.

ANSWERS 1. Five percent dextrose in normal saline 2. 175 mL 3. 125 mL/h 4. 6 h 5. 56 gtt/min 6. 63 mL/h 7. 8 mEq 8. 61 mL/h 9. 24 mg; 400 mcg 10. 66 gtt/min

EXERCISES FOR EXTRA PRACTICE

Exercises 1–5. Find the flow rate.

1. 150 mL to infuse in 75 min
2. 250 mL to infuse in 3 h
3. 500 mL to infuse in 4 h
4. 1000 mL to infuse in 4 h
5. 1000 mL to infuse in 24 h

Exercises 6–10. Determine the total infusion time.

6. 250 mL at 75 mL/h
7. 500 mL at 65 mL/h
8. 500 mL at 80 mL/h
9. 1000 mL at 45 mL/h
10. 1000 mL at 55 mL/h

Exercises 11–15. Find the minute volume.

11. 250 mL at 75 mL/h
12. 500 mL at 125 mL/h
13. 1000 mL at 55 mL/h
14. 100 mL in 30 min
15. 150 mL in 90 min

Exercises 16–20. Calculate the drip rate.

16. 250 mL at 75 mL/h (DF = 10)
17. 500 mL at 125 mL/h (DF = 15)
18. 1000 mL at 55 mL/h (DF = 60)
19. 100 mL in 30 min (DF = 20)
20. 150 mL in 90 min (DF = 15)

Exercises 21–25. Compute the amount of drug delivered each hour.

21. 1000 mL 5%D/NS with 20 mEq of potassium at 50 mL/h
22. 1000 mL NS with 100 U regular insulin to infuse in 12 h
23. 250 mL 5%D/W with 400 mg lidocaine at 40 mL/h
24. 1000 mL 5%D/W with 32,000 U of heparin at 30 mL/h
25. 1000 mL 5%D/W with 1 g of aminophylline at 35 mL/h

Exercises 26–30. Calculate the drip rate for these IV medications when microdrip tubing is used.

26. Give 500 mg of dobutamine in 250 mL 5%D/W at 5 mcg/kg/min for a client weighing 182 lb.
27. Give dopamine 400 mg in 250 mL 5%D/W at 6 mcg/kg/min for a client weighing 133 lb.
28. Give dobutamine 1000 mg in 500 mL 5%D/W at 6 mcg/kg/min for a client weighing 116 lb.
29. Give amrinone 250 mg in 250 mL normal saline at 3 mcg/kg/min for a client weighing 227 lb.
30. Give Nipride 50 mg in 250 mL 5%D/W at 3 mcg/kg/min for a client weighing 195 lb.

ANSWERS 1. 120 mL/h 3. 125 mL/h 5. 42 mL/h 7. 7.7 h 9. 22.2 h 11. 1.3 mL 13. 0.9 mL 15. 1.7 mL 17. 31 gtt/min 19. 67 gtt/min 21. 1 mEq 23. 64 mg 25. 35 mg 27. 14 gtt/min 29. 19 gtt/min

CHAPTER TEST

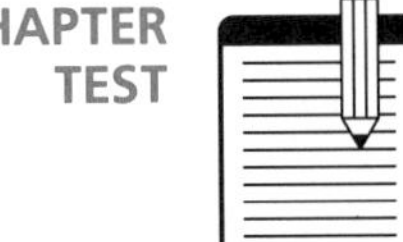

1. Write this abbreviation for an IV solution in words:

   5%D/NS 1. ____________

2. How many milliliters have infused from this 500-mL bag of IV solution? 2. ____________

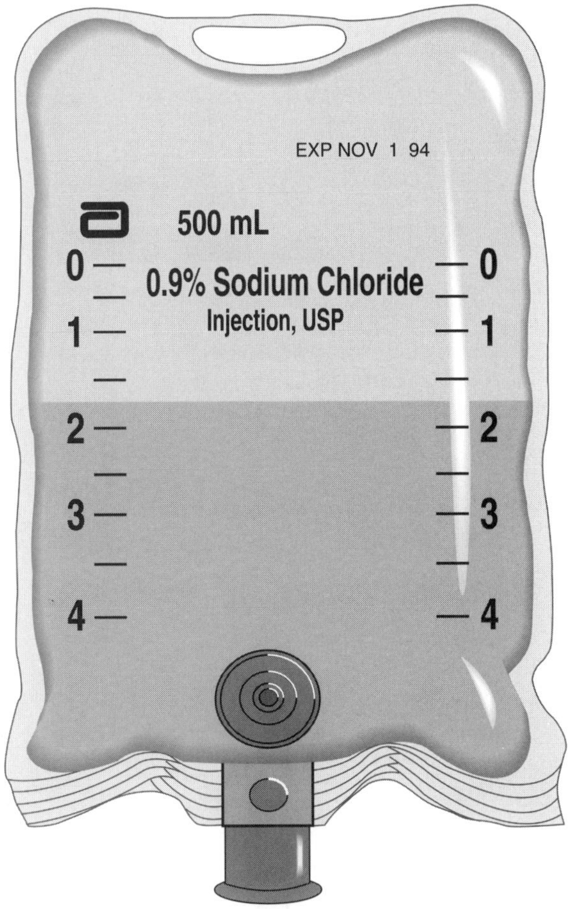

EXP NOV 1 94

500 mL

0.9% Sodium Chloride Injection, USP

3. The physician orders 1000 mL of Ringer's lactate to infuse in 8 h. What should the flow rate be? 3. ____________

4. If a 1000-mL bag of IV solution infuses at 167 mL/h, what is the total time of the infusion? 4. ____________

5. Calculate the drip rate needed to provide the amount of IV fluid ordered in Problem 4 if the drop factor is 20 gtt = 1 mL. 5. ____________

6. The nurse administers IV ACTH in 250 mL of 5%D/W in a 4-h period. What is the flow rate (mL/h)? 6. ____________

7. The physician's order is: 1000 mL 5%D/NS with 40 mEq of potassium at 200 mL/h. How many mEq of potassium does the client receive each hour? 7. ____________

8. The physician orders IV heparin at 1530 U/h. The solution available is 25,000 U of heparin in 1000 mL 5%D/W. What should the flow rate of the solution be to deliver the prescribed amount of heparin? 8. ____________

9. The physician orders IV dopamine to run at 30 mL/h. The available solution is 500 mL 5%D/W with 400 mg dopamine. Calculate in milligrams the amount of drug that the client is receiving each hour and each minute. 9. ____________

10. The physician orders 50 mg of Nipride in 250 mL 5%D/W to infuse at 3 mcg/kg/min. The client weighs 160 lb. Calculate the drip rate using microdrip tubing. 10. ____________

NINE

Individualized Drug Therapy

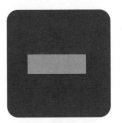

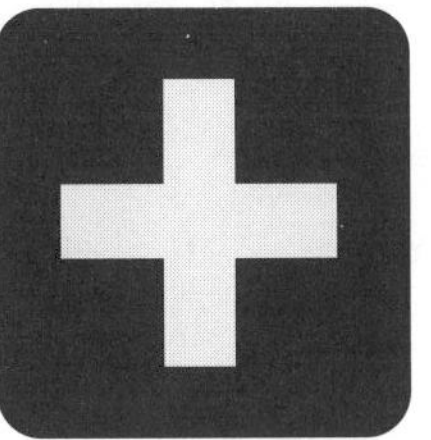

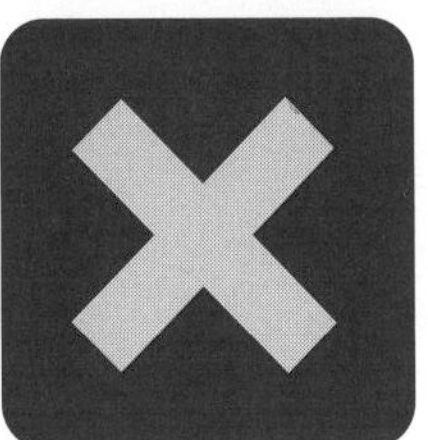

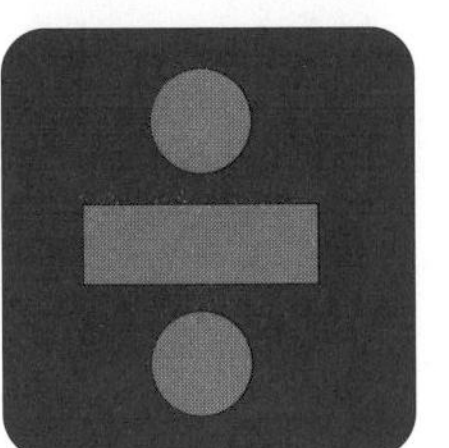

▶ OUTLINE

9-1. INTRODUCTION
9-2. SOURCES OF INFORMATION FOR INDIVIDUALIZED DRUG THERAPY
9-3. HEALTH STATUS AS A BASIS FOR INDIVIDUALIZED DRUG THERAPY
9-4. BODY WEIGHT AND BODY SURFACE AREA AS A MEANS OF INDIVIDUALIZING DRUG THERAPY
9-5. DRUG THERAPY AND CHILDREN
9-6. INTRAVENOUS THERAPY AND CHILDREN
9-7. DRUG THERAPY AND THE ELDERLY
9-8. DRUG THERAPY AND PREGNANCY
9-9. AVOIDING ERRORS: ADHERING TO SAFE DRUG DOSAGE PARAMETERS
9-10. SUMMARY

▶ OBJECTIVES

After studying this chapter, you will be able to:

1. Identify the factors that determine drug dosages.
2. State the sources of information used to determine drug dosages.
3. Calculate drug dosages based on body weight.
4. Calculate drug dosages based on body surface area.
5. Use a child's body surface area to find a child's dosage based on the recommended adult dosage.
6. Identify three common systems used to provide intravenous (IV) fluids and medications for children.
7. Use body weight to calculate the safe dosage range for children and adults, compare the range with the ordered amount, and decide whether to give the drug as ordered.
8. Calculate the drip rate for IV medications, using a Buretrol or similar device.
9. State the special precautions used when giving drugs to the elderly.
10. Calculate drug dosages for pregnant women.
11. Check drug dosages to avoid errors in medication administration.

9-1. INTRODUCTION

Why is drug therapy individualized? Although certain drug dosage ranges are recommended by drug companies, each person is an individual with different characteristics that can affect drug therapy. For example, the amount of drug needed for a one-year-old baby is very different from the amount of the same drug used for a 50-year-old adult. Factors such as age, sex, size (height and weight), culture, and health status all affect the type of drug and the dosage of drug that the physician prescribes.

The nurse's role is to calculate the safe dosage range for each prescribed drug and compare the safe range with the ordered dose. The nurse verifies any unusual drug orders with the physician *before* giving the drug.

Examples

1. The usual dosage of amoxicillin for adults with lower respiratory tract infection is 500 mg every 8 hours. The recommendation for children is 40 mg/kg/day. Children weighing 20 kg or more should be dosed according to adult recommendations.
2. When Ancef is administered to clients with low urinary output because of renal disease, lower daily drug dosage is required.
3. Septra IV infusion is not recommended for infants younger than two months of age.

Proficiency Gauge

You may already understand the principles underlying individualized drug dosages and know the precautions used when administering medications to the elderly and to pregnant women. Complete the following exercises to determine how much you understand. Compare your answers with the answer section only after you have completed the exercises.

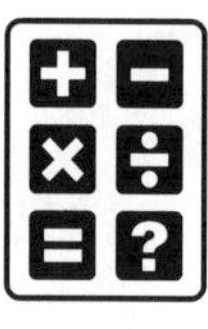

EXERCISES

1. What is the *Physicians' Desk Reference (PDR)* used for? 1. ______________
2. For a client receiving Dilantin, the therapeutic range (desired blood level) of the drug is 10–20 mcg/mL. The client's recent lab test shows the level at 8 mcg/mL. What conclusion should the nurse make and what action should he or she take? 2. ______________
3. Find the number of kilograms in 33 lb. 3. ______________
4. The recommended adult dose of a drug is 500 mg. If Suzie's body surface area (BSA) is 1.3 m^2, what is the recommended dose for her? 4. ______________
5. The physician orders 100 mg of an antibiotic for Stephie. The oral suspension reads: "125 mg/5 mL." How many milliliters should the nurse give her? 5. ______________

6. The physician orders a drug to be diluted in 25 mL of 5%D/W. The volume of undiluted drug needed is 4 mL. How much of the IV solution is needed to achieve the drug dilution? 6. ____________

7. The physician orders 1 g of Zinacef in 50 mL 5%D/NS to infuse via Buretrol over 75 min followed by a 15-mL flush. Calculate the IV drip rate (DF: 1 mL = 60 gtt). (*Note:* Add the drug volume and flush volume together before calculating the drip rate.) 7. ____________

8. The physician orders 20 mEq of potassium qd for Mr. Watson, an elderly man living alone at home. The medication comes in liquid form as 15 mEq/5 mL. How many milliliters should he take? 8. ____________

9. The physician orders a terbutaline sulfate infusion to start at 10 mcg/min. The concentration of the drug in solution is 5 mcg/mL. What IV rate (in milliliters per minute) is needed to provide the prescribed drug? 9. ____________

10. The physician orders magnesium sulfate for a woman with pregnancy-induced hypertension in labor. The IV bag reads "20 g magnesium sulfate in 1000 mL 5%D/W." What is the concentration of the drug in the IV solution (in milligrams per milliliter)? 10. ____________

ANSWERS 1. The *PDR* contains information from drug companies on drug dosages, chemical structure, actions, indications and usages, contraindications, and side effects and toxic reactions. 2. Since the client's level is below the therapeutic range, the nurse should notify the physician of the result. 3. 15 kg 4. 375.7 mg 5. 4 mL 6. 21 mL 7. 52 gtt/min 8. 6.7 mL 9. 2 mL/min 10. 20 mg/mL

9-2. SOURCES OF INFORMATION FOR INDIVIDUALIZED DRUG THERAPY

The physician, pharmacologist (or clinical pharmacist), and/or nurse in most health care settings assess each client for individual factors that may affect drug selection and dosage. These factors, especially age, body size and weight, and health state, are then compared with guidelines recommended by the pharmaceutical company for a given drug.

These recommendations are based on comprehensive research on the drug and its effects. In the United States, the Food and Drug Administration (FDA) carefully monitors the development and use of new drugs and controls their release to the public. A new drug typically takes 6 to 12 years to develop and another 5 to 9 years for clinical trials before FDA approval. In other countries, the process for controlling and releasing new drugs is often less stringent.

Physician's Drug Reference

Physicians obtain most of their information regarding drug dosing from the *Physicians' Desk Reference (PDR).* The *PDR* is an annually published compilation of inserts accompanying each drug that are provided by the manufacturer. In addition to dosing information, the *PDR* provides data about indications and usage, contraindications, precautions, warnings, dosage, and clinical data about the results of drug studies.

Drug Updates

The *PDR* is only published annually, but various newsletters are available from the FDA, the American Medical Association, and other medical and pharmaceutical organizations to provide health care professionals with updated information on new drugs.

Formulary

Each health care facility has its own resource, called a formulary, which contains more specific information on techniques for drug administration. A formulary is used primarily by pharmacy personnel and physicians to determine drug substitutions. For example, cefuroxime axetil (Ceftin) is a very expensive antibiotic. Because of similar chemical structure and drug actions, cefadroxil (Duricef) may be substituted for Ceftin. The nurse needs to be aware when substitute drugs are approved in his or her health care agency.

Nursing Drug References

In addition to these sources, there are numerous drug references with specific information about usual dose ranges, side effects and toxic reactions, and the nursing interventions needed for particular drugs. Some references are books and others are drug cards. Examples of these resources include the *1993 Drug Handbook* (Springhouse), the *Nurses' Drug Reference* (Mosby), and the *Nurse's Drug Handbook* (Saunders). (See Chapter 6 for an excerpt.)

Updates about new drugs are published in nursing journals or are presented in continuing-education programs.

Clinical Pharmacologist

Most hospitals have full-service pharmacy departments that include clinical pharmacologists (Pharm. D.), or pharmacists, who are excellent resources for both physicians and nurses. In some hospitals, the pharmacist writes the protocol for dosing a drug or selects the appropriate drug to be used at the physician's request.

Examples

1. The physician writes an order on the chart for IV gentamicin sulfate "per pharmacy protocol." On the basis of an assessment of the client, the clinical pharmacist then writes an order for gentamicin 80 mg IVPB every 8 h.
2. On the basis of the results of the client's partial thromboplastin time (PTT) (blood-clotting time), the pharmacologist increases the amount of client's IV heparin infusion from 1100 U/h to 1200 U/h and requests a repeat of the laboratory study to monitor changes.

Computer DataBases

Many hospitals have a drug data base available to health care professionals as part of the their hospital information system. Although they differ from place to place, most data bases contain information on generic drug equivalents, available drug forms, side effects and toxic reactions, and client teaching for discharge planning.

Nurse's Responsibility

Although the physician and pharmacologist select the appropriate drugs for each client and prescribe the dose to be given, the nurse is responsible for (1) checking that the drug and dose are reasonable for the individual client and (2) monitoring for therapeutic and side effects. If the nurse has any question or doubt about the drug or its prescribed dosage, he or she contacts the physician or pharmacologist *before* giving the drug to the client. The nurse is the last safety check for drug errors before the client receives the drug. If the dose is too low, the client's health problem may not resolve. More important, if the dose is too high, the client may experience signs of drug toxicity or possibly die.

In rare instances, the nurse may refuse to administer a drug if the drug dose is too high. The nurse notifies the physician and nursing supervisor if this decision is made.

Examples

1. The physician orders a drug to combat tuberculosis for a client. The nurse finds no evidence of this disease on the client's medical record and calls the physician before administering it.
2. The recommended maintenance dose of digoxin (Lanoxin) for an adult is 0.125–0.25 mg every day. The physician prescribes 0.375 mg twice a day. The nurse verifies the prescribed dose with the physician before giving the drug.

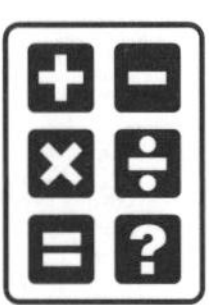

EXERCISES

Exercises 1–4. From the drug insert for fluorouracil injection (Fig. 9–1) answer the following questions:

1. Is this drug intended for clients who can be cured by surgery? (Refer to indications.)
2. Is this drug intended for clients with potentially serious infections? (Refer to contraindications.)
3. What is the maximum daily dosage? (Refer to warnings.)
4. What is the minimum white blood count (WBC) below which therapy should be discontinued? (Refer to precautions.)

Exercises 5–10. From the drug insert for Benadryl (Fig. 9–2) answer the following questions:

5. Is this drug recommended for oral therapy?
6. Is this drug recommended for treatment of motion sickness?
7. Is this drug recommended for treatment of parkinsonism?
8. Is this drug recommended for use in newborn infants?
9. Is this drug recommended as a local anesthetic?
10. What information should be provided to clients about this drug?
11. The *PDR* is published annually. What sources do health care professionals use to keep up with new information that becomes available during the year?
12. What is the primary function of the formulary in a health care facility?
13. What are examples of additional sources of drug information for the nurse?
14. After the physician has prescribed a certain drug for a client, does the nurse then decide on the appropriate dosage?
15. The physician orders trimethoprim–sulfamethoxazole (Bactrim), a sulfa drug, for a client with a known allergy to sulfa. Should the nurse check with the physician before giving the prescribed drug?
16. The recommended maximum daily dose of chlorpromazine hydrochloride (Thorazine) is 2 g/day for a psychiatric disorder and 400 mg/day for nausea. The physician orders 450 mg qid for a client with a psychiatric disorder. On the basis of the recommendations, should the nurse check the dose with the physician before giving it?

Exercises 17–20. Maximum daily dosage instructions for dextromethorphan hydrobromide (Benylin DM) are as follows:

adults: 120 mg/day
children 6–12 years old: 60 mg/day
children 2–6 years old: 30 mg/day

On the basis of this information, which of the following orders should the nurse check with the physician?

17. Mr. Jones, 40 years old, 30 mg q4h
18. Maureen, 7 years old, 7.5 mg q6h
19. Carolann, 5 years old, 2.5 mg qid
20. Gary, 3 years old, 7.5 mg q4h

A.H.F.S. Category 10:00

FLUOROURACIL
INJECTION

WARNING
It is recommended that FLUOROURACIL be given only by or under the supervision of a qualified physician who is experienced in cancer chemotherapy and who is well versed in the use of potent antimetabolites. Because of the possibility of severe toxic reactions, it is recommended that patients be hospitalized at least during the initial course of therapy.

DESCRIPTION: FLUOROURACIL INJECTION/Roche, an antineoplastic antimetabolite, is a sterile, nonpyrogenic injectable solution for intravenous administration. Each 10-mL contains 500 mg fluorouracil; pH is adjusted to approximately 9.2 with sodium hydroxide.

Chemically, fluorouracil, a fluorinated pyrimidine, is 5-fluoro-2,4 (1*H*,3*H*)-pyrimidinedione. It is a white to practically white crystalline powder which is sparingly soluble in water. The molecular weight of fluorouracil is 130.08 and the structural formula is:

H N O NH F O

CLINICAL PHARMACOLOGY: There is evidence that the metabolism of fluorouracil in the anabolic pathway blocks the methylation reaction of deoxyuridylic acid to thymidylic acid. In this manner, fluorouracil interferes with the synthesis of deoxyribonucleic acid (DNA) and to a lesser extent inhibits the formation of ribonucleic acid (RNA). Since DNA and RNA are essential for cell division and growth, the effect of fluorouracil may be to create a thymine deficiency which provokes unbalanced growth and death of the cell. The effects of DNA and RNA deprivation are most marked on those cells which grow more rapidly and which take up fluorouracil at a more rapid rate.

Following intravenous injection, fluorouracil distributes into tumors, intestinal mucosa, bone marrow, liver and other tissues throughout the body. In spite of its limited lipid solubility, fluorouracil diffuses readily across the blood-brain barrier and distributes into cerebrospinal fluid and brain tissue.

Seven to twenty percent of the parent drug is excreted unchanged in the urine in six hours; of this over 90% is excreted in the first hour. The remaining percentage of the administered dose is metabolized, primarily in the liver. The catabolic metabolism of fluorouracil results in degradation products (*e.g.*, CO_2, urea and α-fluoro-ß-alanine) which are inactive. The inactive metabolites are excreted in the urine over the next 3 to 4 hours. When fluorouracil is labeled in the six carbon position, thus preventing the ^{14}C metabolism to CO_2, approximately 90% of the total radioactivity is excreted in the urine. When fluorouracil is labeled in the two carbon position approximately 90% of the total radioactivity is excreted in expired CO_2. Ninety percent of the dose is accounted for during the first 24 hours following intravenous administration.

Following intravenous administration of fluorouracil, the mean half-life of elimination from plasma is approximately 16 minutes, with a range of 8 to 20 minutes, and is dose dependent. No intact drug can be detected in the plasma three hours after an intravenous injection.

INDICATIONS AND USAGE: Fluorouracil is effective in the palliative management of carcinoma of the colon, rectum, breast, stomach and pancreas.

CONTRAINDICATIONS: Fluorouracil therapy is contraindicated for patients in a poor nutritional state, those with depressed bone marrow function, those with potentially serious infections or those with a known hypersensitivity to Fluorouracil.

WARNINGS: THE DAILY DOSE OF FLUOROURACIL IS NOT TO EXCEED 800 MG. IT IS RECOMMENDED THAT PATIENTS BE HOSPITALIZED DURING THEIR FIRST COURSE OF TREATMENT.

Fluorouracil should be used with extreme caution in poor risk patients with a history of high-dose pelvic irradiation or previous use of alkylating agents, those who have a widespread involvement of bone marrow by metastatic tumors or those with impaired hepatic or renal function.

Pregnancy: Teratogenic effects: Pregnancy category D. Fluorouracil may cause fetal harm when administered to a pregnant woman. Fluorouracil has been shown to be teratogenic in laboratory animals. Fluorouracil exhibited maximum teratogenicity when given to mice as single intraperitoneal injections of 10 to 40 mg/kg on day 10 or 12 of gestation. Similarly, intraperitoneal doses of 12 to 37 mg/kg given to rats between days 9 and 12 of gestation and intramuscular doses of 3 to 9 mg given to hamsters between days 8 and 11 of gestation were teratogenic. Malformations included cleft palates, skeletal defects and deformed appendages, paws and tails. The dosages which were teratogenic in animals are 1 to 3 times the maximum recommended human therapeutic dose. In monkeys, divided doses of 40 mg/kg given between days 20 and 24 of gestation were not teratogenic.

There are no adequate and well-controlled studies with Fluorouracil in pregnant women. While there is no evidence of teratogenicity in humans due to Fluorouracil, it should be kept in mind that other drugs which inhibit DNA synthesis (*e.g.*, methotrexate and aminopterin) have been reported to be teratogenic in humans. Women of childbearing potential should be advised to avoid becoming pregnant. If the drug is used during pregnancy, or if the patient becomes pregnant while taking the drug, the patient should be told of the potential hazard to the fetus. Fluorouracil should be used during pregnancy only if the potential benefit justifies the potential risk to the fetus.

Combination Therapy: Any form of therapy which adds to the stress of the patient, interferes with nutrition or depresses bone marrow function will increase the toxicity of Fluorouracil.

PRECAUTIONS: *General:* Fluorouracil is a highly toxic drug with a narrow margin of safety. Therefore, patients should be carefully supervised, since therapeutic response is unlikely to occur without some evidence of toxicity. Severe hematological toxicity, gastrointestinal hemorrhage and even death may result from the use of Fluorouracil despite meticulous selection of patients and careful adjustment of dosage. Although severe toxicity is more likely in poor risk patients, fatalities may be encountered occasionally even in patients in relatively good condition.

Therapy is to be discontinued promptly whenever one of the following signs of toxicity appears:

Stomatitis or esophagopharyngitis, at the first visible sign.

Leukopenia (WBC under 3500) or a rapidly falling white blood count.

Vomiting, intractable.

Diarrhea, frequent bowel movements or watery stools.

Gastrointestinal ulceration and bleeding.

Thrombocytopenia (platelets under 100,000).

Hemorrhage from any site.

The administration of 5-fluorouracil has been associated with the occurrence of palmar-plantar erythrodysesthesia syndrome, also known as hand-foot syndrome. This syndrome has been characterized as a tingling sensation of hands and feet which may progress over the next few days to pain when holding objects or walking. The palms and soles become symmetrically swollen and erythematous with tenderness of the distal phalanges, possibly accompanied by desquamation. Interruption of therapy is followed by gradual resolution over 5 to 7 days. Although pyridoxine has been reported to ameliorate the palmar-plantar erythrodysesthesia syndrome, its safety and effectiveness have not been established.

Information for Patients: Patients should be informed of expected toxic effects, particularly oral manifestations. Patients should be alerted to the possibility of alopecia as a result of therapy and should be informed that it is usually a transient effect.

Laboratory Tests: White blood counts with differential are recommended before each dose.

Drug Interactions: Leucovorin calcium may enhance the toxicity of fluorouracil.

Also see WARNINGS section.

Carcinogenesis, Mutagenesis, Impairment of Fertility: Carcinogenesis: Long-term studies in animals to evaluate the carcinogenic potential of fluorouracil have not been conducted. However, there was no evidence of carcinogenicity in small groups of rats given fluorouracil orally at doses of 0.01, 0.3, 1 or 3 mg per rat 5 days per week for 52 weeks, followed by a six-month observation period. Also, in other studies, 33 mg/kg of fluorouracil was administered intravenously to male rats once a week for 52 weeks followed by observation for the remainder of their lifetimes with no evidence of carcinogenicity. Female mice were given 1 mg of fluorouracil intravenously once a week for 16 weeks with no effect on the incidence of lung adenomas. On the basis of the available data, no evaluation can be made of the carcinogenic risk of fluorouracil to humans.

Mutagenesis: Oncogenic transformation of fibroblasts from mouse embryo has been induced *in vitro* by fluorouracil, but the relationship between oncogenicity and mutagenicity is not clear. Fluorouracil has been shown to be mutagenic to several strains of *Salmonella typhimurium*, including TA 1535, TA 1537 and TA 1538, and to *Saccharomyces cerevisiae*, although no evidence of mutagenicity was found with *Salmonella typhimurium* strains TA 92, TA 98 and TA 100. In addition, a positive effect was observed in the micronucleus test on bone marrow cells of the mouse, and fluorouracil at very high concentrations produced chromosomal breaks in hamster fibroblasts *in vitro*.

Impairment of fertility: Fluorouracil has not been adequately studied in animals to permit an evaluation of its effects on fertility and general reproductive performance. However, doses of 125 or 250 mg/kg, administered intraperitoneally, have been shown to induce chromosomal aberrations and changes in chromosomal organization of spermatogonia in rats. Spermatogonial differentiation was also inhibited by fluorouracil, resulting in transient infertility. However, in studies with a

Figure 9–1 Fluorouracil injection package insert. (Courtesy of Hoffmann-La Roche, Inc., Nutley, NJ.)

AHFS Category 4:00

Benadryl®

(Diphenhydramine Hydrochloride Injection, USP)

DESCRIPTION

Benadryl (diphenhydramine hydrochloride) is an antihistamine drug having the chemical name 2-(Diphenylmethoxy)-N,N-dimethylethylamine hydrochloride. It occurs as a white crystalline powder, is freely soluble in water and alcohol and has a molecular weight of 291.82. The molecular formula is $C_{17}H_{21}NO \cdot HCl$.

$$\left[(C_6H_5)_2CH{-}O{-}CH_2CH_2\overset{H^+}{N}(CH_3)_2 \right] Cl^-$$

Benadryl in the parenteral form is a sterile, pyrogen-free solution available in two concentrations: 10 mg and 50 mg of diphenhydramine hydrochloride per mL. The solutions for parenteral use have been adjusted to a pH between 5.0 and 6.0 with either sodium hydroxide or hydrochloric acid. The multidose Steri-Vials® contain 0.1 mg/mL benzethonium chloride as a germicidal agent.

CLINICAL PHARMACOLOGY

Diphenhydramine hydrochloride is an antihistamine with anticholinergic (drying) and sedative side effects. Antihistamines appear to compete with histamine for cell receptor sites on effector cells.

Benadryl in the injectable form has a rapid onset of action. Diphenhydramine hydrochloride is widely distributed throughout the body, including the CNS. A portion of the drug is excreted unchanged in the urine, while the rest is metabolized via the liver. Detailed information on the pharmacokinetics of Diphenhydramine Hydrochloride Injection is not available.

INDICATIONS AND USAGE

Benadryl in the injectable form is effective for the following conditions when Benadryl in the oral form is impractical.

Antihistaminic: For amelioration of allergic reactions to blood or plasma, in anaphylaxis as an adjunct to epinephrine and other standard measures after the acute symptoms have been controlled, and for other uncomplicated allergic conditions of the immediate type when oral therapy is impossible or contraindicated.

Motion sickness: For active treatment of motion sickness.

Antiparkinsonism: For use in parkinsonism, when oral therapy is impossible or contraindicated, as follows: parkinsonism in the elderly who are unable to tolerate more potent agents, mild cases of parkinsonism in other age groups, and in other cases of parkinsonism in combination with centrally acting anticholinergic agents.

CONTRAINDICATIONS

Use in Newborn or Premature Infants

This drug should *not* be used in newborn or premature infants.

Use in Nursing Mothers

Because of the higher risk of antihistamines for infants generally, and for newborns and prematures in particular, antihistamine therapy is contraindicated in nursing mothers.

Use as a Local Anesthetic

Because of the risk of local necrosis, this drug should not be used as a local anesthetic.

Antihistamines are also contraindicated in the following conditions: Hypersensitivity to diphenhydramine hydrochloride and other antihistamines of similar chemical structure.

WARNINGS

Antihistamines should be used with considerable caution in patients with narrow-angle glaucoma, stenosing peptic ulcer, pyloroduodenal obstruction, symptomatic prostatic hypertrophy, or bladder-neck obstruction.

Use in Children

In infants and children, especially, antihistamines in *overdosage* may cause hallucinations, convulsions, or death.

As in adults, antihistamines may diminish mental alertness in children. In the young child, particularly, they may produce excitation.

Use in the Elderly (approximately 60 years or older)

Antihistamines are more likely to cause dizziness, sedation, and hypotension in elderly patients.

PRECAUTIONS

General: Diphenhydramine hydrochloride has an atropine-like action and therefore, should be used with caution in patients with a history of bronchial asthma, increased intraocular pressure, hyperthyroidism, cardiovascular disease or hypertension. Use with caution in patients with lower respiratory disease including asthma.

Information for Patients: Patients taking diphenhydramine hydrochloride should be advised that this drug may cause drowsiness and has an additive effect with alcohol.

Patients should be warned about engaging in activities requiring mental alertness such as driving a car or operating appliances, machinery, etc.

Drug Interactions: Diphenhydramine hydrochloride has additive effects with alcohol and other CNS depressants (hypnotics, sedatives, tranquilizers, etc).

MAO inhibitors prolong and intensify the anticholinergic (drying) effects of antihistamines.

Carcinogenesis, Mutagenesis, Impairment of Fertility: Long-term studies in animals to determine mutagenic and carcinogenic potential have not been performed.

Benadryl®
(Diphenhydramine Hydrochloride Injection, USP)

Pregnancy: Pregnancy Category B. Reproduction studies have been performed in rats and rabbits at doses up to 5 times the human dose and have revealed no evidence of impaired fertility or harm to the fetus due to diphenhydramine hydrochloride. There are, however, no adequate and well-controlled studies in pregnant women. Because animal reproduction studies are not always predictive of human response, this drug should be used during pregnancy only if clearly needed.

ADVERSE REACTIONS

The most frequent adverse reactions are underscored.

1. *General:* Urticaria, drug rash, anaphylactic shock, photosensitivity, excessive perspiration, chills, dryness of mouth, nose, and throat
2. *Cardiovascular System:* Hypotension, headache, palpitations, tachycardia, extrasystoles
3. *Hematologic System:* Hemolytic anemia, thrombocytopenia, agranulocytosis
4. *Nervous System:* <u>Sedation, sleepiness, dizziness, disturbed coordination,</u> fatigue, confusion, restlessness, excitation, nervousness, tremor, irritability, insomnia, euphoria, paresthesia, blurred vision, diplopia, vertigo, tinnitus, acute labyrinthitis, neuritis, convulsions
5. *GI System:* <u>Epigastric distress</u>, anorexia, nausea, vomiting, diarrhea, constipation
6. *GU System:* Urinary frequency, difficult urination, urinary retention, early menses
7. *Respiratory System:* <u>Thickening of bronchial secretions</u>, tightness of chest and wheezing, nasal stuffiness

OVERDOSAGE

Antihistamine overdosage reactions may vary from central nervous system depression to stimulation. Stimulation is particularly likely in children. Atropine-like signs and symptoms, dry mouth; fixed, dilated pupils; flushing, and gastrointestinal symptoms may also occur.

Stimulants should not be used.

Vasopressors may be used to treat hypotension.

DOSAGE AND ADMINISTRATION

Benadryl in the injectable form is indicated when the oral form is impractical. Parenteral drug products should be inspected visually for particulate matter and discoloration prior to administration, whenever solution and container permit.

DOSAGE SHOULD BE INDIVIDUALIZED ACCORDING TO THE NEEDS AND THE RESPONSE OF THE PATIENT.

Children: 5 mg/kg/24 hr or 150 mg/m²/24 hr. Maximum daily dosage is 300 mg. Divide into four doses, administered intravenously or deeply intramuscularly.

Adults: 10 to 50 mg intravenously or deeply intramuscularly, 100 mg if required; maximum daily dosage is 400 mg.

Benadryl®
(Diphenhydramine Hydrochloride Injection, USP)

HOW SUPPLIED

Benadryl in parenteral form is supplied as:
Benadryl Steri-Vials®—sterile, pyrogen-free solution containing 10 mg diphenhydramine hydrochloride in each milliliter of solution with 0.1 mg/mL benzethonium chloride as a germicidal agent. Available in 10-mL (N 0071-4015-10) and 30-mL (N 0071-4015-13) Steri-Vials (rubber-diaphragm-capped vials).

Sterile, pyrogen-free solution containing 50 mg diphenhydramine hydrochloride in each milliliter of solution with 0.1 mg/mL benzethonium chloride as a germicidal agent. Available in 10-mL (N 0071-4402-10) Steri-Vials.

Benadryl Steri-Dose®—sterile, pyrogen-free solution containing 50 mg diphenhydramine hydrochloride in a 1-mL disposable syringe (Steri-Dose). Available in packages of ten individually cartoned syringes (N 0071-4259-40) and in packages of two trays of 5 syringes (N 0071-4259-41).

Benadryl Ampoule—sterile, pyrogen-free solution containing 50 mg diphenhydramine hydrochloride in a 1-mL ampoule. Available in packages of ten (N 0071-4259-03).

STORAGE CONDITIONS

Store at controlled room temperature 15°–30° C (59°–86° F). Protect from freezing and light.

Caution—Federal law prohibits dispensing without prescription.

Figure 9–2 Benadryl package insert. (Courtesy of Parke-Davis, Morris Plains, NJ.)

ANSWERS 1. No, the drug is effective in "patients who are considered incurable by surgery." 3. 800 mg 5. It can be 7. Yes 9. No 11. Newsletters from the FDA, the American Medical Association, and other organizations 13. Drug references written especially for nurses, such as *Nurses' Drug Handbook,* clinical pharmacologists, computer data bases 15. Yes 17. Yes, daily dose is 30 mg × 6 = 180 mg > 120 mg (maximum dose recommended). 19. No check is needed; 2.5 mg × 4 = 10 mg < 30 mg.

9-3. HEALTH STATUS AS A BASIS FOR INDIVIDUALIZED DRUG THERAPY

One of the most important factors in determining drug dosage is the client's general health and the presence or absence of disease or illness. The physician and pharmacologist use this information to decide on the drug dosage. However, there are times when the nurse questions whether the ordered dose is correct or if a drug should be given at all on the basis of guidelines provided by the physician.

Examples

1. After receiving a morphine injection, the client's respiratory rate decreases to 8/min. The normal respiratory rate for an adult is 12–20. The physician's order states to administer Narcan if respirations fall below 10. In this case, the nurse's assessment findings help determine whether and when the prescribed drug is given.
2. A client's pulse is 54/min. The nurse knows that digoxin is not given without notifying the physician unless the pulse is at least 60. The nurse contacts the physician regarding the low pulse before giving the drug.

SAMPLE EXERCISES

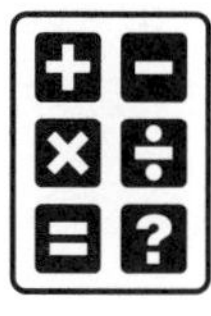

1. The physician's order states that she is to be notified for a systolic blood pressure below 100 before a client is given Inderal. The client's systolic pressure is 98. What should the nurse do?
2. A client is receiving regular insulin for diabetes on a sliding scale schedule as follows:
   If blood sugar (BS) > 400, give 12 U regular insulin
   If BS = 300–400, give 8 U regular insulin
   If BS = 200–299, give 4 U regular insulin
   If BS < 200, do not give insulin
   At 11:30 AM, the client's BS was 358. How much insulin should the nurse give?
3. The physician prescribes 2 tablets of Tylenol for the client when his temperature is above 101°F. The nurse finds that the client's temperature is 100.2°F. Should the nurse give the Tylenol for this elevated temperature?

ANSWERS 1. Call the physician before giving the drug. 2. 8 U regular insulin 3. no

The physician often adjusts drug dosage during the course of drug therapy. Some common reasons for changing the dose are the following:

Not enough drug is being given to achieve the therapeutic or desired level in the blood stream.
The effect of the drug is less than or more than what is desired.
The client's health problem is not responding to the drug.

Examples

1. For a client receiving phenytoin (Dilantin), the desired level in the blood is 10–20 μg/mL. The client's recent laboratory test shows the blood level at 6 μg. As a result, the physician increases the client's daily dose of Dilantin.
2. For a client receiving warfarin (Coumadin), the physician usually maintains the prothrombin time (PT) (blood-clotting factor) at 1.5–2 times the normal value. The client's recent PT is 47; the normal or control value is 13.5. As a result, the physician decreases the daily dose of Coumadin to prevent complications.

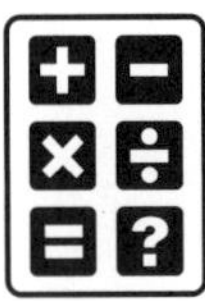

EXERCISES

Exercises 1–4. A client receives insulin for diabetes on a sliding scale as follows:

If blood sugar > 400, give 12 U regular insulin
$= 300–500$, give 8 U regular insulin
$= 200–299$, give 4 U regular insulin
< 200, do not give insulin

For the following levels of blood sugar, how much insulin should the nurse give? (Complete the table.)

	Blood Sugar	Insulin Amount
1.	220	
2.	188	
3.	462	
4.	314	

Exercises 5–8. When administering carmustine, the nurse must assess the client's white blood cell (WBC) and platelet count weekly. The nurse should withhold the drug and notify the physician when the WBC < 4000 or the platelet count $< 75{,}000$.

For each of the following clients, state whether the nurse should withhold the drug.

5. Angela: WBC = 4200, platelets = 80,000
6. Cary: WBC = 3600, platelets = 76,000
7. Ezra: WBC = 4800, platelets = 57,000
8. Gregory: WBC = 6000, platelets = 40,000

Exercises 9–12. When administering an antihypertensive drug, the nurse takes vital signs every 4 h. If systolic blood pressure (SBP)

drops more than 20 mm Hg, the nurse withholds the drug and notifies the physician. For each of the following cases, state whether the nurse should withhold the drug.

Client	First SBP Reading (mm Hg)	Second SBP Reading (mm Hg)
9. Ira	120	140
10. Karen	140	118
11. Martin	160	144
12. Olivia	116	138

ANSWERS 1. 4 U 3. 12 U 5. no 7. yes 9. no 11. no

9-4. BODY WEIGHT AND BODY SURFACE AREA AS A MEANS OF INDIVIDUALIZING DRUG THERAPY

A number of methods are commonly used to determine the correct drug dosage. Using age alone as a factor is unreliable for computing drug dosage because people vary tremendously, particularly children. For example, one 2-year-old may weigh 35 lb and be over 3 ft tall, whereas another weighs 20 lb and is 2 ft tall.

Two of the most common determinants for drug dosing are body weight and body surface area. Although weight is used primarily when determining dosages for children, it may also be considered when prescribing medication for adults, particularly those who are very small, grossly underweight, or very old. Body surface area is used for all age groups, especially in the administration of cancer drugs.

Body Weight

Most recommendations for drug dosage are based on weight in kilograms. For instance, the prescribed dosage of cefazolin sodium (Ancef) for a child may be 50 mg/kg of body weight. If body weight is measured in pounds, the nurse must convert pounds to kilograms. At those times when dosage recommendations are based on weight in pounds, the nurse may need to convert from kilograms to pounds. (Refer to Chapters 4 and 5 for complete discussions of conversions.)

CONVERSIONS

2.2 lb = 1 kg

To convert from pounds to kilograms, divide by 2.2.
To convert from kilograms to pounds, multiply by 2.2.
Round kilograms to the nearest **tenth.**
Round pounds to the nearest **unit.**

Example

Find the number of kilograms in 98 lb. To fix this conversion in your mind, use a table and a proportion.

Table: x kg in 98 lb
1 kg in 2.2 lb

Proportion: $\frac{x}{1} = \frac{98}{2.2} = 44.5$

Result: 98 lb = 44.5 kg

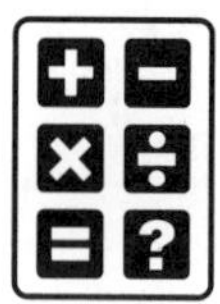

SAMPLE EXERCISES

Exercises 1–5. Find the number of kilograms in each of the weights below.

1. 66 lb
2. 23 lb
3. 5.4 lb
4. 220 lb
5. 2 lb

Exercises 6–8. Find the number of pounds in each of the weights below.

6. 70 kg
7. 16.8 kg
8. 110 kg

ANSWERS 1. $\frac{66 \text{ lb}}{2.2 \text{ lb}} \times 1 \text{ kg} = 30 \text{ kg}$ 2. 10.5 kg 3. 2.5 kg 4. 100 kg 5. 0.9 kg 6. 70×2.2 lb = 154 lb 7. 16.8×2.2 lb = 37 lb 8. 110×2.2 lb = 242 lb

The nurse's responsibility is to ensure the weight is accurate so the physician or pharmacologist can make the correct determination of drug dosage. The *PDR* and other references provide guidelines for assisting the physician in prescribing the correct amount of drug.

Examples

1. A total daily dosage of 25–50 mg/kg of body weight of cefazolin sodium (Ancef) divided into three or four equal doses is recommended for children. For a child weighing 20 kg and receiving 50 mg/kg, the total daily drug amount is 20×50 mg = 1000 mg of Ancef. When divided into 4 equal doses, each dose given to the child is 1000 mg/4 = 250 mg.
2. The recommendation for nitrofurantoin (Macrodantin) dosing is 5–7 mg/kg/day in 4 equally divided doses. This same recommendation may be stated as 5–7 mg/kg/day in divided doses every 6 h. For a child weighing 6.3 kg and receiving 5 mg/kg, the total daily drug amount is 6.3×5 mg = 31.5 mg. Each dose of the drug is $\frac{31.5 \text{ mg}}{4} = 7.88$ mg.

Although the nurse does not make the decision about drug dosage, he or she needs to be aware of the usual dosage range for each drug so errors can be detected. If the child's weight is recorded in pounds, the nurse must first convert pounds to kilograms before doing the calculations in the examples given above.

SAMPLE EXERCISES

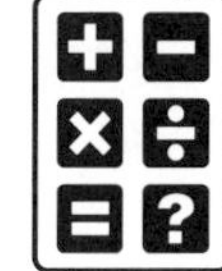

Exercises 1–3. The recommended loading dose for digoxin for a child between 1 month and 2 years old is 0.03 mg/kg. Using this age range and recommendation, answer the following questions. (*Note:* Pediatric doses are usually calculated to the nearest hundredth.)

1. A child weighs 3.6 kg. How much digoxin should the child receive?
2. A child weighs 18 lb. How much digoxin should the child receive?
3. A child weighs 25 lb. How much digoxin should the child receive?

ANSWERS 1. 3.6 × 0.03 mg = 0.11 mg 2. First, divide by 2.2 to change pounds to kilograms.

18 lb = 8.2 kg.

Then multiply: 8.2 × 0.03 mg = 0.25 mg. 3. Again, change pounds to kilograms:

25 lb = 11.4 kg

Then multiply: 11.4 × 0.03 mg = 0.34 mg.

For infants 0–4 weeks old (neonates) and premature infants, the weight may be given in grams, rather than kilograms. If a gram weight is given, first convert grams to kilograms before calculating the correct dosage. Dosage recommendations are most commonly given for weights in kilograms. As discussed in Chapter 4, to change grams to kilograms divide by 1000 (there are 1000 g in 1 kg). Simply move the decimal point in the gram weight three places to the left.

SAMPLE EXERCISES

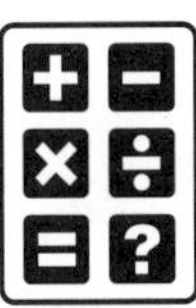

Exercises 1–3. Change the gram weights below to kilograms.

1. 4000 g
2. 2800 g
3. 1250 g

Exercises 4–6. The recommended dosage for neonates receiving ceftazidime (Tazidime) is 30 mg/kg. For each of the weights above, calculate the amount of drug that should be prescribed.

ANSWERS 1. 4 kg 2. 2.8 kg 3. 1.25 kg, or 1.3 kg (rounded)
4. 4 × 30 mg = 120 mg 5. 2.8 × 30 mg = 84 mg
6. 1.3 × 30 mg = 39 mg

Body Surface Area

Another way to calculate drug dosages, particularly in children, is to use body surface area. Body surface area is the preferred method when administering potent or potentially toxic drugs, such as chemotherapy (cancer drugs). **Body surface area (BSA)** is determined by using a preestablished nomogram such as the West nomogram for infants and children shown in Figure 9-3. A similar nomogram is available for prescribing medication to adolescents and adults.

Although the West nomogram for infants and children may look rather confusing, it is fairly simple to use. The boxed area in the middle is used for children of normal height for their weight. To find the BSA in square meters

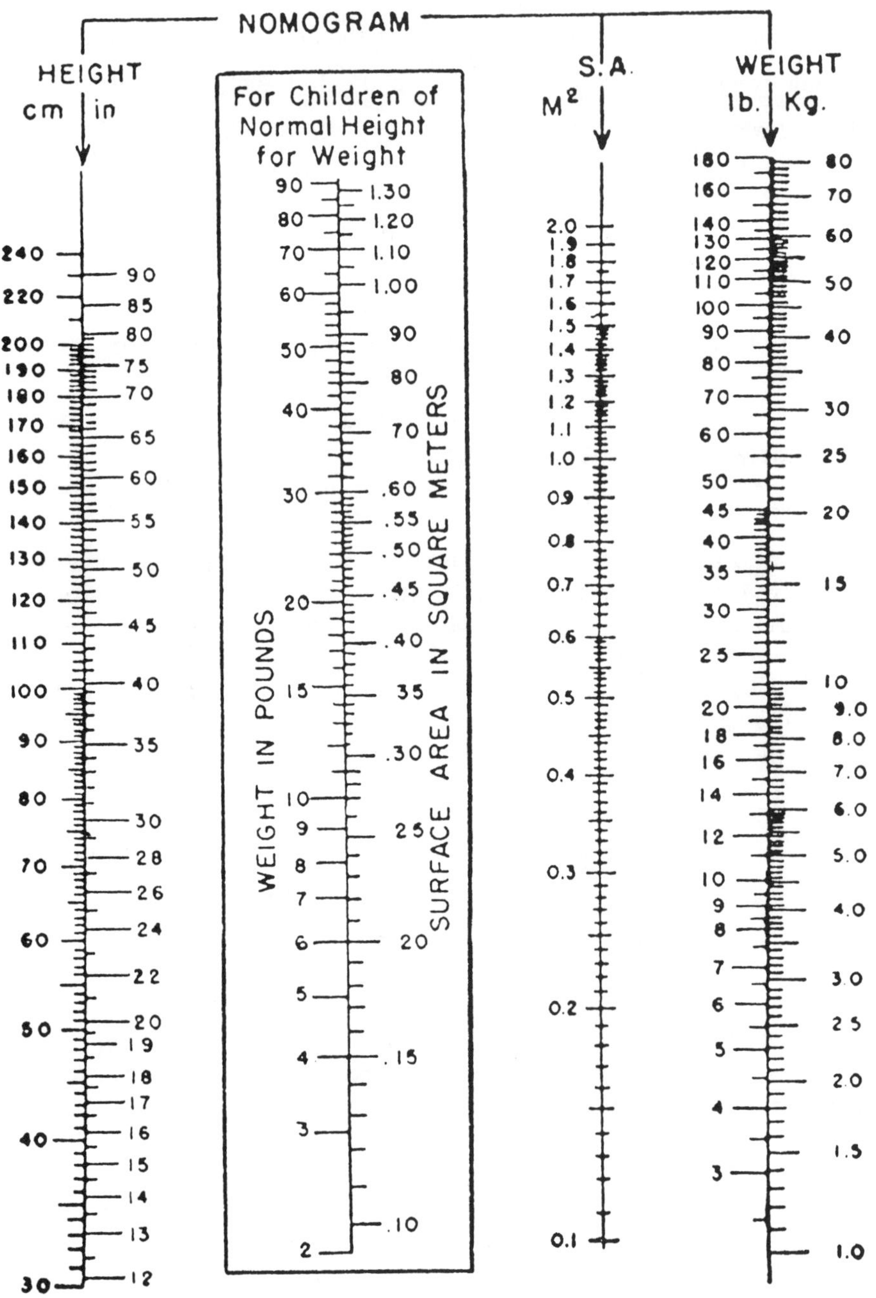

Figure 9–3 West nomogram for infants and children.

(m^2), we must first know the child's weight in pounds. The weight is located on the left side of the middle nomogram, and the corresponding BSA is read on the right side.

Examples

1. A child weighing 44 lb has a BSA of 0.80 m^2
2. An infant who weighs 11 lb has a BSA of 0.29 m^2

Note: The calibrations change along the scale. At the top of the scale, between 80 and 90 lb, there is only 1 marking. Between 40 and 50, there are 5 markings; and between 30 and 40, there are 10 markings.

SAMPLE EXERCISES

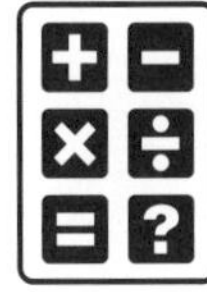

1. Using the part of the nomogram for a child of normal height and weight, find the BSA for Dana, who weighs 70 lb.
2. Corey weighs 29.5 kg and is of normal height and weight. What is Corey's BSA?

ANSWERS 1. 1.10 m^2 2. 29.5 kg = 65 lb; BSA = 1.04 m^2

For children who are not of normal height for their weight, the scales at the far left (height) and far right (weight) are used. Both of these scales have two measurements: centimeters and inches for height, and pounds and kilograms for weight. To find BSA using these two parts of the nomogram, we locate the weight on one scale and the height on the other. A ruler is placed on both measurements and the BSA for that child is the point where the ruler intersects the BSA scale.

Examples

1. A child who weighs 60 lb and who is 39 in. tall has a BSA of 0.9 m^2.
2. For a baby who weighs 13 lb and who is 19 in. long, we read a BSA of 0.3 m^2.

SAMPLE EXERCISES

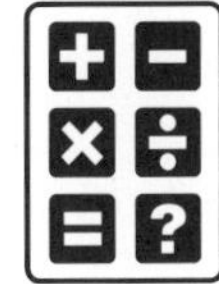

1. Using the far right and left scales for a child who does not have normal height for weight, find the BSA for Maryjo, who weighs 70 lb and is 45 in. tall.
2. Using the far right and left scales, find the BSA for a child who weighs 50 lb and is 36 in. tall.

ANSWERS 1. 1.0 m^2 2. 0.8 m^2

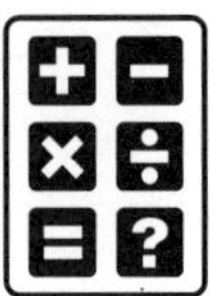

EXERCISES

Exercises 1–10. As a first step in dosage calculations, it is sometimes necessary to convert from one unit of weight to another. Fill in the blanks in the following table by carrying out the appropriate conversion.

	Name of Child	Weight (lb)	Weight (kg)
1.	Elisha	14	
2.	Max	43	
3.	Terence		25.5
4.	Patty		16.8
5.	Barbara	28	
6.	Jack	18	
7.	Vera	50	
8.	Quincy		14.5
9.	Shari	47	
10.	Albert		10.5

Exercises 11–20. Find the BSA for each of the children listed above. Each child is of normal height for weight.

Exercises 21–25. For each child in Exercises 1–5, calculate the correct dosage of theophylline if the recommended maintenance dose is 3 mg/kg q6h. (Calculate for a single dose.)

Exercises 26–30. For each child in Exercises 6–10, calculate the recommended daily dosage of carbamazepine (Tegretol) each child should receive if the recommended daily dose is 10 mg/kg in 2–4 divided doses. (Calculate for a daily dose.)

ANSWERS

	Name of Child	Weight (lb)	Weight (kg)
1.	Elisha	14	6.4
3.	Terence	56	25.5
5.	Barbara	28	12.7
7.	Vera	50	22.7
9.	Shari	47	21.4

11. 0.34 m² 13. 0.95 m² 15. 0.57 m² 17. 0.87 m²
19. 0.83 m² 21. 19.2 mg 23. 76.5 mg 25. 38.1 mg
27. 227 mg 29. 214 mg

9-5. DRUG THERAPY AND CHILDREN

Drug therapy for infants and children is often referred to as pediatric drug therapy. The recommendations for drug dosing for infants and children use several different individual factors. Some drug dosages are based on weight and some on age. Still others are based on body surface area. In most cases, dosages are calculated to the nearest hundredth because such small doses of medication are required.

Examples

1. (Example of *weight* as a basis for dosing) Usual dosages of amoxicillin pediatric drops for infections of the lower respiratory tract are as follows:

    Less than 6 kg: 1.25 mL q8H
    6–7 kg: 1.75 mL q8h
    8 kg: 2.25 mL q8h

2. (Example of *weight* as a basis for dosing) The usual dosage for amoxicillin–clavulanic acid (Augmentin) for a child is 20 mg/kg/day. If Alice weighs 15 kg, she needs 15 × 20 mg/day = 300 mg/day. If the physician orders Alice's daily dosage of Augmentin to be divided into three doses (or every 8 h), then each 8-h dose for Alice should be $\frac{300 \text{ mg}}{3}$ = 100 mg.
3. (Example of *age* as a basis for dosing) The usual dosage for Robitussin-DM is as follows:
    Children 12 years and older: 2 tsp q4h
    Children 6–12 years: 1 tsp q4h
    Children 2 to under 6 years: $\frac{1}{2}$ tsp q4h
    Children younger than 2: Consult your physician.
4. (Example of *body surface area* as a basis for dosing) The recommended dose of lomustine is 130 mg/m^2. A child with a BSA of 1.2 m^2 needs 130 mg × 1.2 = 156 mg of the drug.

SAMPLE EXERCISES

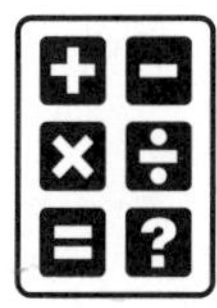

1. If the usual dosages of amoxicillin pediatric drops are as given in Example 1, find the correct dosage for a baby weighing 6.2 kg.
2. If the recommended dosage of lomustine is 130 mg/m^2, find the dose for a child who weighs 34 lb and has a normal height for weight.
3. For Kesia, who weighs 39 lb, the physician orders chlorpromazine hydrochloride 0.25 mg/lb PO q4–6 h prn. Find the number of milligrams she should receive in each dose.

ANSWERS 1. 1.75 mL q8h 2. BSA = 0.66 m^2; dose = 0.66 × 130 mg = 85.8 mg 3. 39 × 0.25 mg = 9.75 mg

When drug dosage recommendations are specified only for adults, the nurse should question the physician regarding why the drug is being used for a child. Most drugs used for children have pediatric dosage recommendations that are calculated by the drug manufacturer.

If the nurse must calculate a corresponding recommended dose for a child, several formulas can be used. One formula is based on BSA.

CALCULATING PEDIATRIC DOSAGES BY SURFACE AREA

$$\text{Child's dosage} = \frac{\text{Child's BSA}}{1.73\ \text{m}^2} \times \text{Adult dosage}$$

The 1.73 m^2 value in the denominator is the average adult BSA. To use the formula above, the nurse must know the child's BSA and recommended adult dosage.

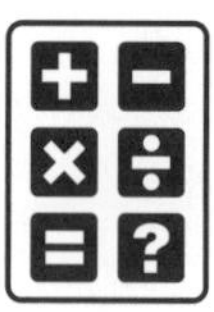

SAMPLE EXERCISES

1. The recommended adult dose of ampicillin is 500 mg given 4 times a day. If the child's BSA is 1.3 m^2, what is the recommended dose? (Rounding to the nearest tenth is appropriate for this situation.)
2. The recommended adult dose of a drug is 120 mg. Clark is of normal height for weight, weighing 70 lb. Using the nomogram to find BSA, calculate the recommended dose for this child.
3. The recommended adult dose of a drug is 25 mg. Jason is 28 in. tall and weighs 30 lb. Using the correct scales (far right and left) to find BSA, calculate the recommended dose for this child. (Round to two decimal places.)

ANSWERS 1. $\frac{1.3}{1.73} \times 500 \text{ mg} = 375.7 \text{ mg}$

2. $\frac{1.10}{1.73} \times 120 \text{ mg} = 76.3 \text{ mg}$ 3. $\frac{0.55}{1.73} \times 25 \text{ mg} = 7.95 \text{ mg}$

Another formula is based on weight.

CLARK'S RULE

$$\text{Child's dosage} = \frac{\text{Child's weight in pounds}}{150 \text{ lb}} \times \text{Adult dosage}$$

This method of determining drug dosages for children is being phased out in the United States because the average adult weight is greater than 150 lb.

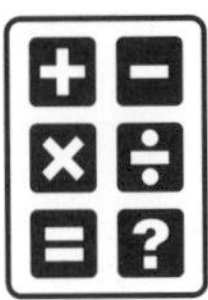

SAMPLE EXERCISES

1. The recommended initial adult dosage for phenoxybenzamine hydrochloride (Dibenzyline) is 10 mg PO daily. What is a safe dosage for Johnny, who weighs 26 lb?
2. The recommended maintenance adult dosage for zidovudine (Retrovir) is 100 mg q4h around the clock. What is a safe single dosage for Cherise, who weighs 41 lb?
3. The recommended adult dosage for naloxone (Narcan) is 0.1 mg IV. What is a safe dosage for Dennis, who weighs 57 lb?

ANSWERS 1. $\frac{26}{150} \times 10 \text{ mg} = 1.7 \text{ mg}$

2. $\frac{41}{150} \times 100 \text{ mg} = 27.3 \text{ mg}$ 3. $\frac{57}{150} \times 0.1 \text{ mg} = 0.04 \text{ mg}$

Oral Medications

Most oral drugs for infants and small children come in liquid form so that they can be easily swallowed. As described in Chapter 6, various measuring devices are used to give these medications, such as medicine droppers, special spoons, and medicine cups.

Calculating oral medications for children is the same process as that described in Chapters 6 and 7.

SAMPLE EXERCISES

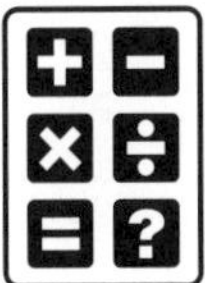

1. The physician orders 50 mg of Ceclor for Suzie. The oral suspension is available as 125 mg/5 mL. How many milliliters of Ceclor should the nurse give her?

2. The physician orders 125 mg of Keflex for Donald. The oral suspension is available as 250 mg/5 mL. How many milliliters of Keflex should the nurse give him?

3. The physician orders 20 mg of Dilantin for Debbie. The oral suspension is available as 30 mg/5mL. How many milliliters of Dilantin should the nurse give her?

4. The physician orders 6 mg/kg of cephradine q6h for Bruce, who weighs 47 lb.
   (a) How many milligrams should the nurse administer?
   (b) If the strength of the oral suspension is 125 mg/5 mL, how many milliliters should the nurse administer?

5. Sulfisoxazole 2 g/m^2 PO is prescribed for Laura (weight 7.2 kg, height 36 cm).
   (a) How many milligrams should the nurse administer?
   (b) If the strength of the oral suspension to be used is 500 mg/5 mL, how many milliliters should the nurse administer?

ANSWERS 1. $\frac{50}{125} \times 5 \text{ mL} = 2 \text{ mL}$ 2. 2.5 mL 3. 3.3 mL

4. (a) 47 lb = 21.4 kg; dose = 21.4 × 6 mg = 128.4 mg (b) volume of suspension = $\frac{128.4}{125} \times 5 \text{ mL} = 5.14$, or 5.1 mL 5. (a) BSA = 0.3 m^2; dose = 0.3 × 2 g = 0.6 g = 600 mg (b) $\frac{600}{500} \times 5 \text{ mL} = 6 \text{ mL}$

Parenteral Medications

Medications for infants and children are given most commonly by mouth or intravenously. However, a subcutaneous or intramuscular injection is sometimes required. We use the same process for calculating parenteral medications as we do for oral liquid medications.

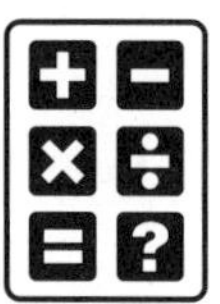

SAMPLE EXERCISES

1. The physician orders Cefadyl 320 mg IM q6h. The available vial of Cefadyl reads 1.2 mL = 500 mg. How many milliliters should the nurse give?
2. The physician orders Demerol 20 mg IM as a preoperative medication. The available ampule reads 1 mL = 50 mg. How many milliliters should the nurse give?
3. The physician orders Omnipen-N 75 mg IM. The available vial reads 1 mL= 125 mg. How many milliliters should the nurse give?

ANSWERS 1. 0.8 mL 2. 0.4 mL 3. 0.6 mL

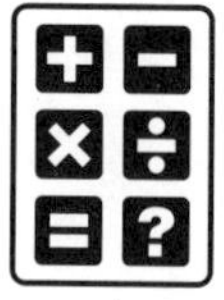

EXERCISES

Exercises 1–4. Pediatric doses may be divided into classes based on body weight. Dosage recommendations for a drug are as follows:

If child's weight <20 kg, give 12 mg/kg.
If child's weight ≥20 kg, give 250 mg.

What should the dosage be for each of these children?

1. Anita (22 kg)
2. Richard (17.6 kg)
3. Helen (32 lb)
4. Howard (50 lb)

Exercises 5–8. Maximum daily dosage for a drug may be given as follows:

Age <9 years old: give 24 mg/kg.
9–12: give 20 mg/kg.
12–16: give 18 mg/kg.
>16: give 13 mg/kg, or 900 mg, whichever is less.

According to the above recommendations, what is the maximum recommended daily dose for each child?

5. Juan, who weighs 30 kg and is 8 years old
6. Pearl, who is 10 years old and weighs 30 kg
7. Robin, who is 17 and weighs 70 kg
8. Jack, who weighs 80 lb and is 14 years old

Exercises 9–12. Akiretta weighs 30 lb and is 42 in. tall. The physicians' orders for Akiretta include

daunorubicin 25 mg/m^2
vincristine 1.5 mg/m^2
prednisone 40 mg/m^2

9. What is Akiretta's BSA?

10. How many milligrams of daunorubicin should Akiretta receive?

11. How many milligrams of vincristine should she receive?

12. How many milligrams of prednisone should she receive?

Exercises 13–16. Using the formulas in the boxes "Calculating Pediatric Dosages" and "Clark's Rule," calculate a child's dose from a typical adult dosage.

13. The recommended adult dose of a drug is 850 mg. If Sandy's BSA is 0.82 m^2, what is the recommended dosage for Sandy?

14. The recommended adult dose of a drug is 275 mg. Aubrey is of normal height for his weight (48 lb). Using the nomogram in Figure 9–3, calculate his BSA and the recommended dosage for him based on his BSA.

15. The recommended adult dose of a drug is 75 mg. Kazimir weighs 19 lb. Calculate the recommended dosage for this child, using Clark's rule.

16. The recommended adult dose of a drug is 1.5 g. Elise weighs 16.2 kg. Calculate the recommended dose for Elise, using Clark's rule.

Exercises 17–20. Amoxicillin trihydrate (Amoxil) is available as an oral suspension in two strengths: (a) 125 mg/5 mL and (b) 250 mg/mL. The physician orders 40 mg/kg/day for Norman (weight 16 kg) and Martina (weight 27 lb).

17. How many milligrams of Amoxil does Norman receive per day?

18. How many milliliters of each type of Amoxil suspension delivers the correct daily amount?

19. How many milligrams should Martina receive per day?

20. How many milliliters of each type of Amoxil suspension delivers the correct daily amount?

ANSWERS 1. 250 mg 3. 174 mg 5. 720 mg 7. 900 mg 9. 0.62 m^2 11. 0.9 mg 13. 399.5 mg 15. 9.5 mg 17. 640 mg/day 19. 492 mg/day

---

9-6. INTRAVENOUS THERAPY AND CHILDREN

In many ways, the calculations for intravenous fluids and medication and the method for their administration in children are very similar to that discussed in Chapter 8. The biggest difference is that microdrip sets that deliver 60 gtt/mL are used for infants and small children. In addition, because of the small size of the clients, electronic devices to control the rate of fluid delivery are typically used.

For intermittent medication administration, several methods of delivery are used. First, if the child has a primary IV line running continuously, an intravenous piggyback method with a secondary tubing set may be used (see Chapter 8). In this method, the drug may be prepared by the agency's pharmacy in small-volume bags.

Another option is the use of special IV sets that connect to an IV bag and are called by their specific trade names, such as Buretrol, Volutrol, or Soluset. Figure 9–4 shows a typical system, which consists of a calibrated chamber

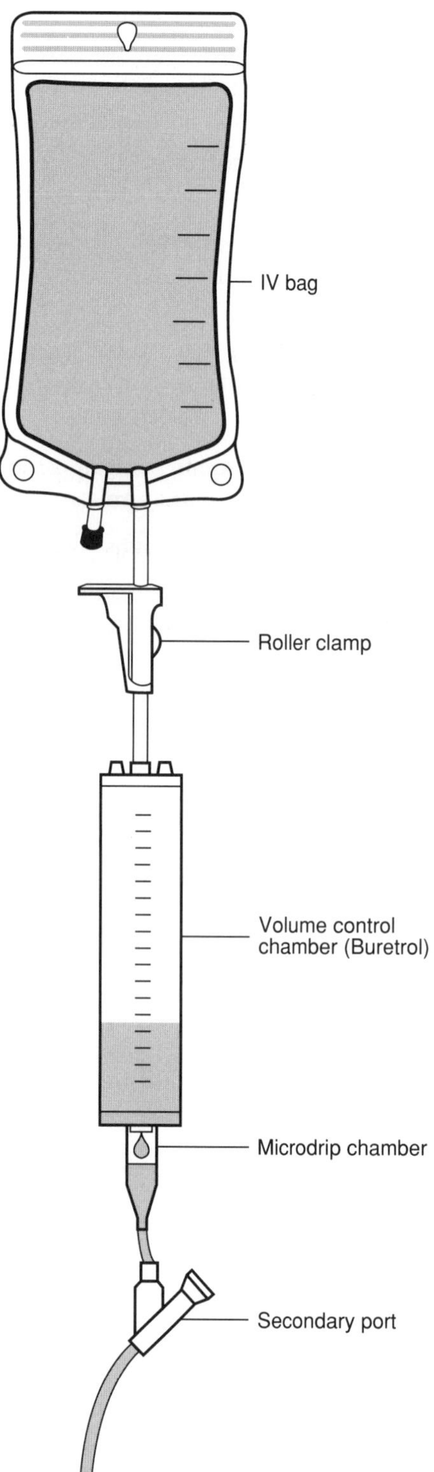

Figure 9–4 Intravenous administration set.

that can hold a maximum of 100–150 mL of fluid. The scale is calibrated in 1-mL increments to increase accuracy and assist in the measurement of often very small amounts of fluid. These devices may be used for continuous or intermittent IV drug infusions. The nurse usually prepares medications for delivery in the Buretrol system.

With these methods of IV drug delivery for children, a solution to flush the IV tubing is given after the medication. For peripheral IVs, the amount of flush solution is typically 15 mL. For central IVs, 20 mL is typically used.

These amounts and the procedures for giving them vary by institution, and the nurse must check to ensure that the correct procedure and amount of flush solution are used.

For older children, intermittent drug administration may be accomplished through a heparin or saline lock, as described in Chapter 8. In this system, the cannula remains in the vein for use only as needed. The amount of flush solution may be as little as 1–2 mL, depending on agency policy. Calculations for administering drugs using this system are the same as discussed in Chapter 8.

Calculation of IV Medication via a Buretrol

When calculating the amount of fluid necessary to deliver a medication, add the flush amount to the drug volume *before* calculating the drip rate (in drops per minute).

CALCULATION OF IV MEDICATION VIA A BURETROL

$$\text{Drip rate} = \frac{\text{Total volume of fluid (in mL)} \times 60 \text{ (drop factor)}}{\text{Time in minutes}}$$

In this formula, as in other IV calculation formulas, the drop factor (sometimes called set calibration) is the number of drops per milliliter that the IV tubing set delivers. The time in minutes in the denominator refers to the amount of time over which the total fluid volume infuses.

Some agencies prefer that only the volume of fluid containing the drug be used to calculate the drip rate, followed by another calculation for the flush solution. Either method is acceptable as long as it complies with agency policy.

Examples

1. The physician orders Zinacef 750 mg in 50 mL of 5%D/W to infuse via Buretrol over 60 min. A 15-mL flush is to follow. Calculate the IV drip rate. Using the formula above, we have

$$\frac{[50 \text{ mL (Diluted drug)} + 15 \text{ mL (Flush)}] \times 60 \text{ gtt/mL}}{60 \text{ min}} = 65 \text{ gtt/min}$$

2. A child is to receive 10 U of medication in 25 mL of fluid to be infused over 40 min. If a 20-mL flush follows, what should the drip rate be? Using the formula above, we have

$$\frac{[25 \text{ mL (Diluted drug)} + 20 \text{ mL (Flush)}] \times 60 \text{ gtt/mL}}{40 \text{ min}} = 68 \text{ gtt/min}$$

($\frac{1}{2}$ gtt cannot be counted.)

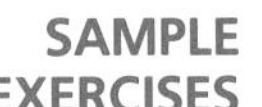

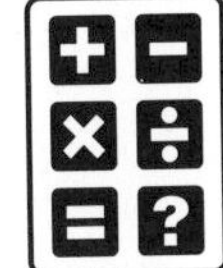

Exercises 1–3. Find the drip rate for each of these situations, using a Buretrol.

1. A dosage of 1 g of an antibiotic has been diluted in 40 mL to be infused over 45 min. A 15-mL flush follows.

2. The physician orders 25 mg of a drug in 50 mL to run in over 60 min. A 20-mL flush follows.
3. A dosage of 300 mcg is ordered in 40 mL of 5%D/W to run in over 1 h. A 15-mL flush follows.

ANSWERS 1. 73 gtt/min 2. 70 gtt/min 3. 55 gtt/min

The actual procedure for adding the medication to the diluent also requires a calculation.

Examples

1. The physician orders an antibiotic dosage of 100 mg diluted in 20 mL of 5%D/NS to run over 30 min. A 15-mL flush follows.

   Step 1. The nurse notes that the drug vial label indicates that 100 mg is contained in 2 mL.
   Step 2. The nurse runs 18 mL of 5%D/NS into the Buretrol, then adds the 2 mL of the drug for a total dilution of 20 mL:

$$18 \text{ mL (Solution)} + 2 \text{ mL (Concentrated drug)} = 20 \text{ mL (Diluted drug)}$$

   The nurse rolls the Buretrol between the hands to thoroughly mix the drug with the solution, and the Buretrol is labeled to indicate what drug is infusing.

   Step 3. The formula on p. 321 is used to calculate the drip rate.

$$\frac{[20 \text{ mL (Diluted drug)} + 15 \text{ mL (Flush)}] \times 60 \text{ gtt/mL}}{30 \text{ min}} = 70 \text{ gtt/min}$$

   Step 4. After the 20 mL of diluted drug has infused, the nurse adds the 15 mL of flush to the Buretrol for infusion.

2. The physician orders a medication dosage of 500 mg in a volume of 3 mL to be diluted to 30 mL and run over 50 min. A 20-mL flush follows.

   Step 1. The drug is contained in 3 mL.
   Step 2. 3 mL Drug + 27 mL Diluent = 30 mL Diluted drug
   Step 3. $\frac{[30 \text{ mL} + 20 \text{ mL}] \times 60 \text{ gtt/mL}}{50 \text{ min}} = 60$ gtt/min
   Step 4. After the drug has infused, start the 20 mL of flush.

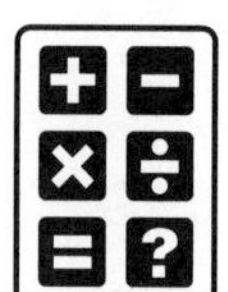

EXERCISES

1. What is a Buretrol?
2. How is the Buretrol calibrated?
3. What is a typical amount of flush solution used for (a) peripheral IV medications and (b) central IV medications?

Exercises 4–7. Complete the table on p. 323 to calculate the amount of IV solution needed to provide the prescribed total dilution of drug in each question.

	Total Dilution (mL)	Volume of Drug (mL)	Volume of IV Solution Added
4.	25	3	
5.	40	5	
6.	20	1	
7.	30	2	

Exercises 8–15. Find the Buretrol IV drip rate in each of the following cases. (Remember to use a drop factor of 60.)

	Drug Dosage (mg)	Volume after Dilution (mL)	Infusion Time	Flush (mL)
8.	250	80	1 hr	15
9.	450	80	1.5 hr	20
10.	150	45	45 min	15
11.	2.25	20	20 min	15
12.	15	50	45 min	15
13.	40	40	50 min	15
14.	90	35	50 min	15
15.	100	60	30 min	20

ANSWERS 1. A Buretrol or similar device is used to deliver small amounts of IV fluids or medication to infants and children.
3. (a) 15 mL (b) 20 mL 5. 35 mL 7. 28 mL 9. 67 gtt/min
11. 105 gtt/min 13. 66 gtt/min 15. 160 gtt/min

9-7. DRUG THERAPY AND THE ELDERLY

The number of people older than 65 years old is increasing rapidly. As a result of longer life expectancy and better treatment for illness, older adults typically have one or more chronic diseases that often require drug therapy. Unlike drug therapy for children, there are no set rules or standard ways to adjust drug dosages based on the special needs of the elderly. Some drug companies, however, have begun to publish recommendations for drugs given to older adults.

Normal physiologic changes associated with aging affect how a drug is used and eliminated from the body. The principle that many physicians use to prevent drug overdose or some of the adverse effects of drugs in the elderly is "start low; go slow."

One of the major changes that occur with age is a decrease in the ability of the kidneys to eliminate waste and, sometimes, the toxic metabolites of a drug. The test that physicians use to measure the ability of the kidneys to remove these products is called **creatinine clearance.** The higher the creatinine clearance, the better the function of the kidneys. Conversely, a low creatinine clearance indicates poorly functioning kidneys and a risk from high doses of drugs.

Some drug dosages for the elderly and other clients with decreased kidney function are based on the client's creatinine clearance value. In some cases, drug companies issue precautions for use of certain drugs in the elderly.

Examples

1. A drug recommendation reads "Needs a creatinine clearance of 50 mL/min" to receive this drug.
2. For clients with actual renal disease, the recommendations for IV Septra are:

Creatinine Clearance	Dosage Recommendation
Above 30	Use the standard amount
15–30	Half the standard amount
Below 15	Use not recommended

3. The precaution for Actifed with codeine reads: "The ingredients in Actifed with Codeine Cough Syrup are more likely to cause adverse reactions in elderly clients."

The actual drug dosage ordered for an elderly client is determined by the physician. The dosage calculation for determining the amount of a drug needed to deliver the prescribed dosage is the responsibility of the nurse. Some clients who cannot swallow tablets or capsules may need a liquid form of the ordered drug. The nurse notifies the physician that an alternative form of the medication is needed. Dosage calculation of solids or liquids for an older adult is no different from the calculation procedure described in Chapters 6 and 7.

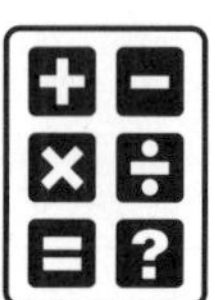

SAMPLE EXERCISES

1. The physician orders aprobarbital (Alurate) 15 mg PO tid for sedation for Mr. Aland. If Alurate elixir 40 mg/5 mL is available, what is the volume of each dose? (Round to the nearest tenth.)
2. The physician orders Alurate 60 mg PO hs. If Alurate elixir 40 mg/5 mL is available, how much elixir should the nurse give and when?
3. Ms. Giotanni's physician orders secobarbital (Seconal) 5.5 mg/kg IV q4h for acute psychotic agitation. She weighs 85 lb. If Seconal 50 mg/mL is to be used,
   (a) How much drug (in milligrams) does she need per dose?
   (b) What volume should the nurse give?

ANSWERS 1. 1.9 mL 2. 7.5 mL at bedtime
3. (a) 212.3 mg (b) 4.2 mL every 4 h

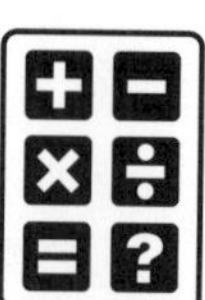

EXERCISES

Exercises 1–2. The physician orders acetazolamide (Diamox) 500 mg bid for Ms. Lamorr, who has glaucoma.

1. How often should she take the medication?
2. If Diamox 250 mg tablets are available, how many tablets should she take for each dose?

Exercises 3–6. Depression is one of the most common mental health problems in the elderly. The physician has prescribed antidepressants for the following clients, who will be started on a regimen (that is one-third the recommended adult dose) and observed carefully. Using the information in the following table, find the number of tablets or milliliters corresponding to one-third the recommended adult dose that each client should receive.

	Client	Recommended Adult Dose	Available Form
3.	Mr. Kinjet	imipramine PO 75 mg/day	Tablets 25 mg
4.	Ms. Mauret	nortriptyline PO 25 mg tid	Solution 10 mg/5 mL
5	Ms. Garvic	doxepin PO 75 mg/day	Solution 10 mg/mL
6.	Mr. Herbley	trazodone PO 150 mg/day	Tablets 50 mg

Exercises 7–8. Ms. Anderry takes digoxin (Lanoxin) elixir 0.125 mg PO qd for congestive heart failure. The strength of the elixir is 50 mcg/mL.

7. How often should she take her medication?
8. How much elixir (in milliliters) should she be taking?

Exercises 9–12. Potassium supplements to prevent or treat low potassium levels are very important for the elderly. Calculate the appropriate dose in each of the following cases.

9. Ordered: potassium bicarbonate 50 mEq PO in water qd
   Available: tablets 25 mEq
10. Ordered: potassium acetate 20 mEq PO bid
    Available: elixir, 6.7 mEq/5 mL
11. Ordered: potassium chloride 20 mEq IV over 4 h
    Available: IV solution of 40 mEq/L
12. Ordered: potassium chloride 40 mEq IV over 10 h
    Available: IV solution of 40 mEq/L

Exercises 13–16. Isoproterenol hydrochloride (Isuprel) may be prescribed for a number of health problems that affect the elderly. Calculate the appropriate dose in each of the following cases.

13. Ordered: 20 mg SL q6h for bronchospasm
    Available: glossets (tablets) 10 mg
14. Ordered: 0.4 mg SC for cardiac dysrhythmias
    Available: solution 1:5000
15. Ordered: 0.05 mg IV for heart block
    Available: solution 1:5000
16. Ordered: 0.2 mg IV for cardiac standstill
    Available: solution 1:50,000

Exercises 17–18. One of the uses for thiopental sodium (Pentothal) is induction anesthesia before other anesthetics are given. Mr. Gemonic weighs 130 lb and is to receive 3 mg/kg IV. If a solution of 500 mg/20 mL is used, then

17. How much drug (in milligrams) is given?
18. What volume is given?

Exercises 19–20. For Ms. Nortan (weight 118 lb), the physician ordered Ismotic 1.5 g/kg PO qid. Ismotic solution 45% is available.

19. How much solution (in milliliters) should she take per dose?
20. How many doses should she take each day?

ANSWERS 1. twice a day 3. 1 tablet 5. 2.5 mL 7. once a day 9. 2 tablets 11. 500 mL 13. 2 tablets 15. $\frac{0.05}{1000} \times 5000\text{ mL} = 0.25\text{ mL}$ 17. 177.3 mg 19. $\frac{80.4}{45} \times 100\text{ mL} = 178.7\text{ mL}$

9-8. DRUG THERAPY AND PREGNANCY

To prevent possible harm to the developing fetus, drugs are not routinely used when a woman is pregnant. The main exceptions are vitamins and iron, which are typically given to help both the mother and baby meet the additional nutritional demands of pregnancy. When other drugs are needed to treat or maintain disease control, the mother and baby are carefully monitored for adverse effects. Manufacturers of drugs make recommendations for use of specific drugs during pregnancy.

Examples

1. A warning in the *PDR* states that "Aminoglycosides [a type of antibiotic] can cause fetal harm when administered to a pregnant woman."
2. Another example of a warning is "Entex should be given to a pregnant woman only if clearly needed."
3. Another such warning is "Septra IV infusion should be used during pregnancy only if the potential benefit justifies the potential harm to the fetus."

The dosage calculations for drugs given to the pregnant woman are similar to dosage calculations for any adult.

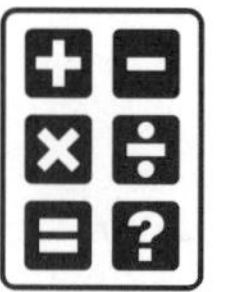

SAMPLE EXERCISES

Exercises 1–4. The physician orders the following dosages of iron for four women who are pregnant. Compute the number of tablets or milliliters for each dose.

1. Ordered: 300 mg/day in 3 divided doses
   On hand: 100-mg tablets
2. Ordered: 300 mg/day in 3 divided doses
   On hand: Oral suspension 100 mg/5 mL
3. Ordered: 450 mg/day in 3 divided doses
   On hand: Oral suspension 100 mg/5 mL
4. Ordered: 600 mg/day in 3 divided doses
   On hand: Oral suspension 45 mg/0.6 mL

ANSWERS 1. 1 tablet 2. 5 mL 3. 7.5 mL 4. 2.7 mL

At the time of labor and delivery, certain intravenous medications may be administered to help facilitate labor, to slow or prevent labor, or to treat a medical complication. Women in labor typically have a continuous IV infusion. Medications are usually added to a secondary IV bag and monitored by an electronic device, such as that described in Chapter 8.

When a drug is added to the IV solution, the first step in drug calculation is determining the concentration (strength) of the solution, usually specified per milliliter. To find the concentration of a drug in solution, we can use a ratio or this formula initially shown in Chapter 7:

STRENGTH (CONCENTRATION)

$$\frac{\text{Total amount of drug}}{\text{Total amount of IV solution (in mL)}} = \text{Drug concentration}$$

Examples

1. Magnesium sulfate ($MgSO_2$) 10 g is added to 500 mL 5%D/W. What is the concentration of this drug in the IV solution? To avoid decimals, we first change 10 g to milligrams: 10 g = 10,000 mg. Using the formula, we obtain

$$\frac{\text{10,000 mg (Amount of drug)}}{\text{500 mL (Amount of solution)}} = \text{20 mg/mL}$$

   The resulting concentration of the drug is 20 mg/mL.

2. Terbutaline sulfate (Brethine) 5 mg is added to 1000 mL of normal saline. What is the concentration of the drug? To avoid decimals, we must first change milligrams to micrograms: 5 mg = 5000 mcg. Using the formula, we obtain

$$\frac{\text{5000 mcg (Amount of drug)}}{\text{1000 mL (Amount of solution)}} = \text{5 mcg/mL}$$

SAMPLE EXERCISES

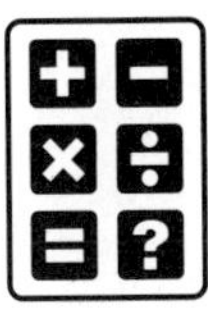

1. Ritodrine hydrochloride (Yutopar) 150 mg is diluted in 500 mL 5%D/W. What is the concentration of the drug?
2. Oxytocin with chlorobutanol (Pitocin) 10 U (1 mL) is added to 1000 mL normal saline. There are 1000 milliunits (mU) in one unit (U) of oxytocin. What is the concentration of the drug in milliunits?

ANSWERS 1. $\frac{\text{150,000 mcg}}{\text{500 mL}} = \text{300 mcg/mL}$

2. $\frac{\text{10,000 mU}}{\text{1000 mL}} = \text{10 mU/mL}$

Once the concentration of the drug has been determined, the calculation of the IV fluid rate needed to deliver the required amount of drug is the same procedure as that used in Chapter 8.

Examples

1. The physician orders terbutaline sulfate IV infusion to start at 10 mcg/min. The concentration of the drug in solution is 5 mcg/mL. We can use either ratio and proportion or the formula $\frac{D}{H} \times Q$ (Chapters 5, 6, and 7) for determining the amount of IV fluid to deliver:

$$\frac{D}{H} \times Q = \frac{10 \text{ mcg}}{5 \text{ mcg}} \times 1 \text{ mL}$$
$$= 2 \text{ mL}$$

To find the hourly IV rate needed, we multiply:

$$2 \text{ mL/min} \times 60 \text{ min/h} = 120 \text{ mL/h}.$$

2. The physician orders $MgSO_2$ 2 g/h. The concentration of the drug in solution is 20 mg/mL. The amount of IV fluid to deliver is:

$$\frac{2000 \text{ mg (2 g)}}{20 \text{ mg}} \times 1 \text{ mL} = 100 \text{ mL}$$

Note: In this case, we do not need to multiply by 60 to find the flow rate because the dose was ordered per hour, rather than per minute.

3. Ritodrine hydrochloride 50 mcg/min is ordered by the physician. The available concentration of the drug is 300 mcg/mL.

Amount to deliver: $\frac{50 \text{ mcg}}{300 \text{ mcg}} \times 1 \text{ mL} = 0.17 \text{ mL};$

Flow rate: $0.17 \text{ mL/min} \times 60 \text{ min/h} = 10 \text{ mL/h}$

4. The physician orders oxytocin to infuse at 2 mU/min. The concentration on hand is 10 mU.

Amount to deliver: $\frac{2 \text{ mU}}{10 \text{ mU}} \times 1 \text{ mL} = 0.2 \text{ mL};$

Flow Rate: $0.2 \text{ mL/min} \times 60 \text{ min/h} = 12 \text{ mL/h}$

The nurse needs to know the hourly rate of IV infusion for setting the electronic pump. In some cases, the hourly rate is too high for the pump, and the nurse must calculate and monitor the drip rate for an IV infusion by gravity as described in Chapter 8.

Although the calculation procedures for finding the concentration of the drug and the amount of IV fluid to deliver were discussed separately here, most often the nurse needs to do both steps for a single situation.

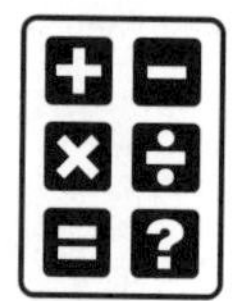

SAMPLE EXERCISES

1. The physician orders terbutaline sulfate 15 mcg/min by continuous IV infusion. The IV bag reads "Terbutaline sulfate 10 mg in 1000 mL 5%D/W." At what rate should the IV pump be set to deliver the prescribed amount of medication?

2. The physician orders an initial (loading) dose of magnesium sulfate IV of 4 g over 15 min. The IV bag reads "$MgSO_2$ 20 g in 1000 mL 5%D/W." How

much IV solution is needed to deliver 4 g of medication? (In this case, it is not necessary to calculate the amount of drug per milliliter because the physician has ordered a specific one-time dosage.)

3. The physician orders ritodrine hydrochloride 40 mcg/min by continuous IV infusion. The IV bag reads "Ritodrine hydrochloride 150 mg in 500 mL NS." What should the hourly IV rate be to deliver the prescribed amount of medication?

ANSWERS

1. Step 1. Find the concentration of the drug.

   10,000 mcg/1000 mL = 10 mcg/mL (Drug concentration on hand)

   Step 2. Find the volume of solution to infuse per hour.

$$\frac{15 \text{ mcg}}{10 \text{ mcg}} \times 1 \text{ mL} = 1.5 \text{ mL; } 1.5 \text{ mL/min} \times 60 \text{ min/h} = 90 \text{ mL/h}$$

2. $$\frac{x \text{ mL}}{1000 \text{ mL}} = \frac{4 \text{ g}}{20 \text{ g}}$$
$$x = 200$$

   200 mL must infuse to deliver 4 g of the drug.

3. Step 1. Find the concentration of the drug.

$$\frac{150{,}000 \text{ mcg}}{500 \text{ mL}} = 300 \text{ mcg/mL}$$

   Step 2. Find the volume of solution to infuse.

$$\frac{40 \text{ mcg}}{300 \text{ mcg}} \times 1 \text{ mL} = 0.13 \text{ mL; } 0.13 \text{ mL} \times 60 = 8 \text{ mL}$$

EXERCISES

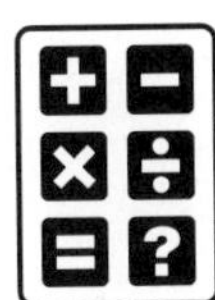

Exercises 1–5. A variety of iron salts is available to treat iron deficiency in pregnant women. It is important to teach the client not to substitute one iron tablet for another because of differences in the actual amount of iron (elemental iron). Some examples of iron salts are

Ferrous fumarate: contains 33% elemental iron
Ferrous gluconate: contains 12% elemental iron
Ferrous sulfate: contains 20% elemental iron

Find the amount of elemental iron in each of the following doses:

1. Ferrous fumarate 300 mg
2. Ferrous gluconate 300 mg
3. Ferrous sulfate 600 mg
4. Ferrous fumarate 600 mg
5. Ferrous gluconate 600 mg

Exercises 6–9. Pregnant women need twice the usual requirements of folic acid. If the following doses have been ordered, state the number of tablets or volume of injection for each dose.

6. Ordered: folic acid 0.8 mg PO
   Available: Apo-Folic tablets, 0.4 mg

7. Ordered: folic acid 0.8 mg SC
   Available: Apo-Folic injection, 5 mg/mL
8. Ordered: folic acid 1 mg IM
   Available: Folvite injection, 5 mg/mL
9. Ordered: folic acid 0.8 mg IM
   Available: Folvite injection, 10 mg/mL
10. Methylergonovine (Methergine) is a drug commonly given after childbirth to stimulate expulsion of the placenta (afterbirth). The physician orders 0.4 mg PO q6h. The tablets available are 0.2 mg. How many tablets should the nurse give for each dose?
11. Terbutaline sulfate 5 mg is mixed in 500 mL 5%D/W. What is the concentration of drug in solution in micrograms per milliliter?

Exercises 12–14. Calculate the infusion rate needed to provide the following doses of terbutaline sulfate using the drug concentration in Exercise 11. (Complete the table.)

	Dose	Volume per Minute	Volume per Hour
12.	5 mcg/min		
13.	10 mcg/min		
14.	15 mcg/min		

15. Magnesium sulfate 15 g is diluted in 1000 mL 5%D/W. What is the concentration of the drug in milligrams per milliliter?

Exercises 16–20. Calculate the infusion rate needed to provide the following doses of magnesium sulfate using the drug concentration available in Exercise 15. (Complete the table.)

	Dose	Volume per Hour
16.	500 mg/h	
17.	1 g/h	
18.	2 g/h	
19.	3 g/h	
20.	3.5 g/h	

ANSWERS 1. 99 mg 3. 120 mg 5. 72 mg 7. 0.2 mL 9. 0.1 mL 11. 10 mcg/mL

	Dose	Volume per Minute	Volume per Hour
13.	10 mcg/min	1 mL/min	60 mL/h

15. 15 mg/mL

	Dose	Volume per Hour
17.	1 g/h	67 mL/h
19.	3 g/h	200 mL/h

9-9. AVOIDING ERRORS: ADHERING TO SAFE DRUG DOSAGE PARAMETERS

Throughout this chapter we have presented numerous examples of how nurses can help avoid drug errors, even though they do not usually prescribe medication. All drug errors are significant, but those involving infants or small children are probably the most important. A small dosage error that might have little or no effect in an adult can kill or seriously disable an infant or small child.

The nurse is responsible for calculating the safe dosage ranges for all clients. If there is *any* doubt about the drug or its prescribed dosage, the nurse notifies the physician or clinical pharmacist before administering the drug.

9-10. SUMMARY

1. WHY IS DRUG THERAPY INDIVIDUALIZED?

   Drug dosages are individualized, depending on a number of factors, such as age, sex, weight, and health status. The physician or clinical pharmacologist determines the drug dosage to be administered.

2. SOURCES OF INFORMATION FOR INDIVIDUALIZING DRUG THERAPY

   There are several references that the physician uses to determine the correct drug to prescribe and the correct drug dosage. Some common examples are the *Physicians' Desk Reference* and the institution's formulary. References providing drug information and nursing interventions are also available.

3. HEALTH STATUS AS A BASIS FOR INDIVIDUALIZING DRUG THERAPY

   Drugs are prescribed on the basis of the health status of the client. Dosages are also altered depending on the specific needs of each individual. For example, a diabetic with a very high blood sugar level receives a higher dose of insulin than the diabetic with a lower blood sugar level.

4. BODY WEIGHT AND BODY SURFACE AREA AS A MEANS OF INDIVIDUALIZING DRUG THERAPY

   Many drug manufacturers recommend dosages that are based on the client's weight or body surface area to prevent drug overdose. This practice is especially common in drug administration for infants and children, as well as for very potent intravenous medications, such as chemotherapeutic agents. Body surface area is determined by using the appropriate nomogram to locate the client's height and weight.

5. DRUG THERAPY AND CHILDREN

   Drug therapy for children, or pediatric drug therapy, is a specialized area requiring careful calculation and monitoring. Drug dosages may be based on age, weight, or body surface area. The nurse may need to convert a weight from pounds to kilograms or vice versa, depending on how the drug is ordered. Most drugs are given either orally or intravenously. Because they cannot swallow tablets or capsules, infants and small children require liquid medication.

6. INTRAVENOUS THERAPY AND CHILDREN

Intravenous medications may be given either intermittently or continuously. Intermittent drug administration systems include IV piggyback with a secondary set, a heparin or saline lock, and the use of a Buretrol or similar device to accurately measure the amount of medication and fluid given. When drugs are given via a Buretrol, a flush solution of 15 or 20 mL is usually administered in addition to the diluted medication. Most drug delivery is monitored by an electronic device to prevent drug overdose or fluid overload.

7. DRUG THERAPY AND THE ELDERLY

There are few recommendations for drug dosing for elderly clients. Because of the physiologic changes associated with aging, drugs may not be used effectively by or eliminated properly from the body. As a result, drugs tend to stay in the body longer, causing adverse effects. The general principle for geriatric drug therapy is "start low; go slow."

8. DRUG THERAPY AND PREGNANCY

Pregnant women receive as few drugs as possible to avoid possible harm to the fetus. At the time of labor and delivery, intravenous drugs may be given to induce or slow labor. Other drugs may be given to treat medical complications associated with labor and delivery. Drug calculations are the same as for other intravenous drugs except that the drugs may change frequently as the client's condition changes.

9. AVOIDING ERRORS: ADHERING TO SAFE DRUG DOSAGE PARAMETERS

Although the physician is responsible for prescribing drug dosages, the nurse is responsible for knowing or determining the safe dosage ranges for drugs that he or she administers. Any doubt about drug therapy needs to be directed to the physician before the drug is given.

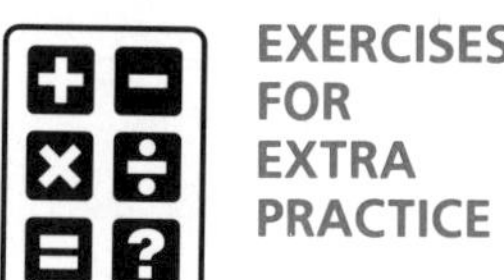

EXERCISES FOR EXTRA PRACTICE

Exercises 1–4. For each of the children below, calculate the dosage based on body weight and the recommended adult dosage.

	Name of Child	Weight	Recommended Adult Dosage (mg)
1.	Jean	25 lb	40
2.	Lee	78 lb	200
3.	George	16.7 kg	150
4.	Holly	4.2 kg	25

Exercises 5–8. For each of the children below, calculate the dosage based on BSA and the recommended adult dosage.

	Name of Child	BSA (m^2)	Recommended Adult Dosage
5.	Peter	0.23	75 mg
6.	Molly	0.95	750 mg
7.	Ruth	1.02	1 g
8.	Ezra	0.16	125 mg

Exercises 9–12. The recommended maintenance dose of digoxin for a child is 0.012 mg/kg PO daily in divided doses q12h. For each of the children below, indicate whether the ordered daily dose is within a safe dosage range.

	Name of Child	Weight	Ordered Dosage (mg)
9.	Erica	10 kg	0.175
10.	Tanya	6.3 kg	0.075
11.	Samuel	47 lb	0.25
12.	Donna	68 lb	0.50

Exercises 13–16. Find the Buretrol IV drip rate in each of the following cases (DF = 60).

	Amount of Drug (mg)	Volume after Dilution (mL)	Infusion Time	Flush (mL)
13.	125	75	1 h	20
14.	12	15	20 min	15
15.	8.1	30	45 min	20
16.	72	55	75 min	15

Exercises 17–20. Ritodrine is ordered for a woman in labor. For each of the following cases, calculate the infusion rate in milliliters per minute and milliliters per hour. (Complete the table.) The concentration of the drug is 300 mcg/mL.

	Ordered Dose	Milliliters per Minute	Milliliters per Hour
17.	100 mcg/min		
18.	50 mcg/min		
19.	0.15 mg/min		
20.	0.35 mg/min		

ANSWERS 1. 6.67 mg 3. 36.74 mg 5. 9.97 mg 7. 0.59 g, or 590 mg 9. no 11. yes 13. 95 gtt/min 15. 67 gtt/min

	Ordered Dose	Milliliters per Minute	Milliliters per Hour
17.	100 mcg/min	0.33	20
19.	0.15 mg/min	0.5	30

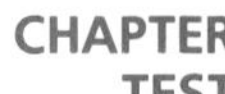

CHAPTER TEST

1. A physician orders 25 mg of Inderal for a client if her diastolic blood pressure (denominator) goes above 95. Her blood pressure today is 178/92. Should the nurse give the medication? 1. ____________
2. Convert 44 lb to kilograms. 2. ____________
3. The physician orders Tylenol 650 mg for Dorothy. Tablets on hand are 325 mg each. How many tablets should the nurse give? 3. ____________

4. The physician orders 50 mg of Omnipen-N IM for Diane. The available vial reads 1 mL = 125 mg. How many milliliters should the nurse give? 4. ____________

5. The recommended drug dosage for a child is 3 mg/kg/day in 4 divided doses. What is a safe *daily* dosage for a child who weighs 9.6 kg? 5. ____________

6. The physician orders a drug dosage of 150 mg diluted in 50 mL 5%D/W to run over 60 min. A 20-mL flush follows. If a Buretrol with a DF of 60 is used, what should the drip rate be? 6. ____________

7. The recommended adult dosage for an antibiotic is 500 mg. 7. ____________

   (a) What is the safe dosage for a child weighing 18 lb? (Use Clark's rule.)
   (b) What is the safe dosage for a child with a BSA of 0.55 m^2?

8. An elderly client has a prescription for furosemide (Lasix) 20 mg qd. The pharmacist gave her Lasix tablets 40 mg. How many tablets should she take to have the correct dose? 8. ____________

9. Ritodrine is given to a client in labor. The nurse mixes 150 mg in 500 mL 5%D/W. What is the concentration of the drug in micrograms per milliliter? 9. ____________

10. Terbutaline sulfate IV is started at 20 mcg/min. The concentration of the drug in solution is 5 mcg/mL. What is the hourly rate needed to provide the prescribed medication? 10. ____________

ANSWERS 1. no 2. 20 kg 3. 2 tablets 4. 0.4 mL 5. 28.8 mg 6. 70 gtt/min 7. (a) 60 mg (b) 159 mg 8. $\frac{1}{2}$ tablet 9. 300 mcg/mL 10. 240 mL/h

---

TEN

Documentation

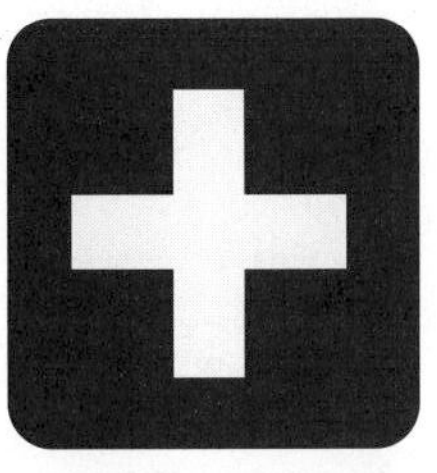

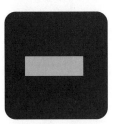

▶ OUTLINE

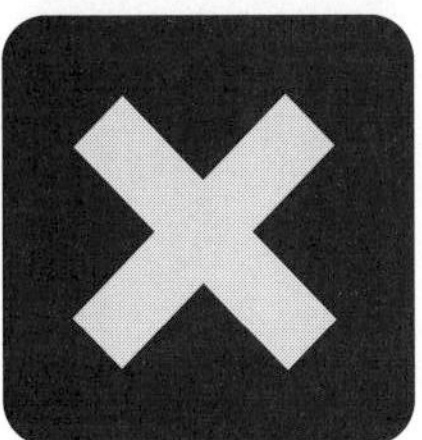

▶ OBJECTIVES

After studying this chapter, you will be able to:

1. State why accurate documentation is important.
2. Record a client's fluid intake and output.
3. Compute an average, or arithmetic mean.
4. Graph vital signs on a graphic chart.
5. Identify the advantages of using flow sheets for documentation.
6. Interpret the 24-h clock.
7. Record medication administration on a medication administration record (MAR).
8. Identify the advantage of using computers for clinical documentation of drug therapy.
9. Avoid errors in medication administration by checking and rechecking.

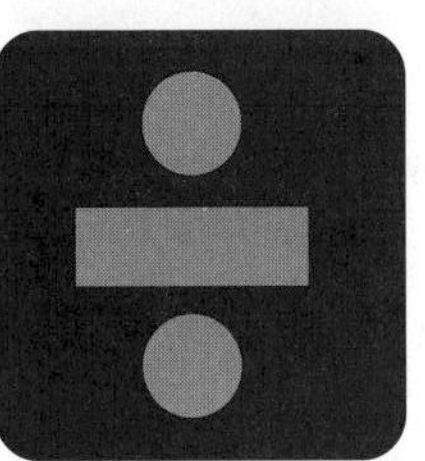

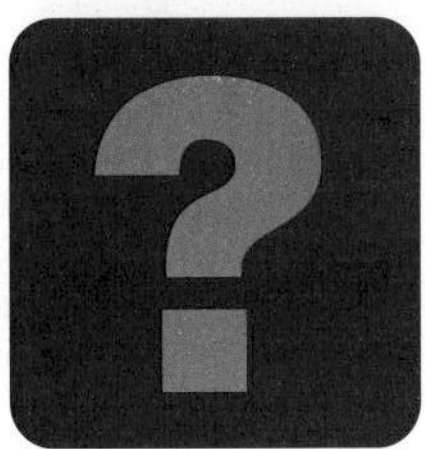

10-1. INTRODUCTION

Throughout this book, we've mentioned physicians' orders and documenting drug and intravenous therapy. Every health care setting—whether a hospital, nursing home, home health agency, or clinic—has its own policies for documentation, or charting, on the client's record. Some of these policies are mandated by state and federal regulations or accrediting agencies. Others are individualized for the needs of each setting and the type of client being served.

This chapter presents examples of several forms to illustrate the types of charting that accompany drug and intravenous therapy. Most health care settings have similar charting forms.

Why Document?

Documentation is important for a number of reasons:

1. Providing a legal record of care given to a client
2. Providing a communication tool for all members of the health care team
3. Validating care for reimbursement by third-party payors, such as insurance companies and Medicare
4. Providing information for quality improvement studies and clinical research

Proficiency Gauge

You may already understand the processes of documentation. To determine the level of your understanding, complete the following exercises and compare your answers with those at the end only after you've completed the exercises.

1. A client drinks 6 oz of coffee and 4 oz of prune juice. How many milliliters should be recorded on an intake and output record? 1. ____________
2. A nurse records the following information about a client's intake and output:

   200 mL urine
   35 mL wound drainage
   50 mL vomitus
   240 mL milk
   120 mL tea

   What is the total amount of the client's output? 2. ____________
3. A client voids 480 mL in an 8-h period. What is the average hourly amount of urine voided? 3. ____________
4. Using the graphic chart in Figure 10–1, graph a temperature of 100.2°F at 0800 on August 20. 4. ____________
5. What advantage does a flow sheet have over other forms for charting? 5. ____________
6. What is 7 PM in 24-hour clock, or military, time? 6. ____________

GRAPHIC CHART

Last Name	First Name	Attending Physician	Room or Ward No.	Bed	Hospital No.

Date								
Day in Hospital								
Day P.O. or P.P.								

	Hour	A.M.			P.M.			A.M.			P.M.			A.M.			P.M.			A.M.			P.M.			A.M.			P.M.			A.M.			P.M.			A.M.			P.M.			A.M.			P.M.		
		4	8	12	4	8	12	4	8	12	4	8	12	4	8	12	4	8	12	4	8	12	4	8	12	4	8	12	4	8	12	4	8	12	4	8	12	4	8	12	4	8	12	4	8	12	4	8	12
TEMPERATURE	106°																																																
	105°																																																
	104°																																																
	103°																																																
	102°																																																
	101°																																																
	100°																																																
	99° Normal																																																
	98°																																																
	97°																																																
	96°																																																
PULSE	150																																																
	140																																																
	130																																																
	120																																																
	110																																																
	100																																																
	90																																																
	80																																																
	70																																																
RESPIRATION	60																																																
	50																																																
	40																																																
	30																																																
	20																																																
	10																																																

Blood Pressure								
Fluid Intake								
Urine								
Defecation								
Weight								

Form 2501 BRIGGS, Des Moines, IA 50306 PRINTED IN U.S.A. **GRAPHIC CHART**

Figure 10–1 Sample graphic chart. (From Briggs, Des Moines, IA 50306.)

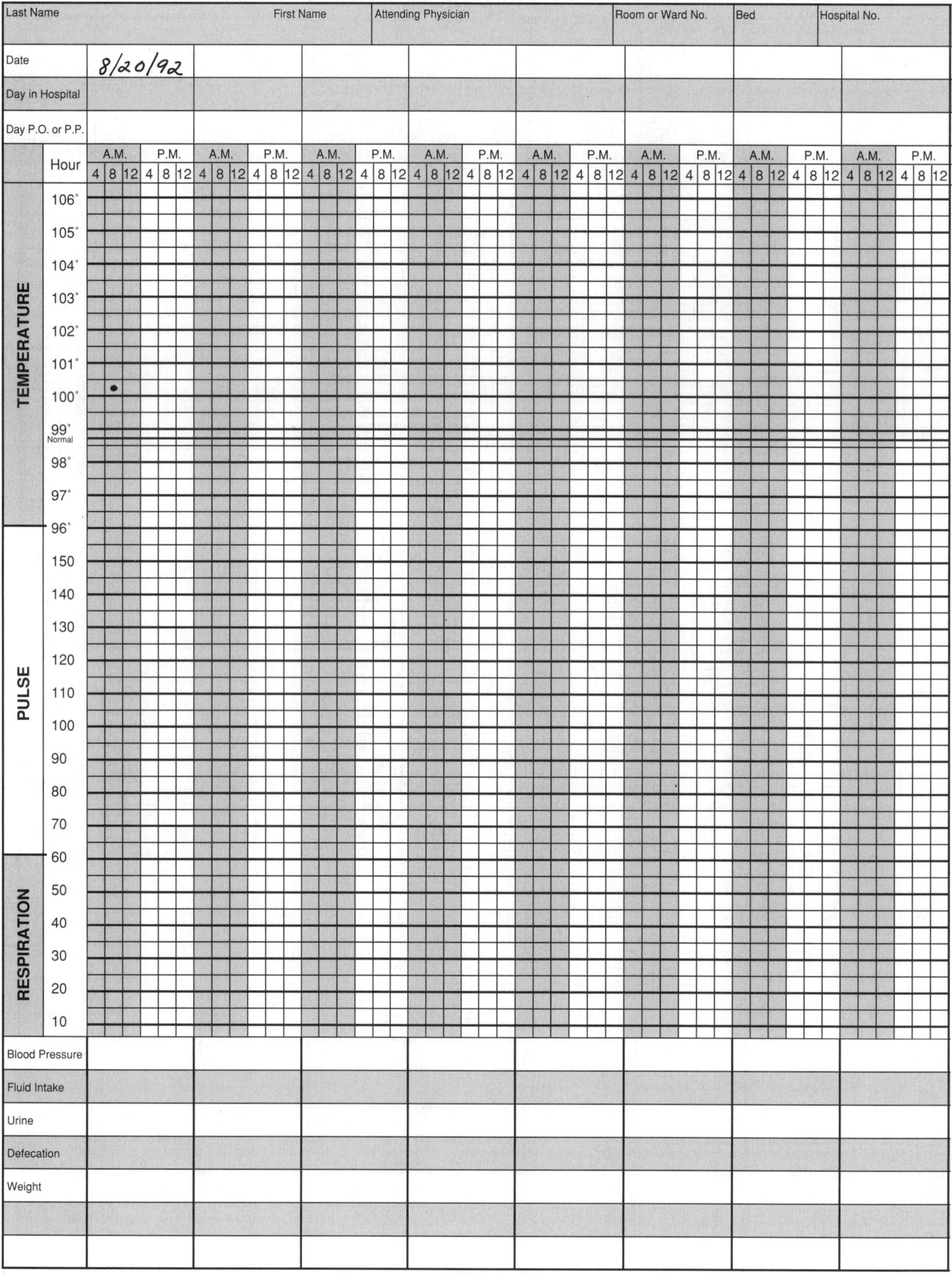

Figure 10–2 Answer to question 4 of Proficiency Gauge. (From Briggs, Des Moines, IA 50306.)

7. What time is 0255? 7. ____________
8. What is an MAR used for? 8. ____________
9. State one way that computers can help prevent documentation errors. 9. ____________
10. State one common medication error. 10. ____________

ANSWERS 1. 300 mL 2. 285 mL 3. 60 mL 4. see Figure 10–2 5. Accessibility, convenience, time saver (any one) 6. 1900 7. 2:55 AM 8. To record medications that are administered 9. Any one of the following: prevents transcription errors, saves time, avoids errors associated with illegible handwriting 10. Any one of the following: wrong medication, wrong dosage, transcription errors, failure to record medications or discontinue medications as ordered

---

10-2. INTAKE AND OUTPUT RECORD

In the hospital and long-term care setting, many clients require monitoring and recording of their fluid intake and output (I & O). This monitoring is sometimes referred to as the client being "on I & O." The purpose of measuring I & O is to compare the client's intake with his or her output. This is particularly important when the client is receiving diuretics (fluid pills) to increase urinary output.

Fluid Intake

All fluids taken by mouth, by feeding tube, or intravenously are recorded in milliliters. Usually at the end of each 8-h shift, the fluid amounts are added for a shift total. Then, at the end of the day, or 24-hour period, the total amount of fluid taken in is computed and recorded.

The I & O sheet is often left at the client's bedside for convenience in recording. Oral fluids are recorded in milliliters, but the containers may be labeled in ounces. Both the type and the amount of fluid are recorded. Recording intake is especially important when the client has a fever and needs to receive increased fluids. The sample shown here indicates how the nurse records this information.

ORAL FLUIDS

Time	Type of fluid	Amount of fluid
4 pm	Water	150 mL

In some cases, the nurse needs to convert from one measurement system to another, most commonly from the household system to the metric system as discussed in Chapter 5.

Examples

1. Mr. Jones drank 8 oz of milk and 4 oz of orange juice for breakfast at 8 AM. How many milliliters of each fluid did he consume?

$$30 \text{ mL} = 1 \text{ oz}$$
$$8 \times 30 \text{ mL} = 240 \text{ mL (milk)}$$
$$4 \times 30 \text{ mL} = 120 \text{ mL (juice)}$$

2. Ms. Bordinski drank $\frac{1}{4}$ c coffee (8-oz cup), $\frac{1}{2}$ bowl broth (10-oz bowl), and 1 glass (6 oz) of cranberry juice for lunch at 12:30 PM. How many milliliters of each fluid did she take in?

$$\frac{1}{4} \times 8 \text{ oz} = 2 \text{ oz} = 60 \text{ mL (coffee)}$$
$$\frac{1}{2} \times 10 \text{ oz} = 5 \text{ oz} = 150 \text{ mL (broth)}$$
$$6 \times 30 \text{ mL} = 180 \text{ mL (juice)}$$

If the client receives intravenous therapy, the amount of fluid given is also recorded. (Chapter 8 discusses IV fluid calculations in detail.) When a bag or bottle is hung or added, the nurse records the time and the type and amount of fluid in the appropriate column on the I & O sheet. When the IV fluid has infused, the nurse records the *actual* amount of fluid infused, or *absorbed.*

Recording IV solution intake is made easier and more accurate if the IV is regulated by an electronic controller or pump. In this case, the nurse records the volume infused as indicated on the pump and "clears" this number from the device so that the oncoming shift begins at zero.

Examples

1. The nurse hangs a 1000-mL bag of 5%D/W at 3 AM. The fluid was absorbed at 11 AM when a second bag of the same solution was hung. How is this information recorded on the input part of the I & O sheet shown below?

PARENTERAL FLUIDS

Time	Amount/Type of Fluid	Amount Absorbed
3 AM	1000 mL D5/W	
11 AM		1000 mL
11 AM	1000 mL D5/W	
1 PM	1000 mL D5/W	
6 PM	IV D/C'd	550 mL

2. The nurse discontinues an IV at 6 PM with 450 mL remaining in a 1000-mL bag that was hung at 1 PM. How is this information recorded on the above form?

If a bag or bottle of fluid is not complete by the end of the nurse's shift, he or she may alert the oncoming nurse to how much fluid is left in the bag.

Examples

1. If 375 mL of a 1000-mL bag of IV solution is absorbed on the 3–11 shift, the nurse records that 375 mL was absorbed and 625 mL is left in the bag (LIB).
2. If 900 mL of a 1000-mL bag of 5%D/1/2NS is absorbed during the 7–3 shift, the nurse records 900 mL absorbed and 100 mL LIB.

Every agency is a little different about I & O charting. The nurse always checks the policies to ensure that he or she complies with the requirements of a particular health care setting and that abbreviations being used are acceptable in that setting.

Output

The same basic procedure for intake is used when charting output. The type and amount of fluid are recorded and is usually added for 8-h and 24-h totals. The most commonly measured fluid output is urine. Urine can be either amounts from the spontaneous voiding (the client goes to the bathroom and voids) or amounts taken from a urinary catheter. The drainage bag from the catheter is emptied, and the urine is measured at specified intervals. In a critical care unit, urine amounts may be recorded every hour. On a general hospital unit or in a nursing home, the urine is usually measured and recorded at 8-h intervals.

Other output includes liquid stool, vomitus, and any type of drainage from the body or from tubes in the body, such as nasogastric drainage. The nurse records these amounts in the section of the form for output and under the appropriate heading.

SAMPLE EXERCISES

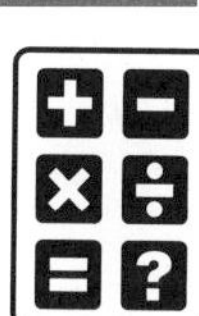

1–4. Record the following outputs during the 3–11 shift on the output section of the I & O form provided in the form below.

OUTPUT

Time	Urine	NG Drainage	Wound Drainage	Vomitus	Misc.

1. 325 mL of urine at 4 PM
2. 36 mL of wound drainage at 11 PM
3. 75 mL of vomitus at 7 PM
4. 200 mL of nasogastric (NG) drainage at 11 PM
5. What was the total output for the 3–11 shift for this client?

ANSWERS

1–4.

OUTPUT

Time	Urine	NG Drainage	Wound Drainage	Vomitus	Misc.
4 pm	325 mL				
7 pm				75 mL	
11 pm		200 mL	36 mL		

5. 325 + 36 + 75 + 200 = 636 mL

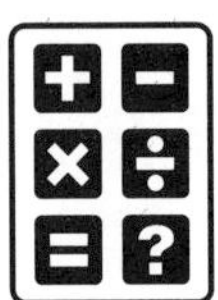

EXERCISES

Exercises 1–5. Convert the following amounts of fluid to milliliters.

1. 3.5 oz
2. 8 oz
3. $\frac{3}{4}$ c (8-oz cup)
4. $\frac{1}{3}$ c (6-oz cup)
5. 3 tsp

Exercises 6–10. Compute how much IV fluid has absorbed from a 1000-mL bag if the following amounts are left in the bag:

6. 275 mL
7. 550 mL
8. 130 mL
9. 890 mL
10. 75 mL
11. State three types of fluid output that the nurse measures and records.

ANSWERS 1. 105 mL 3. 180 mL 5. 15 mL 7. 450 mL 9. 110 mL 11. Any three of the following: urine, vomitus, liquid stool, any type of drainage from the body

10-3. AVERAGES

After a client's output is recorded, it is often important to find some average measurements. The most important average that the nurse computes in most settings is the hourly urine output, which should be 30 mL or more for an adult. The amount of urine a client produces indicates how well his or her kidneys are functioning; adequate kidney function is needed to maintain health. The **average** is the arithmetic mean, or the sum of all measurements divided by the number of measurements.* The formula for the arithmetic mean follows.

* Other types of averages are the median and the mode.

COMPUTING THE AVERAGE

$$\text{Average (mean)} = \frac{\text{Sum of all the measurements}}{\text{Number of measurements}}$$

Examples

1. A client's urinary output was recorded during the 7–3 shift as:

   8 AM: 200 mL
   1 PM: 175 mL
   3 PM: 125 mL

   To find the average amount of urine voided each time, use the formula above:

   $$x = \frac{200 \text{ mL} + 175 \text{ mL} + 125 \text{ mL}}{3} = \frac{500 \text{ mL}}{3} = 167 \text{ mL}$$

2. In most cases, the amount of urine for each voiding is not as significant as the hourly amount. To find the hourly average for the 7–3 shift (an 8-h period), use the following:

   $$\frac{500 \text{ mL}}{8 \text{ h}} = 63 \text{ mL of urine/h}$$

   This amount is above the minimum hourly average (30 mL/h) for healthy kidney function.

3. The amount of wound drainage in a Jackson-Pratt surgical drain during a 24-h period was recorded as follows:

   3 PM: 50 mL
   11 PM: 30 mL
   7 AM: 10 mL

   To find the average amount of drainage per 8-h shift (three shifts), we use the following:

   $$\frac{50 \text{ mL} + 30 \text{ mL} + 10 \text{ mL}}{3} = \frac{90 \text{ mL}}{3} = 30 \text{ mL}$$

   The hourly rate of drainage over 24 h is obtained as follows:

   $$\frac{90 \text{ mL}}{24 \text{ h}} = 3.8 \text{ mL/h}$$

EXERCISES

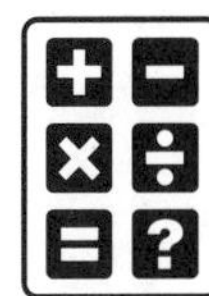

Exercises 1–5. Compute the average hourly amount of output in each of the following situations.

1. 250 mL in 8 h
2. 640 mL in 24 h
3. 1240 mL in 24 h
4. 195 mL in 8 h
5. 80 mL in 6 h

Exercises 6–10. If each of the outputs in Exercises 1–5 was urine, state whether the averages are above the expected hourly average for an adult.

ANSWERS 1. 31.25 mL 3. 51.67 mL 5. 13.33 mL 7. no 9. no

10-4. GRAPHS

In some cases, data are placed on a graph to quickly identify trends, or changes over time. The most common example of graphing is the graphic chart for recording vital signs—temperature, pulse, respiration (TPR), and blood pressure (BP) (Fig. 10–3).

In many cases, taking vital signs is part of medication administration or calculation. For example, if a client is receiving antibiotics, the temperature is usually monitored during drug therapy. If a client's temperature exceeds a certain limit, the physician may order another drug, such as acetaminophen (Tylenol), to lower it. Because of their side effects, other drugs can be given only if the pulse and blood pressure are within acceptable limits.

Examples

1. The chart in Figure 10–3 has three separate grids for graphs of temperature, pulse, and respiration. The top graph shows Mr. Michal's temperatures for 1 week. The graph makes it easy to see that his temperature rises in the afternoon, remains steady for the evening, and falls during the night.
2. From the graph, we can easily read the highest temperatures (°F) that Mr. Michal reached and when they were first recorded:

   104°F at 4 PM on January 10, 1993
   103.5°F at 4 PM on January 8, 1993

3. The middle graph shows that Mr. Michal's pulse follows the same general trends as his temperature, except for the last day, when the pulse was steady despite the rise in temperature.
4. To read the details of the chart, we read the values that correspond to each point, that is, the date and time (indicated at the top of each column), and the measurement of temperature, pulse, or respiration (indicated on the left of each row). Thus, on January 8, at 12 AM (noon) Mr. Michal's

   Temperature was 101.5°F
   Pulse rate was 80 bpm (beats/min)
   Respiration rate was 25 breaths/min

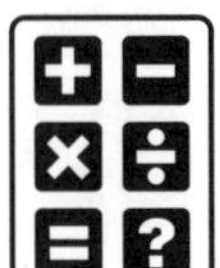

SAMPLE EXERCISES

Exercises 1–3. Figure 10–4 is a graphic chart showing Ms. Halow's temperature and pulse measurements for 3 days.

1. When was Ms. Halow's temperature below normal?
2. What is the difference between Ms. Halow's highest and lowest recorded pulse rate?
3. What was Ms. Halow's average temperature on day 1?
4. What was Ms. Halow's average pulse rate for the 3 days?

GRAPHIC CHART

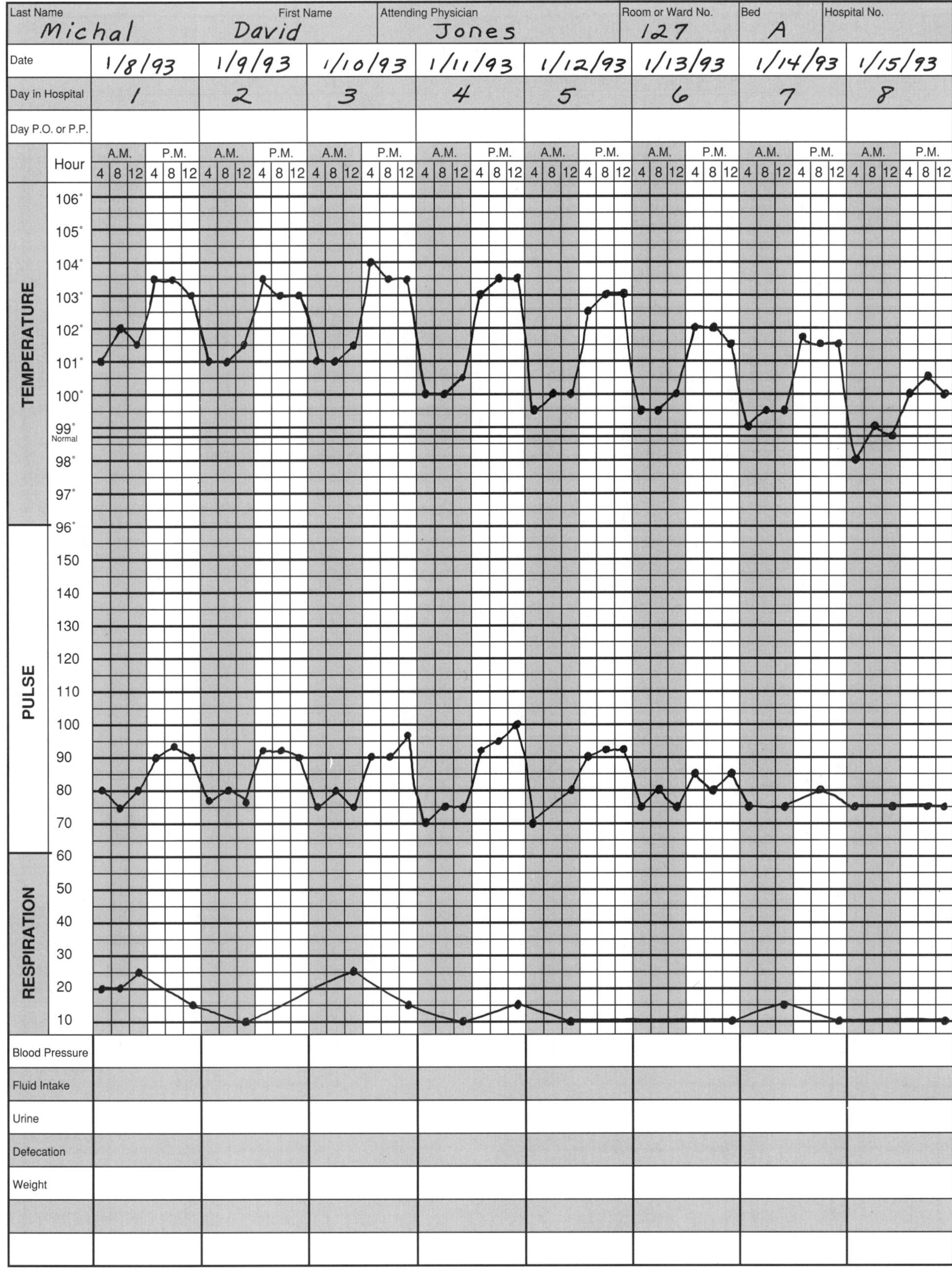

Last Name	First Name	Attending Physician	Room or Ward No.	Bed	Hospital No.
Michal	David	Jones	127	A	

Date	1/8/93	1/9/93	1/10/93	1/11/93	1/12/93	1/13/93	1/14/93	1/15/93
Day in Hospital	1	2	3	4	5	6	7	8
Day P.O. or P.P.								
Hour	A.M. 4 8 12 / P.M. 4 8 12	A.M. 4 8 12 / P.M. 4 8 12	A.M. 4 8 12 / P.M. 4 8 12	A.M. 4 8 12 / P.M. 4 8 12	A.M. 4 8 12 / P.M. 4 8 12	A.M. 4 8 12 / P.M. 4 8 12	A.M. 4 8 12 / P.M. 4 8 12	A.M. 4 8 12 / P.M. 4 8 12
TEMPERATURE (106°, 105°, 104°, 103°, 102°, 101°, 100°, 99° Normal, 98°, 97°, 96°)								
PULSE (150, 140, 130, 120, 110, 100, 90, 80, 70, 60)								
RESPIRATION (60, 50, 40, 30, 20, 10)								
Blood Pressure								
Fluid Intake								
Urine								
Defecation								
Weight								

Form 2501 BRIGGS, Des Moines, IA 50306 PRINTED IN U.S.A.

GRAPHIC CHART

Figure 10–3 Graphic chart for recording vital signs. (From Briggs, Des Moines, IA 50306.)

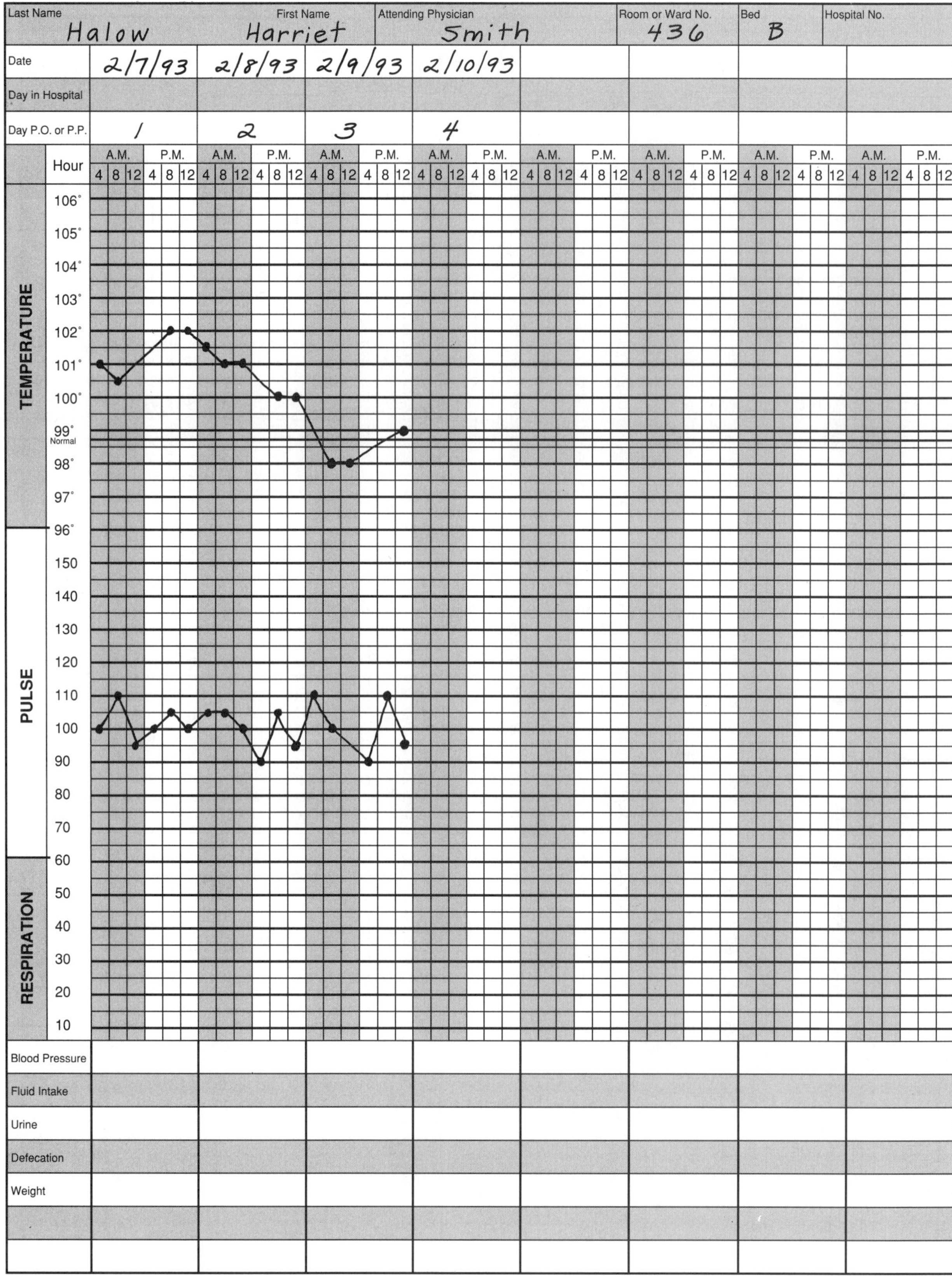

GRAPHIC CHART

Last Name	First Name	Attending Physician	Room or Ward No.	Bed	Hospital No.
Halow	Harriet	Smith	436	B	

Date	2/7/93	2/8/93	2/9/93	2/10/93				
Day in Hospital								
Day P.O. or P.P.	1	2	3	4				

Hour: A.M. 4 8 12, P.M. 4 8 12 (repeated for each day)

TEMPERATURE: 106°, 105°, 104°, 103°, 102°, 101°, 100°, 99° Normal, 98°, 97°, 96°

PULSE: 150, 140, 130, 120, 110, 100, 90, 80, 70, 60

RESPIRATION: 50, 40, 30, 20, 10

Blood Pressure

Fluid Intake

Urine

Defecation

Weight

Form 2501 BRIGGS, Des Moines, IA 50306 PRINTED IN U.S.A.

GRAPHIC CHART

Figure 10–4 Ms. Halow's graphic chart for Sample Exercises 1–4. (From Briggs, Des Moines, IA 50306.)

ANSWERS 1. 8 AM and 12 AM on day 3. 2. 20 bpm 3. 101.4°F 4. 100.9, or 101 bpm

HOW TO DRAW A GRAPH

1. Select the appropriate column for date and time.
2. Move down that column to reach the corresponding measurement.
3. Place a point in the middle of the column.
4. Check that the point indicates both correct time and correct measurement.
5. Draw line segments connecting the points in order.

Example

Temperature measurements recorded for Ms. Chine on the first day in the hospital were as follows:

Time	4 AM	8 AM	12 AM	4 PM	8 PM	12 PM
Temperature (°F)	101	103	101.5	98.6	99.5	100.5

The temperature graph looks like the enlarged illustration in Figure 10–5.

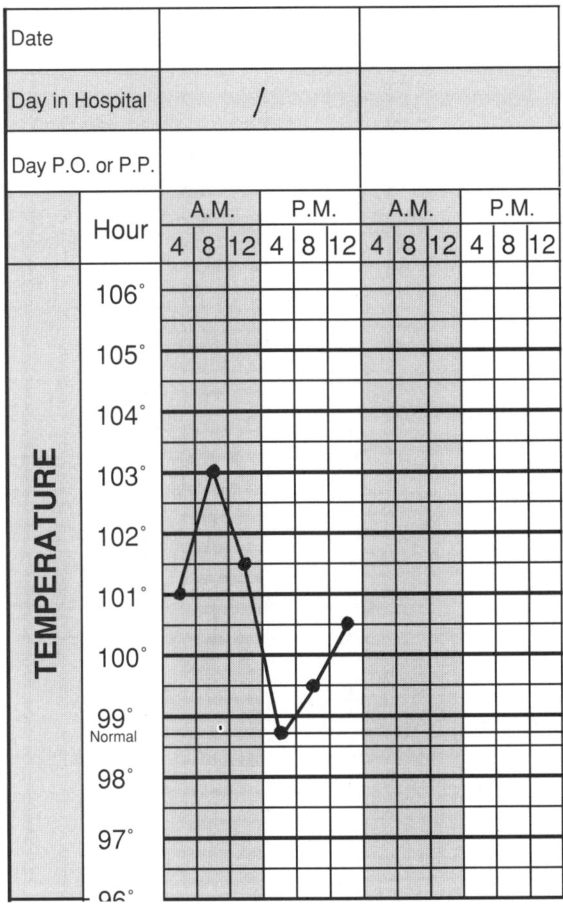

Figure 10–5 Temperature graph for Ms. Chine.

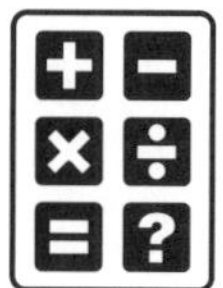

SAMPLE EXERCISES

Pulse and respiration measurements recorded for Ms. Chine on the first day in the hospital were as follows:

Time	4 AM	8 AM	12 AM	4 PM	8 PM	12 PM
Beats per Minute	80	90	85	70	70	75
Respirations per Minute	25	25	25	20	15	15

Draw pulse and respiration graphs on the enlarged graphic chart in Figure 10–6.

ANSWERS (see Fig. 10–7)

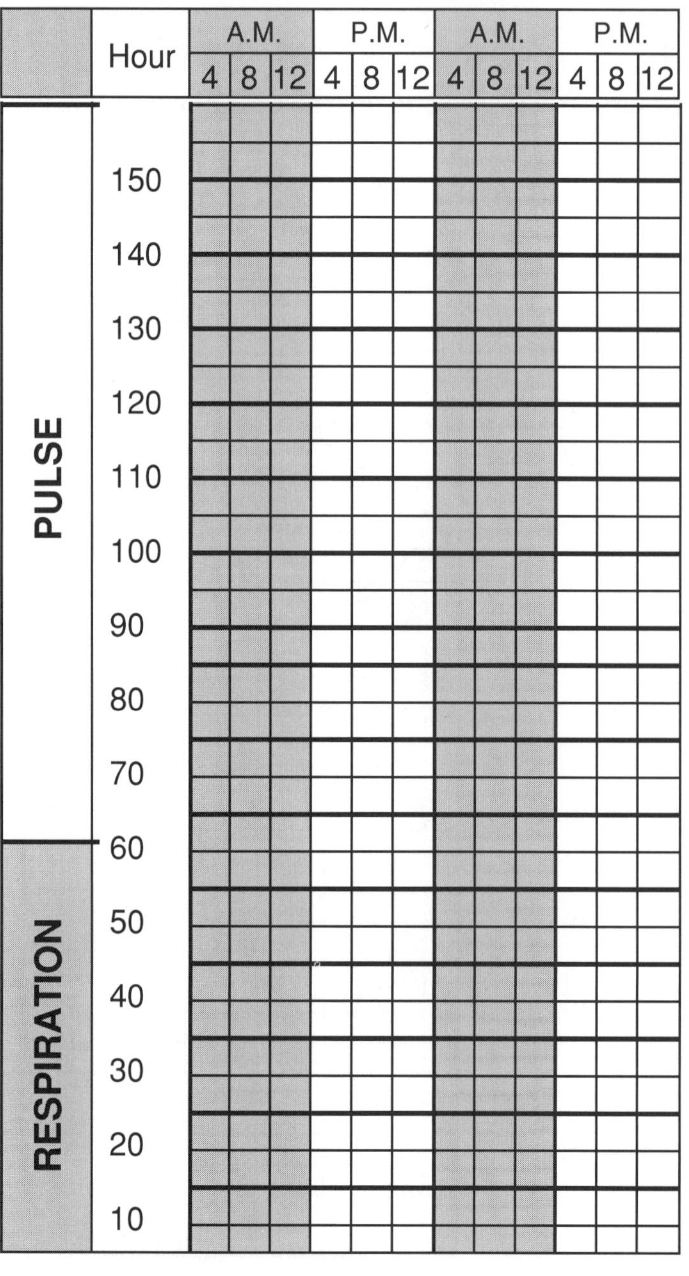

Figure 10–6 Graphic chart for Sample Exercises.

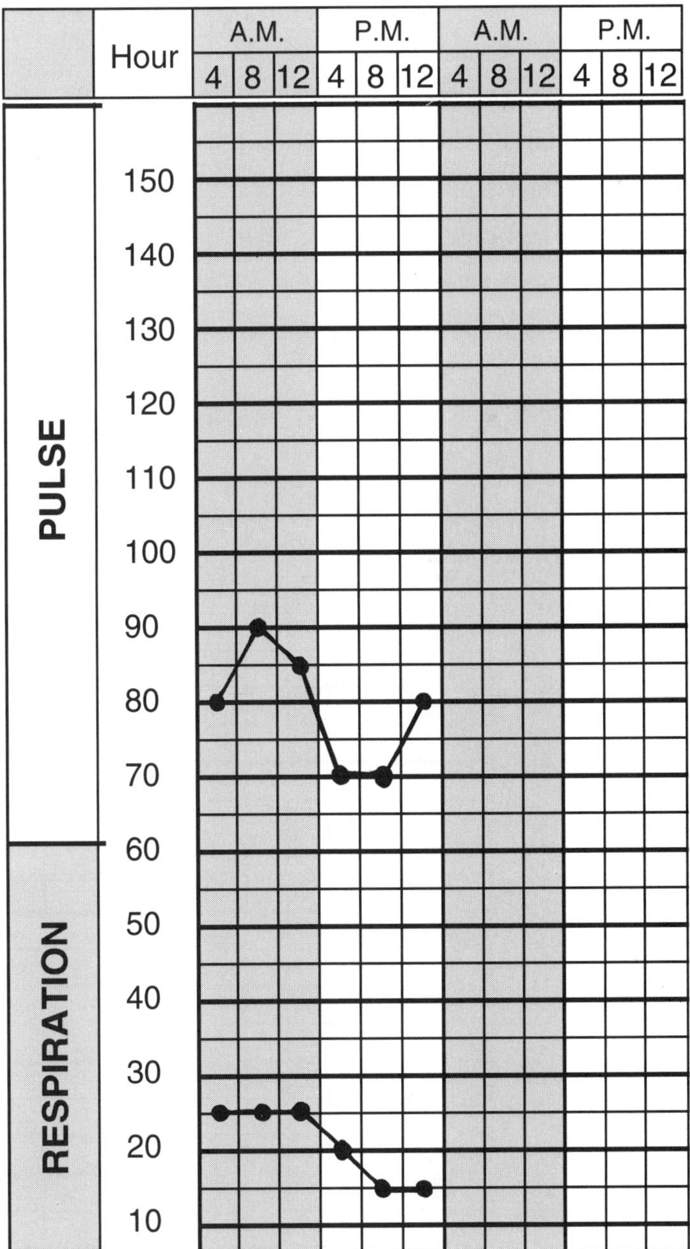

Figure 10–7 Graphic chart answer for Sample Exercises.

EXERCISES

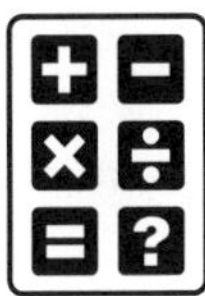

Exercises 1–18. Answer the following questions about the graphs shown for Mr. Michal in Figure 10–3 on p. 345.

1. What were the client's highest and lowest recorded temperatures?
2. What are the highest and lowest temperatures for which space is provided on the grid?
3. When did Mr. Michal reach his highest recorded temperature? His lowest?
4. For what period(s) did his temperature rise regularly? Fall?
5. To the nearest tenth, what was his average temperature on the first day?
6. What was his average temperature on the fourth day?
7. What were his lowest and highest pulse rates?

8. What are the lowest and highest pulse rates for which space is provided on the grid?
9. When did Mr. Michal reach his highest recorded pulse rate? His lowest?
10. Over what period(s) did the greatest fall in pulse rate occur?
11. What was his average pulse rate on the third day?
12. What was his average pulse rate on the sixth day?
13. What was his highest recorded respiration rate?
14. What is the lowest respiration rate for which space is provided on the grid?
15. When did Mr. Michal reach his highest recorded respiration rate?
16. For what period did the respiration rate rise the most?

	Hour	A.M.			P.M.			A.M.			P.M.		
		4	8	12	4	8	12	4	8	12	4	8	12
PULSE	150												
	140												
	130												
	120												
	110												
	100												
	90												
	80												
	70												
RESPIRATION	60												
	50												
	40												
	30												
	20												
	10												

Figure 10–8 Graphic chart for Exercises 19–20.

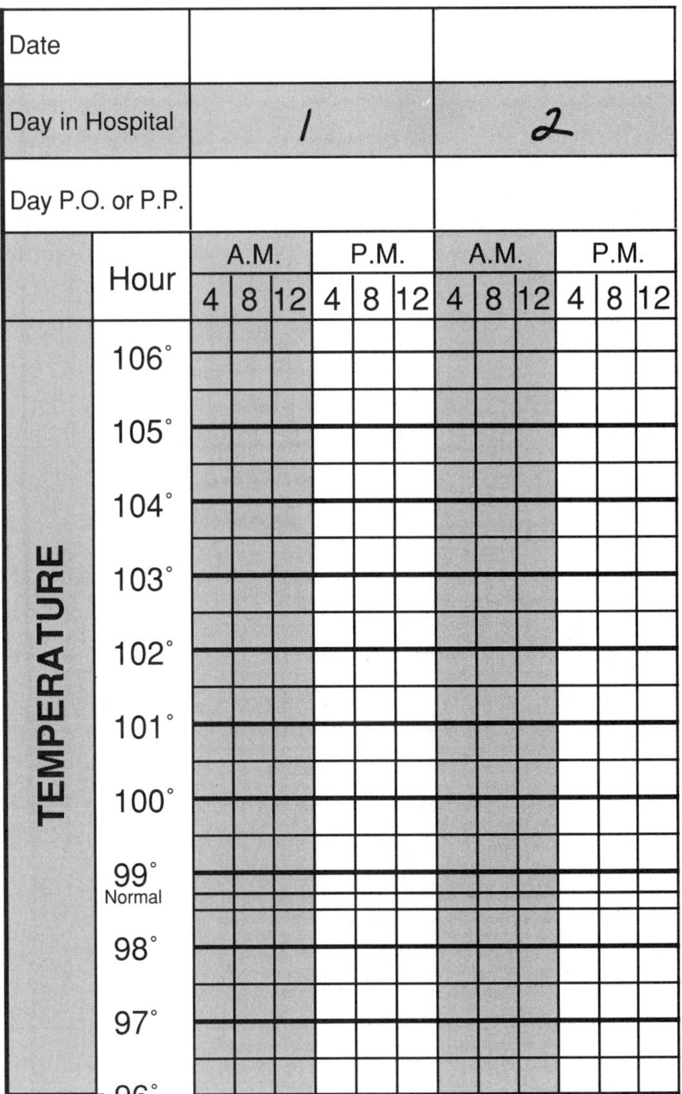

Figure 10–9 Graphic chart for Exercises 21–22.

17. What was the client's average respiration rate recorded for the first 2 days?

18. What was the client's average respiration rate recorded on the last 2 days?

Exercises 19–20. The following measurements have been recorded:

Time	4 AM	8 AM	12 AM	4 PM	8 PM	12 PM
Beats per Minute	60	75	95	80	100	85
Respirations per Minute	25	30	25	15	10	10

On the graphic chart shown in Figure 10–8, draw the indicated graphs.

19. Pulse

20. Respiration

Exercises 21–22. The following measurements have been recorded:

Time	4 AM	8 AM	12 AM	4 PM	8 PM	12 PM
Temperature (°F, day 1)	102	102.5	103	99.5	103.5	102
Temperature (°F, day 2)	103	103.5	102	101.5	100.5	98.6

On the graphic chart in Figure 10–9, draw the indicated graphs.

21. Temperature (Day 1)

22. Temperature (Day 2)

ANSWERS 1. Highest: 104°F; lowest: 98°F 3. Highest: 4 PM on day 3; lowest: 4 AM on day 8 5. $\frac{\text{Sum of temperatures}}{6} = 102.4°\text{F}$ 7. Lowest: 70 bpm; highest: 100 bpm 9. Highest: 12 PM on day 4; lowest: 4 AM on days 4 and 5 11. 84 bpm 13. 25 breaths/min 15. 12 AM on days 1 and 3 17. 18 breaths/min 19. (see Fig. 10–10) 21. (see Fig. 10–11)

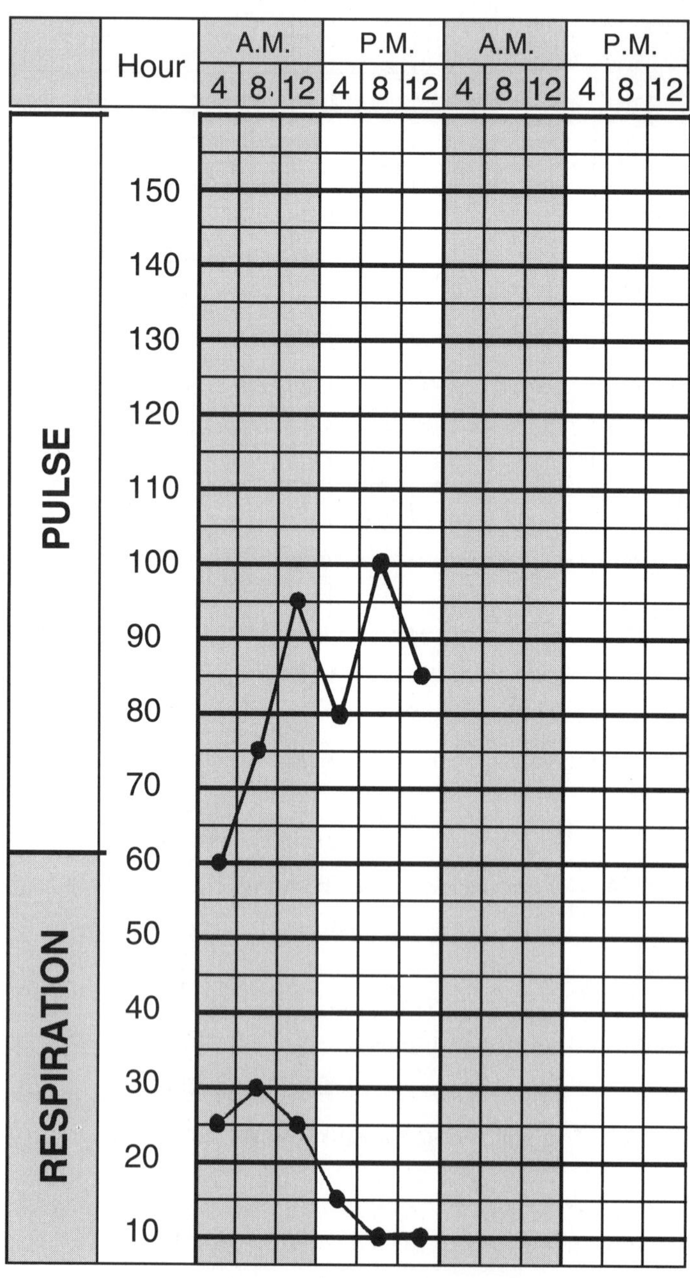

Figure 10–10 Answer for Exercises 19–20.

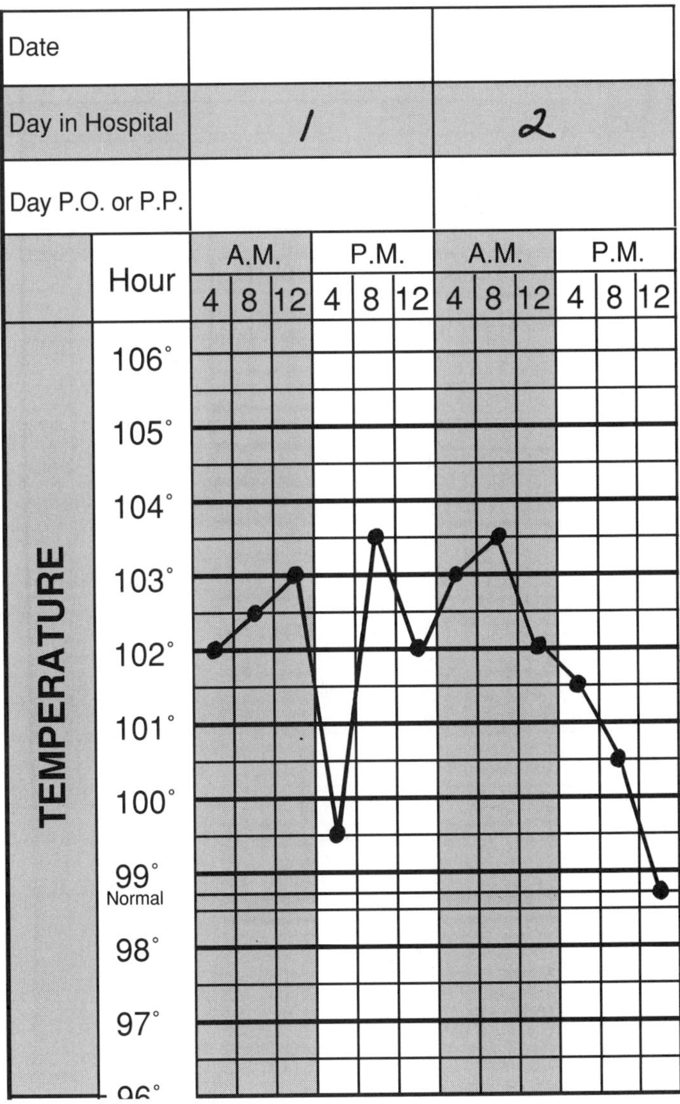

Figure 10–11 Answer for Exercises 21–22.

10-5. FLOW SHEETS

Some health care facilities have eliminated the graphic chart to prevent the data from being written twice—once on the vital signs worksheet and again on the graphic chart. The trend in health care settings today, especially in hospitals, is the use of streamlined forms to allow the nurse to record the critical information only once at the client's bedside.

The development of a multitude of flow sheets has helped to prevent duplication, redundancy, and time in charting. Flow sheets often include information about the client's activities of daily living, vital signs, intake and output, finger stick blood sugars, and physical assessment data (e.g., breath sounds). Having a comprehensive flow sheet that contains the daily routine care keeps all this information together in one place. Figure 10–12 illustrates part of the data that may be found on a nursing flow sheet.

In some instances, particularly on specialty care units, specialized flow sheets are also used. For example, the Glasgow Coma Scale is used to monitor a client's level of consciousness when a head injury or other brain lesion is suspected. As seen in Figure 10–13, the nurse assesses the client and assigns a

RESPIRATORY	
	RESPIRATIONS EASY AND REGULAR
	BREATH SOUNDS CLEAR
	FREQUENT BREATH SOUNDS q__________
	DYSPNEA ON EXERTION
	O_2 __________ L/MIN VIA __________
	O_2 VIA__________ % VENTI-MASK
	POST-OP COUGH & DEEP BREATH
	SUCTIONED VIA__________
	TRACH CARE
	COUGH
	HUMIDIFIER
	ORAL/NASAL AIRWAY UTILIZED

Figure 10–12 Portion of a nursing flow sheet.

		Date											
		Time											
Best eye-opening response	Spontaneously	4											
	To speech	3											
	To pain	2											
	No response	1											
Best verbal response	Oriented x3	5											
	Conversation: confused	4											
	Speech: inappropriate	3											
	Sounds: incomprehensible	2											
	No response	1											
Best motor response to painful stimuli	Obeys verbal command	6											
	Localizes pain	5											
	Flexion – withdrawal	4											
	Flexion – abnormal	3											
	Extension – abnormal	2											
	No response	1											
(T = Tube)	TOTAL	3-15											

Figure 10–13 Glasgow Coma Scale.

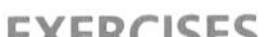

score for each of three types of responses. The scores are added to obtain a total score indicating the client's level of consciousness. A high score of 15 indicates no problem. Smaller numbers reflect more serious problems.

EXERCISES

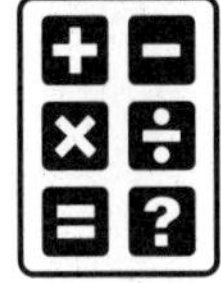

1. Why are flow sheets becoming so popular in health care settings?
2. What are three types of data that may be charted on a flow sheet?
3. (a) What is the total possible score on the Glasgow Coma Scale in Figure 10–13?
   (b) What does a total score of 15 indicate about the client?

ANSWERS 1. Flow sheets prevent duplication and redundancy in charting and save time. 2. Any three of the following: activities of daily living, physical assessment information, vital signs, intake and output, finger stick blood sugars 3. (a) 15 (b) No problem with consciousness level

10-6. THE 24-HOUR CLOCK

In many parts of the world and in the US military, a different system for recording time is used. Some civilian health care facilities in the United States have also adopted this 24-h clock system.

What does the physician mean when he or she says that the client should have IV therapy beginning at 0800 and ending at 1600? The numbers 0800 and 1600 refer to numbers on the 24-h clock, a method of measuring time without using a colon or the symbols AM and PM. The major advantage of this system in health care is that it helps prevent errors. The times 8 AM and 8 PM may look very similar if the A and the P are not clear. If a drug is ordered to be given at 8 AM, it may not be given until 8 PM if the letters are not properly formed.

The 24-h clock is illustrated below.

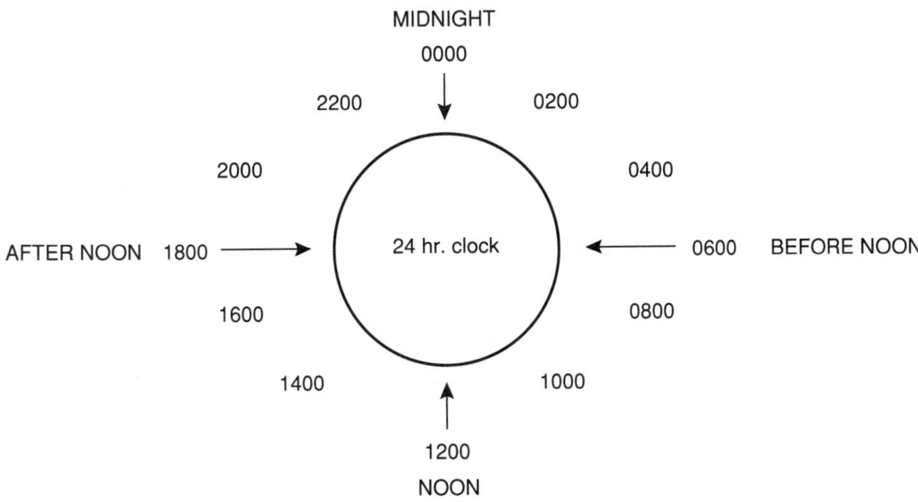

Examples

1. The four-digit number 0830 signifies that 8 h and 30 min have passed since midnight. Any four-digit number represents a point in time if the first two digits on the left (from 00 to 23) is the number of hours since the previous day began (midnight) and the last two digits on the right (from 00 to 59) is the number of additional minutes.

Military Time	Hours Since Midnight	Minutes After the Hour	Regular Clock Time
0830	8 h	30 min	8:30 AM
1200	12 h	0 min	noon, or 12 PM
1625	16 h	25 min	4:25 PM
2359	23 h	59 min	11:59 PM
0000	0 h	0 min	Midnight, the beginning of a new day, or 12 AM
0005	0 h	5 min	5 min after midnight, or 12:05 AM

2. A number less than 1200 represents a time *before* noon because fewer than 12 h have passed since midnight. Thus, 0845 represents 8:45 AM.
3. A number above 1200 represents a time *after* noon because more than 12 h have passed since midnight. Thus, 1605 represents more than 16 h after midnight, or 4:05 PM.

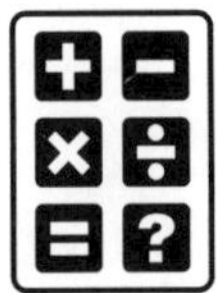

SAMPLE EXERCISES

Exercises 1–2. State whether AM (morning) or PM (afternoon) is represented.

1. 0145
2. 1450

Exercises 3–4. In each of the cases above, how much time has passed since midnight?

Exercises 5–8. For each interval below, how much time has elapsed?

5. From 0100 to 0600
6. From 0325 to 0550
7. From 1100 to 2300
8. From 1500 to 0200

ANSWERS 1. AM 2. PM 3. 1 h and 45 min 4. 14 h and 50 min 5. 5 h 6. 2 h and 25 min 7. 12 h 8. 11 h

Conversions from Ordinary Clock Time

If we wish to record time on official records, we often need to convert ordinary clock time to 24-h clock time.

CONVERSIONS FROM ORDINARY TIME	
From AM	**From PM**
Omit the colon and AM	Omit the colon. Omit PM and add 1200.
6:50 AM = 0650	6:50 PM = 1850

Examples

1. To convert 11:48 AM to 24-h time, simply omit the colon and AM. Thus, 11:48 AM = 1148.
2. To convert 11:48 PM to 24-h time, omit the colon and PM and add 1200. Thus, 11:48 PM = 2348.
3. An appointment for an x-ray at 5:30 PM may be written 1730.

SAMPLE EXERCISES

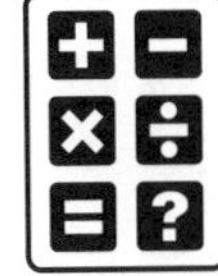

Exercises 1–4. Convert to 24-h time.

1. 4:21 AM
2. 11:13 AM
3. 1:43 PM
4. 7:16 PM

ANSWERS 1. 0421 2. 1113 3. 1343 4. 1916

Conversion to Ordinary Clock Time

To check 24-hour time with a watch, it is necessary to convert 24-hour time back to ordinary time.

CONVERSIONS TO ORDINARY TIME	
To AM	**To PM**
Insert the colon. Insert AM.	Subtract 1200. Insert the colon. Insert PM.
0915 = 9:15 AM	1458 = 2:58 PM

Examples

1. To convert 0243 to ordinary time, insert a colon and AM.

   0243 = 2:43 AM

2. To convert 2109 to ordinary time, subtract 1200, then insert a colon and PM.

   2109 = 9:09 PM

3. To convert 0003 to ordinary time, insert a colon and AM.

$$0003 = 0{:}03 \text{ AM} = 12{:}03 \text{ AM}$$

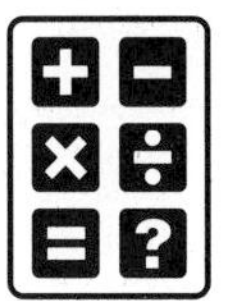

SAMPLE EXERCISES

Exercises 1–5. Convert the following to ordinary time:

1. 0105
2. 0642
3. 1836
4. 2005
5. 0001

ANSWERS 1. 1:05 AM 2. 6:42 AM 3. 6:36 PM 4. 8:05 PM 5. 12:01 AM

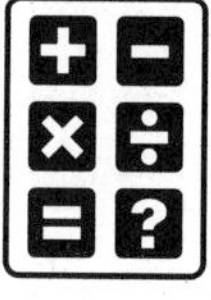

EXERCISES

Exercises 1–4. State whether morning or afternoon is represented.

1. 1014
2. 2350
3. 2159
4. 0955

Exercises 5–8. In each of the cases above, how much time has passed since midnight?

Exercises 9–12. Find the length of time elapsed in each of the following intervals.

9. 0700 to 1900
10. 1140 to 2350
11. 1700 to 0100
12. 2030 to 0230

Exercises 13–22. Convert the following to 24-h time:

13. 6:30 AM
14. 10:21 AM
15. 12 noon
16. 12 midnight
17. 3:54 PM
18. 9:17 PM
19. 2:55 AM
20. 20 min after midnight
21. 4:48 PM
22. 10 min before midnight

Exercises 23–28. Convert the following to ordinary time:

23. 0208
24. 0753
25. 1743
26. 2210
27. 0016
28. 0004

Exercises 29–34. In each of the following cases, find the length of the time interval.

29. From 0300 to 1000
30. From 415 to 1135
31. From 1000 to 1600
32. From 1135 to 2150
33. From 1600 to 0100
34. From 2150 to 0005

Exercises 35–38. If we are to begin IV therapy for Ms. D. at 1400 and to continue for the number of hours given below, when on the ordinary clock should we stop?

35. 3 h
36. 9 h
37. 11 h
38. 12 h

Exercises 39–40. If Ms. A. had IV therapy for 8 h, ending at the time given below, when, on the 24-h clock, was the IV started?

39. 1100
40. 0200

ANSWERS 1. AM 3. PM 5. 10 h, 14 min 7. 21 h, 59 min 9. 12 h 11. 8 h 13. 0630 15. 1200 17. 1554 19. 0255 21. 1648 23. 2:08 AM 25. 5:43 PM 27. 12:16 AM 29. 7 h 31. 6 h 33. 9 h 35. 5:00 PM 37. 1:00 AM 39. 0300

10-7. MEDICATION ADMINISTRATION RECORD

The medication administration record (MAR) is the form used to document that the medications ordered by the physician have been given. Figure 10–14 is an example of a typical MAR. Most health care settings today use an MAR Kardex or chart form, which they carry to the client's room when giving medications. This replaces the older method of using small medication cards for each drug given. In some countries this traditional system is still used, but in the United States most facilities use the more convenient MAR.

Although the actual format varies from facility to facility, the same basic information is included in an MAR. The nurse or unit clerk completes the record for each client by transcribing, or copying, the physician's orders onto the MAR. In some systems, all medication and IV fluid orders are written on one form.

Not all medications are given on a continuous basis. Some drugs are given only as the client needs them, for example, for episodes of pain, or only one time, such as furosemide (Lasix) given IV push for rapidly increasing body fluid. These "as needed," or prn, medications are typically charted on a different part of the MAR from the regimen drugs. For prn or one-time medications, the nurse also documents the reason for the drug and the results of its action, for example, that pain was relieved after receiving the prescribed analgesic.

Figure 10–14, shows the physician's order for five continuing medications to be given to a client at varying times. The nurse checks the MAR to determine what drugs are ordered, how much of each drug, and when and how each is to be given. The nurse also verifies the MAR with the physician's orders. After administering each drug, the nurse signs his or her initials to show that the drug was given. The initials are then written under the Signature/Title section to identify who gave the medication.

For parenteral medications, the nurse indicates the injection site for each dose.

PAGE 1

ORIGINAL DATE ORDERED / INITIALS	DRUGS MODE / DOSE INTERVAL	HOURS	DATE 11/3	DATE 11/4	DATE 11/5	DATE 11/6	DATE	DATE	DATE	DATE	DATE	DATE	DATE	DATE	STOP/DATE TIMES
11/3/92 DI	Allopurinol 300 mg PO bid	10 00 2000													
11/3/92 DI	Ampicillin 500 mg q8h PO	0800 1600 2400													
11/3/92 DI	Digoxin 0.125 mg PO qd	1000 AP													
11/3/92 DI	Lasix 80 mg qd	10 00													
11/3/92 DI	Humulin-N 35 u q AM subq	0730 Site													

INITIAL	SIGNATURE

MEDICATION RECORD

MONTH
YEAR

ROOM	AGE	NAME

Figure 10–14 Medication administration record (MAR).

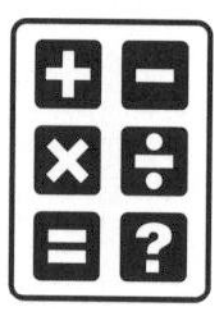

EXERCISES

Exercises 1–4. Using the MAR sample in Figure 10–14, do the following exercises:

1. Show that you gave allopurinol 300 mg at 2000 on November 3.
2. Show that you gave 35 U of Humulin N at 0730 on November 3 in the right thigh.
3. Show that you gave digoxin at 1000 on November 4 and recorded an apical pulse (AP) of 72 before giving the drug.
4. Show that you gave ampicillin at 1600 on November 4.
5. The nurse notes that the physician ordered 80 mg of Lasix qd. How many times a day should the drug be given?
6. When preparing to administer Lasix for the above order, the nurse finds 40-mg tablets. How many should the nurse give to the client for one dose at 1000?
7. What time is 1000?

8. Digoxin 0.125 mg is ordered to be given at 1000. The tablets on hand are 0.25 mg. How many should the nurse give?
9. Humulin N is ordered to be given subq, or SC. By what route is this drug administered?
10. What time is 2400?

ANSWERS 1, 3. Place your initials in the appropriate box; also record pulse and injection site. 5. Once a day 7. 10 AM 9. subcutaneously

---

10-8. COMPUTERS AND DOCUMENTATION

Like other businesses and industries, health care facilities are becoming increasingly aware of the benefits of computers. Many hospitals have hospital-wide information systems that allow one department to communicate with another and have ready access to a large amount of information. Nursing information systems, sometimes referred to as informatics, are being developed in a few hospitals and the trend is growing.

There are a number of ways that computers are being used in nursing. One common way is the entry of physicians' orders into the system to generate computerized MARs. This process prevents transcription errors because the unit clerk or nurse does not need to read the physician's order and copy it onto the MAR. It also saves time because the data are entered once and then printed onto the appropriate forms by the computer. The MAR looks like the sample in Figure 10–14, but the medications are typed instead of handwritten.

In some hospitals, nurses are replacing flow sheets and nurses' notes forms with the computer. In a few settings, a computer terminal is at the bedside so the nurse can document as soon as the care has been provided. Other facilities are experimenting with small, hand-held terminals so that the nurse can enter data anywhere. The advantage of these systems is that the nurse does not need to waste valuable time looking for a chart or form to record information. In a hurry, many nurses grab the first piece of paper, tissue, or napkin they can find to jot down information. Some nurses write on their hands or arms to help remember what to record on the chart later. The problem with illegible handwriting is also eliminated by using bedside or hand-held terminals.

For further information about computers, see Appendix 6.

EXERCISES

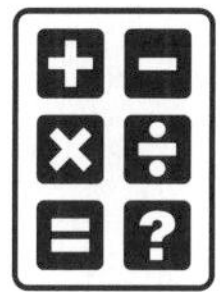

1. State two reasons why computers are beginning to be used for nursing documentation.
2. What are two advantages of bedside or hand-held terminals?

ANSWERS 1. Any two of the following: prevents errors, saves time, prevents duplication 2. Any two of the following: allows the nurse to make entries at any time, avoids the problem of illegible handwriting, saves time

---

10-9. AVOIDING ERRORS: CHECKING AND RECHECKING

When giving medications, the nurse checks and rechecks that the medication, route of administration, time of administration, and dosage of medication are correct. Before giving the medication, the nurse checks to see that the order on the MAR is the same as the physician's order.

Errors in medication administration are a major reason why nurses are sued for malpractice. Some common errors include

1. Failing to give the correct medication
2. Giving the wrong dose of a medication
3. Failing to record medications that have been given
4. Failing to discontinue a medication as ordered
5. Transcribing orders improperly or transcribing improper orders
6. Giving the medication to the wrong person

Examples

1. (Failing to record medications that have been given) An elderly client was experiencing severe surgical pain and received a potent narcotic medication. Because it was near the end of the nurse's shift, she forgot to record what she gave. The oncoming nurse decided to give the pain medication because, according to the MAR, the client had not received a dose for a long time. After the repeated dose, the client experienced respiratory failure.
2. (Transcribing improper orders) The physician ordered 5 mL of atropine for a client on a coronary care unit. He meant to write 0.5 mL, but did not write the zero. The decimal point was hard to see and was omitted on the MAR when the nurse transcribed the order. The nurse thought that this dose was too high but did not want to question a physician.

Even though the physician or clinical pharmacist writes the medication order, the nurse is also responsible for accurate medication administration.

10-10. SUMMARY

1. WHY DOCUMENT?

   Documentation, or record-keeping, is one of the most important functions of the nurse. The client's chart is a legal document that provides communication among all health care team members and serves as a record of client care given in a health care facility. Documentation is required when administering drugs and intravenous fluids.

2. INTAKE AND OUTPUT RECORD

   Intake and output records are used frequently in acute and long-term care settings. The client's fluid intake is measured and recorded and compared with output, primarily urine.

3. AVERAGES

   Sometimes the nurse must compute averages. For example, the nurse may need to determine whether the adult client is voiding at least 30 mL of urine each hour for healthy kidney functioning. The total amount of urine output is divided by the number of hours in which the output was obtained.

4. GRAPHS

Nurses sometimes use graphs for recording data over time to determine trends. For example, some hospitals require graphing of temperature, pulse, respirations, and/or blood pressure.

5. FLOW SHEETS

A popular trend in nursing documentation is the use of a variety of flow sheets. The flow sheet usually saves the nurse time, is convenient, and contains a lot of information in one, easily accessible place. Special flow sheets, such as the Glasgow Coma Scale, may also be used to assess an aspect of client functioning and assign a score.

6. THE 24-HOUR CLOCK

An alternative system for recording time is the 24-h clock. The advantage of this system is its use of numbers exclusively, rather than numbers, colon, and letters. There is also less error in reading 24-h clock time when handwriting is illegible.

7. MEDICATION ADMINISTRATION RECORD (MAR)

The MAR is the chart form used to record medications that are given to a client. The nurse initials the MAR next to each medication after it is administered.

8. COMPUTERS AND DOCUMENTATION

Some health care agencies are beginning to use computerized forms for charting. The most popular are the physicians' orders, MARs, and reports from other departments. A few hospitals are trying data input at the client's bedside or with a hand-held device.

9. AVOIDING ERRORS: CHECKING AND RECHECKING

Medication errors are one of the major reasons why nurses get sued for malpractice. The nurse checks the MAR against the physician's orders and rechecks each step of drug calculation and dosage.

EXERCISES FOR EXTRA PRACTICE

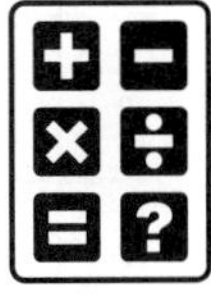

Exercises 1–5. Record the following information on the I & O sheet provided in Figure 10–15 for April 18:

1. 175 mL coffee at 6 PM
2. 30 mL water at 3:30 PM
3. 240 mL iced tea at 7 PM
4. 210 mL voided urine at 9:15 PM
5. 25 mL wound drainage at 11 PM
6. What was the total intake for the 3–11 shift using the information above?
7. What was the average hourly urine output during the 3–11 shift?
8. What was the average fluid intake per hour during the 3–11 shift?

DATE ______________

	Time	Oral Type	Oral Amount	Time	Parenteral Type & Amt	Amount Absorbed	Time	Type Tube Feeding	Rate	Amount Absorbed	Residual	Time	Irrig. Started	Used	Time	Urine	NG/ Vomitus	Chest Tubes	Drains	Other
11-7																				
Stool																Irrig.				
TOTALS																				
7-3																				
Stool																Irrig.				
TOTALS																				
3-11																				
Stool																Irrig.				
TOTALS																				
24 HR. TOTALS																				

Figure 10–15 Intake—output sheet for Exercises 1–5.

GRAPHIC CHART

Last Name	First Name	Attending Physician	Room or Ward No.	Bed	Hospital No.

Date									
Day in Hospital									
Day P.O. or P.P.									
	Hour	A.M. 4 8 12 / P.M. 4 8 12	A.M. 4 8 12 / P.M. 4 8 12	A.M. 4 8 12 / P.M. 4 8 12	A.M. 4 8 12 / P.M. 4 8 12	A.M. 4 8 12 / P.M. 4 8 12	A.M. 4 8 12 / P.M. 4 8 12	A.M. 4 8 12 / P.M. 4 8 12	A.M. 4 8 12 / P.M. 4 8 12
TEMPERATURE	106°								
	105°								
	104°								
	103°								
	102°								
	101°								
	100°								
	99° Normal								
	98°								
	97°								
	96°								
PULSE	150								
	140								
	130								
	120								
	110								
	100								
	90								
	80								
	70								
RESPIRATION	60								
	50								
	40								
	30								
	20								
	10								
Blood Pressure									
Fluid Intake									
Urine									
Defecation									
Weight									

Form 2501 BRIGGS, Des Moines, IA 50306 PRINTED IN U.S.A. **GRAPHIC CHART**

Figure 10–16 Graphic chart for Chapter Test question 4.

Exercises 9–16. Convert the following military times to ordinary time:

9. 0347
10. 1450
11. 2334
12. 2019
13. 0123
14. 1715
15. 1125
16. 1520

ANSWERS 1, 3, 5. Record the I & O as indicated in the examples found earlier in the chapter. 7. 26 mL 9. 3:47 AM 11. 11:34 PM 13. 1:23 AM 15. 11:25 AM

PAGE 1

ORIGINAL DATE ORDERED / INITIALS	DRUGS MODE DOSE INTERVAL	HOURS	DATE 11/3	DATE 11/4	DATE 11/5	DATE 11/6	DATE	DATE	DATE	DATE	DATE	DATE	DATE	DATE	STOP/DATE TIMES
11/3/92 / DI	Allopurinol 300 mg PO bid	1000 2000													
11/3/92 / DI	Ampicillin 500 mg q8h PO	0800 1600 2400													
11/3/92 / DI	Digoxin 0.125 mg PO qd	1000 AP													
11/3/92 / DI	Lasix 80 mg qd	1000													
11/3/92 / DI	Humulin-N 35 u q AM subq	0730 Site													

INITIAL	SIGNATURE

MEDICATION RECORD

MONTH YEAR		
ROOM	AGE	NAME

Figure 10–17 Medication Administration Record for Chapter Test question 7.

CHAPTER TEST

1. Ms. Ignas drinks 2 cartons (8-oz) of milk, $\frac{1}{4}$ c coffee (8-oz cup), and 50 mL of water. What was her total intake? 1. ____________
2. Susan voided 4 times during the day, producing the following amounts: 125 mL, 300 mL, 200 mL, and 150 mL. What was the average amount she voided each time? 2. ____________
3. If Susan voided the amounts above in a 24-h period, what was her average hourly urine output? 3. ____________
4. Using the graphic chart in Figure 10–16, chart the following TPR for 1600: 102.6, 88, 24. 4. ____________
5. What time is 2345? 5. ____________
6. Write 1:45 AM using 24-h clock time. 6. ____________
7. Using the MAR provided in Figure 10–17, record that you gave ampicillin at 0800 on November 3. 7. ____________

8–10. List three types of medication errors that nurses make.

8. ____________

9. ____________

10. ____________

ANSWERS 1. 590 mL 2. 193.8 mL 3. 32.3 mL 4. (see Fig. 10–18) 5. 11:45 PM 6. 0145 7. Initial the correct box.
8–10. Any three of the following: failure to give the correct drug; failure to give the correct dosage; failure to discontinue a drug as ordered; failure to record a drug as given; failure to transcribe the order correctly or transcription of an improper order

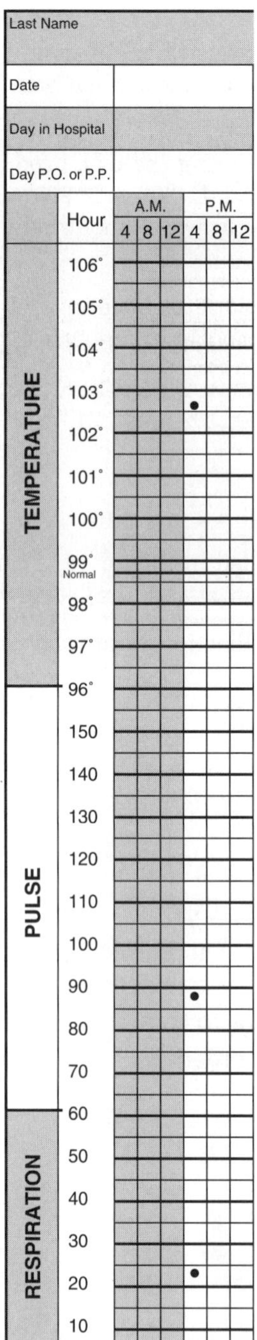

Figure 10–18 Answer to Chapter Test question 4.

APPENDIX 1
Alphabetical List of Useful Measurements

(Including commonly used approximate equivalents)

centimeter (cm) = 0.01 meter (m) = 0.4 inch (in.)
cubic centimeter (cm^3, or cc) = 1 milliliter (mL)
cup (c) = 8 fluid ounces (fl oz)
dram (ʒ) = 60 grains (gr lx) = 4 grams (g)
drop (gtt) = 0.06 milliliter (mL)
fluid dram (ʃʒ) = 60 minims (♏ lx) = 4 milliliters (mL)
fluid ounce (fl oz, ʃ℥) = 30 milliliters (mL)
= 30 cubic centimeters (cc)
= 8 fluid drams (ʃʒ viii)
foot (ft) = 12 inches (in.) = 0.3 meter (m)
gallon (gal) = 4 quarts (qt)
glassful = 1 cup = 8 fluid ounces (fl oz, ʃ℥)
= 240 milliliters (mL)
grain (gr) = 60 milligrams (mg)
gram (g) = 0.001 kilogram (kg) = 15 grains (gr xv)
hour (h, hr) = 60 minutes (min)
inch (in.) = 2.5 centimeters (cm)
kilogram (kg) = 1000 grams (g) = 2.2 pounds (lb)
kilometer (km) = 1000 meters (m) = 0.6 mile
liter (L) = 1 cubic decimeter (dm^3) = 1.1 quart (qt)
= 1 kilogram (kg)
meter (m) = 1.1 yard (yd)
microgram (μg, mcg) = 0.001 milligram (mg)
mile = 1.6 kilometer (km)
milliequivalent (mEq) = 0.001 equivalent (Eq)
milligram (mg) = 0.001 gram (g)
milliliter (mL) = 0.001 liter (L) = 15 minims (♏ xv)
millimeter = 0.001 meter (mm)
millimole = 0.001 mole (mmol)
minim (♏) = 0.06 milliliter (mL)
minute (min) = 60 seconds (s, sec)
ounce (oz) = 30 grams (g) = 8 drams (ʒ viii)
pint (pt) = 16 fluid ounces = 2 cups = 500 milliliters (mL)
pound (lb, avoirdupois) = 16 ounces (oz) = 450 grams (g)
= 0.45 kilogram (kg)
quart (qt) = 2 pints (pt) = 0.9 liter (L)
tablespoon (tbsp) = 15 milliliters (mL)
teaspoon (tsp) = 5 milliliters (mL)
yard (yd) = 3 feet (ft) = 0.9 meter (m)
$yard^2$ (square yard) = 0.8 square meter (m^2)

APPENDIX 2
International System (SI) of Units

A. PRIMARY MEASURES

Length: meter (m)
Area: square meter (m^2)
Volume: cubic meter (m^3)
Mass (Weight): gram (g)
Amount of substance: mole (mol)

B. PREFIXES

(Used as multiplication factors with primary measures given above)

Name	Symbol	Multiplication Factor
giga	G	1,000,000,000
mega	M	1,000,000
kilo	k	1000
hecto	h	100
deka	da	10
deci	d	0.1
centi	c	0.01
milli	m	0.001
micro	μ	0.000001
nano	n	0.000000001
pico	p	0.000000000001

APPENDIX 3
Apothecaries' System

A. WEIGHT

Basic unit: the grain (gr)
60 grains (gr) = 1 dram (ʒ)
8 drams (ʒ) = 1 ounce (oz, ℥)
12 ounces (oz) = 1 pound (lb)

FLUID CAPACITY

Basic unit: the minim (♏)
60 minims (♏) = 1 fluid dram (ʃʒ)
8 fluid drams (ʃʒ) = 1 fluid ounce (ʃ℥)
16 fluid ounces (ʃ℥) = 1 pint (pt, O)
2 pints (pt) = 1 quart (qt)
4 quarts (qt) = 1 gallon (gal, C)

B. ILLUSTRATIVE SYMBOLS AND COMMON CONVERSIONS TO METRIC MEASURES

Symbol	Apothecaries' Measure	Approximate Metric Equivalent
Weight		
gr $\frac{1}{150}$	$\frac{1}{150}$ grain	0.4 milligram
gr $\frac{1}{4}$	$\frac{1}{4}$ grain	15 milligrams
gr ss	$\frac{1}{2}$ grain	30 milligrams
gr i	1 grain	60 milligrams
gr iss	$1\frac{1}{2}$ grain	100 milligrams
gr ii	2 grains	120 milligrams
gr v	5 grains	300 milligrams
gr xv	15 grains	1000 milligrams (1 g)
ʒ i	1 dram	4 grams
℥ i	1 ounce	30 grams
Liquid Capacity		
♏ i	1 minim	0.06 milliliter
ʃʒ i	1 fluid dram	4 milliliters
ʃ℥ i	1 fluid ounce	30 milliliters

APPENDIX 4
Roman Numerals

Hindu-Arabic	Roman	Hindu-Arabic	Roman
1	i	50	l
2	ii	60	lx
3	iii	70	lxx
4	iv	80	lxxx
5	v	90	xc
6	vi	99	xcix
7	vii	100	c
8	viii	150	cl
9	ix	200	cc
10	x	300	ccc
11	xi	400	cd
12	xii	500	d
13	xiii	600	dc
14	xiv	700	dcc
15	xv	800	dccc
16	xvi	900	cm
17	xvii	1000	m
18	xviii	1111	mcxi
19	xix	1500	md
20	xx	2000	mm
29	xxix	10,000	$\overline{x}$
30	xxx	20,000	$\overline{xx}$
40	xl	100,000	$\overline{c}$

APPENDIX 5
How to Deal with Math Anxiety

Math Anxiety: The Symptoms

Math anxiety is that uncomfortable feeling of tension (sometimes even panic) associated with mathematical activities. It stems from a history of old difficulties with math, and can cause new and continued difficulties. Because math education is cumulative, students who miss some basic concepts (for reasons such as illness, inadequate teaching, a move from one school to another, or simply boredom and lack of motivation) find it hard to catch up and suffer a great loss of self-confidence. Women may be troubled by a subconscious fear that math is for men only.

Fear of exhibiting naked incompetence in public causes tension in the classroom, panic during tests, and hatred of assignments. Relatively easy problems suddenly appear to be totally unfamiliar and impossible to solve; problems that are obviously familiar cannot be solved because of mental blocks; juxtaposition of several numbers causes indigestion; and simple operations cause confusion: "Should I multiply or divide?"

The Cure

Is there a cure for this malady? Is it possible to alleviate math anxiety, promote learning, and build self-confidence? For each person, the remedy may be different. To determine your own personal path to a cure for math anxiety, answer the following questions:

1. Are you aware of your own symptoms of math anxiety?
2. Is concentration easy?
3. Do you have an organized way of studying math?
4. Do you use discussion with others and self-talk to strengthen your math power?
5. Do you have techniques for increasing your memory power?
6. Do you have techniques for efficient learning of math?

For each negative response to the questions above, see the following list for related suggestions.

Recommendations

1. Are you aware of your own symptoms of math anxiety?
   (a) Write out your personal math history to pinpoint the causes of your lack of self-confidence.
   (b) Make notes of your negative physical or mental reactions to mathematical activities as you notice them. Greater insight and awareness can help you to gain control over these automatic reactions. Use relaxation techniques and positive thinking to diminish their effect.

2. Is concentration easy?
   (a) Blot out pessimistic thoughts with images of past and future achievement and return to the math.
   (b) Counter feelings of annoyance and impatience with images of future satisfaction to be gained by completing math requirements and making progress towards your goals. Look for present satisfaction in the math itself: find your own patterns and illustrations to help you learn, and watch for useful connections to your other interests. You may become intrigued.
   (c) Consciously postpone extraneous thoughts for another specified time if you cannot eliminate them altogether.
   (d) Use breaks to minimize tension—stretch, exercise, briefly carry out some other activity.
3. Do you have an organized way of studying math?
   (a) Select a quiet spot and a time of day that you have found best for math and adhere to these as much as possible.
   (b) Plan reasonable goals for the amount to be done each day, adhere to the plan, and give yourself rewards.
   (c) Be prepared with lots of scrap paper; write clearly. Allow plenty of space.
   (d) Keep appropriate reference materials at hand.
   (e) Prepare ahead for exams—don't cram!
   (f) Keep records of your progress.
4. Do you use discussion with others and self-talk to strengthen your math power?
   (a) Find congenial classmates and colleagues with whom to discuss math concepts and problems and to discuss the math anxiety that you feel.
   (b) Don't be shy about asking questions and searching for understanding. Make notes with questions for colleagues, instructors, or classmates.
   (c) Be generous in explaining topics you know. When you give an explanation, you increase your own insight and skill.
   (d) Talk to yourself! When working alone, discuss possible solutions with yourself and justify your methods as if you were your own teacher, or a member of a committee.
   (e) Always ask yourself "Is this answer reasonable?" "Does this answer make sense?" Always tabulate, estimate, compute, and check. (TECC!)
   (f) Write to the author of your textbook through the publisher. Enclose a stamped, self-addressed envelope for a reply. To write to the authors of this text, address your questions directly to

       Dr. Sally I. Lipsey
       P.O. Box 207
       Lake Peekskill, NY 10537
5. Do you have techniques for increasing your memory power?
   (a) Make a special effort to remember easy diagrams or pictures that act as reminders of concepts and methods. Use the ones in the text or make up your own.

Examples:

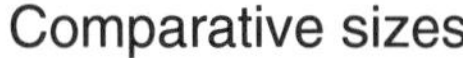

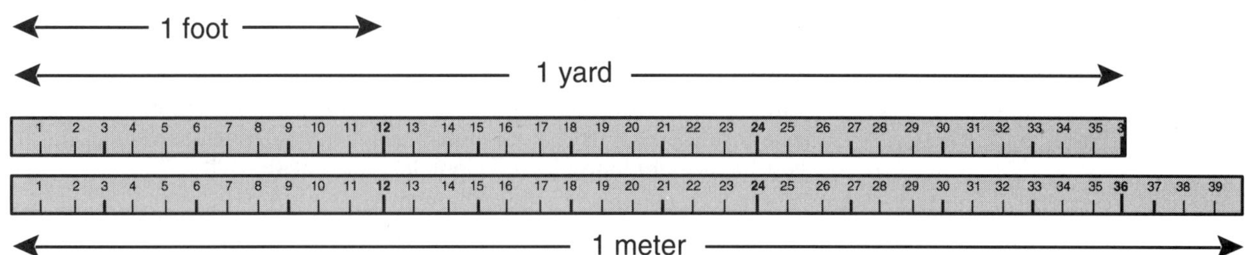

Approximate Thumb Measurements

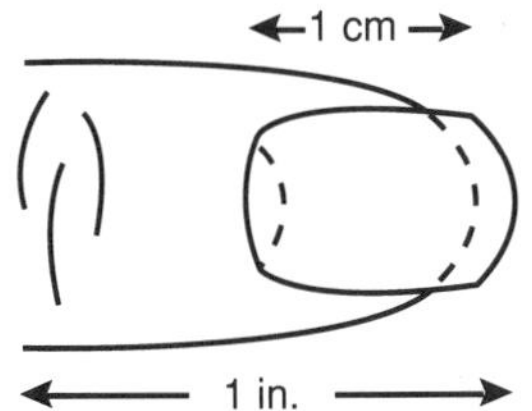

1 liter

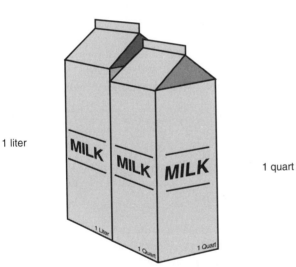

1 quart

(b) Use suggested symbolic devices and make up your own.

Examples:

(i) <eft is <ess
(ii) L C D for sum of fractions
C hange to equivalent fractions
D on't lose the Denominator

(c) Use suggested patterns and look for your own.

Example:

x grams in 10 mL (Desired)
2 grams in 100 mL (Have)

$$\frac{x}{2} = \frac{10}{100}$$

(Students who do not pay attention to patterns make errors, such as $\frac{x}{2} = \frac{100}{10}$.)

(d) Do not depend totally on memory. It is wise to make the best possible use of memory, but as we inevitably find out, memorization is not enough. Many times, we must use our knowledge to figure out something for which memorized rules do not immediately apply. Also, when we are tense, our brains block out just those memories we hoped would substitute for real understanding.

6. Do you have techniques for efficient learning of math?

(a) Refer to a concrete model wherever possible.

Examples: A ruler for fractions, money for decimals, thermometers for comparison of Fahrenheit and Celsius scales.

(b) Use diagrams wherever possible.

Example: How many pieces of tape of length $\frac{3}{4}$ in. can be made from a tape of length 3 in.?

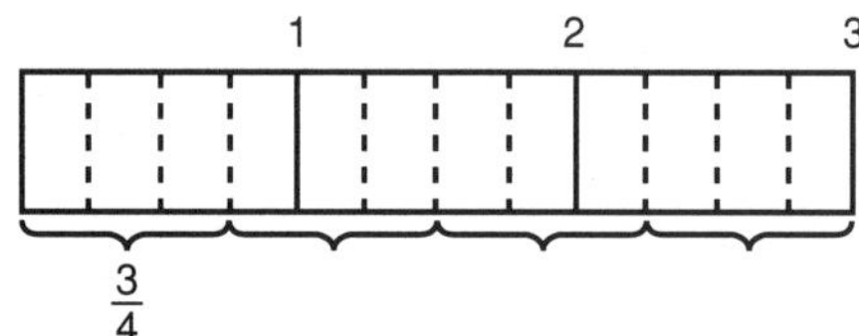

(c) If a problem is confusing, replace the given numbers with simpler numbers.

Examples:

(i) "Convert 0.342 m to centimeters" may be changed to "Convert 1 m to centimeters." Then 1 m = 100 cm reminds us to multiply by 100 for this conversion.
Result: 0.342 m = 34.2 cm

(ii) Change "How many 3.8-mL doses can be poured from 22.8 mL of solution?" to "How many 4-mL doses can be poured from 20 mL?" or "How many 4-oz glasses of orange juice can be poured from 20 oz?) Then it is easy to see that division solves the problem, and it is simple now to estimate the result.
Estimate: $20 \div 4 = 5$ doses
Result: $22.8 \div 3.8 = 6$ doses
Check: $3.8 \times 6 = 22.8$

(d) Enjoy the fact that there are alternative approaches to every problem and choose the one you like the best.

Example:

How many 3.8-mL doses can be made from 22.8 mL of solution?

(i) See easy approach given above.

(ii) Alternative approach:
x doses from 22.8 mL (Desired)
1 dose from 3.8 mL (Have)

$$\frac{x}{1} = \frac{22.8}{3.8} = 6$$

(iii) Alternative approach:

If: 3.8 mL for 1 dose

And: 22.8 mL for x doses

Then: $$\frac{3.8}{22.8} = \frac{1}{x}$$

Cross-multiplying: $3.8\ x = 22.8$

Dividing: $x = 6$

We need to change math anxiety to math power! We **can** change math anxiety to math power by learning how to relax more and yet concentrate better and by learning how to get more satisfaction from both the processes and the results. Then we can enjoy both the beauty and the utility of mathematics.

APPENDIX 6
Basic Aspects of Computers

In the hospital of the future, there will be a computer at each bedside, and nurses will use it routinely. Today most hospitals have computers, but in some cases, they are used only for bookkeeping and specialized medical purposes. Where computers are placed at nurses' stations, many nurses are readily using them for nursing care plans and medical records of clients. Nurses are "designing, developing, and implementing nursing information systems. They are using computers to provide documentation needed for their timely reports and to assist them in providing safe quality care at a reasonable cost."*

The computer, which performs many tasks in addition to computing, is helpful to the nurse in a number of important ways: monitoring, storage and retrieval, calculations and analyses, word processing and communication.

Monitoring Systems

Nurses in intensive care areas or in some other types of nursing units may set computers to ring various types of alarms to alert staff to conditions ranging from slightly abnormal to serious emergency.

Storage and Retrieval

The computer has the capacity to store large amounts of reference material and data in a relatively small space. Computers can hold summaries of information about different diseases, drugs, or diets which can be displayed or printed out when needed. Interdepartmental or interinstitutional information about patients (such as history, medical and nursing interventions, or special diet) may be entered regularly and retrieved easily. This is important in the care of each individual patient and also in the collection of data for nursing research. These uses of the computer are helpful in freeing the nurse for higher priority activities. The uses for the computer are not unlimited, however, because it is difficult to enter all the information needed. For one thing, inputting such data may require too much time, and in some areas of health care, the basic knowledge does not exist.

---

* Saba V and McCormick KA: *Essentials of Computers for Nurses.* Philadelphia: Lippincott; 1986:19.

Calculations and Analyses

The computer also acts as a very fast calculator. It may be programmed to determine quantities such as dosages and IV drip rates. It may also be programmed for analysis of results of diagnostic measures. In the case of electroencephalograms, for instance, computerized analysis can "detect subtle changes in brain activity that are virtually impossible to see in conventional EEG records. Moreover, although the computer cannot diagnose the patient's condition, it can compare a patient's brain activity with other normal or pathological EEGs. . . . "* Computer time is also well spent on the preparation of budgets. Fast, efficient calculations expedite decisions; one may also try out different possible allocations of funds and project the results in each case. For statistical analyses of any large sets of data that are much too time-consuming for any single researcher, the computer is ideal.

Word Processing and Communication

A word processing program may be used to turn the computer into a luxury typewriter. One may, with great efficiency, write, revise, print, and store a great variety of information, including nursing plans, reports, and letters. Communications may be sent from computer to computer whether located in the same building or further apart.

Although some nurses may not yet have access to a computer, everyone should have enough information about the nature of the computer to understand not only the tasks computers can perform but also their limitations. As much as possible, nurses should receive hands-on experience with computers.† Such experience provides familiarity with the two basic aspects of computers: the physical components of the system (hardware) and the programs for operating the computer and processing data (software).

Computer Hardware

Essentially, computer hardware consists of an input unit, a central processing unit, an auxiliary memory unit, and an output unit. The central processing unit (CPU, or processor) contains devices for control of operations, for performance of arithmetic and logic, and for primary storage.

INPUT UNIT (OR TERMINAL) — facilitates entry of data or instructions. Usually it looks like a keyboard of a typewriter with some extra keys. As we type, ordinary language is converted into machine language (a numerical code) and transmitted into a memory device. We see the typed entries by looking at an attached video display terminal (VDT), or cathode ray terminal (CRT). In some cases, we make entries via the screen by means of a pointer (mouse).

CONTROL UNIT — determines the sequence of steps in computer procedures, by connecting and disconnecting circuits in the order needed to carry out a given assignment.

ARITHMETIC AND LOGIC UNIT — carries out addition, subtraction, multiplication, and division, and compares magnitudes. For instance, given data from a patient's blood test, it can (a) use division and subtraction in a formula to calculate the amount of LDL cholesterol in the blood, and (b) use logic to

* Coburn KL, Sullivan CH, and Hundley J: High-tech maps of the brain. *Am J Nurs.* 1988;88(11):1500.

† Nursing students who have practice using computers will feel comfortable with computerized exams (such as State Board Exams) and computer-assisted instruction.

determine whether the result is less than, equal to, or greater than a normal value.

PRIMARY STORAGE UNIT (OR MAIN MEMORY) — stores data and instructions for processing data. These materials are stored by means of electronic circuits etched on silicon chips.

AUXILIARY STORAGE UNIT — stores additional data or instructions in portable devices, such as magnetic tape or disks of various types, which may be connected to the computer. Magnetic tape is plastic ribbon that can be magnetized; disks, hard or floppy, come in different sizes and are like stereo records. These storage devices can be erased easily and reused.

OUTPUT UNIT — delivers material requested such as results of calculations, graphs, charts, or reprints of information. This unit may be a VDT or CRT screen, a printer, magnetic tape, or disks.

Computer Software

Whereas hardware comprises the physical media for data storage and processing, software is sets of instructions for running the machinery and processing the data. A set of instructions is called a computer program.

PROGRAM — detailed instructions for the computer, written in a programming language by a programmer. A programming language is a code that can be "understood" by the machine and translated into electronic responses. The programmer may choose from any of a number of possible languages (BASIC, Fortran, Cobol, PL1, etc.), depending on both the computer and the programmer's goals. Programs can be custom-made or purchased from software companies.

Considerations in Choosing a Computer System

Many hospitals already have terminals at the nurses' station, from which files, such as the hospital information system, the nursing information system, and client records, can be retrieved. A small number of hospitals have bedside computer charting systems, called POC (point-of-care) systems, that enable nurses and physicians to record information only once rather than on a number of different charts. Different health care workers can review the chart at any time, even simultaneously, at different terminals. Point-of-care systems may provide such advantages as automatic transfer of information from one file to another; automatic entry of information from medical appliances; the highlighting of selected data; linkage to the computer at the nurses' station, the lab, and the pharmacy; and a drug calculator.*

Some health-care professionals advocate hand-held computers over bedside terminals. Although bedside terminals have eliminated some of the problems associated with traditional paper charts, they are costly and are not always dependable.†

An effective computer system needs to have many advantages over traditional print systems. Questions to ask in evaluating a computer system include the following:

---

* Meyer C: Bedside computer charting: inching toward tomorrow. *Am J Nurs.* 1992;92(4):38–42.

† Meintz S and Shaha S: Our hand-held computer beats them all. *RN* 1992;55(1):52–57.

1. Is it cost-effective?
2. Does it conform to the needs of our hospital, or can it easily be made to do so?
3. Can it communicate with other agencies at the hospital?
4. Is it fast, easy, and comfortable to use?
5. How much training is necessary?
6. Does it save time over traditional methods?
7. Is it dependable?

Prices are falling, computer systems are improving, and pressure is rising to conform with government and insurance requirements and nursing needs. There will be a steady increase in the use of computers by the health care profession. At the same time, the installation of a computer system in a hospital will inspire changes in nursing practice, especially documentation.*

SUGGESTED EXPLORATIONS

1. On visits to different hospitals, ask for permission to see various samples of computer output wherever computers are used. Note who makes use of computers and how.
2. Evaluate the computer system in at least one hospital by answering the following questions:
   (a) How is it cost-effective?
   (b) Does it conform to the needs of the hospital?
   (c) Does it communicate with other agencies at the hospital? Which ones?
   (d) Is it fast, easy, and comfortable to use?
   (e) How much training is necessary?
   (f) How is time saved over traditional methods?
   (g) Is it dependable? Does it ever break down, or make it difficult to retrieve needed data?
3. Visit different computer stores to inquire about systems recommended for nursing applications. Ask for demonstrations and literature.
4. Attend a computer class in computer literacy and word processing, or take lessons from the computer laboratory at your institution or in the neighborhood library.

* Ibid:41

SELECTED REFERENCES

American Society of Hospital Pharmacists: *American Hospital Formulary Service Drug Information.* Bethesda, MD: American Society of Hospital Pharmacists, 1991.

Coburn K. et al: High-tech maps of the brain. *Am J Nurs.* 1988;88(11):1500.

Cohen MR: *200 Medication Errors and How to Avoid Them.* Springhouse, PA: Springhouse, 1991.

Deglin J and Vallerand AH: *Davis's Drug Guide for Nurses.* 3rd ed. Philadelphia: Davis, 1992.

Gilman A, et al: *Goodman and Gilman's Pharmacological Basis of Therapeutics.* 8th ed. New York: Pergamon, 1990.

Hodgson BB et al.: *Nurse's Drug Handbook.* Philadelphia: WB Saunders, 1993.

Ignatavicius D and Bayne M: *Medical Surgical Nursing, a Nursing Process Approach.* Philadelphia: WB Saunders, 1991.

Institute of Electrical and Electronic Engineers: *American National Standard Metric Practice.* New York: Institute of Electrical and Electronic Engineers, 1982.

Knapp-Spooner C and Brett J: Less is more: A med/surg flow sheet. *RN* 1992;55(3):36–39.

Kogelman S and Warren J: *Mind Over Math.* New York: McGraw-Hill, 1979.

Loebl S and Spratto G: *The Nurse's Drug Handbook.* 5th ed. New York: Delmar, 1989.

Medical Economics: *Physicians' Desk Reference.* 46th ed. Montvale, NJ: Medical Economics, 1992.

Meintz S and Shaha S: Our hand-held computer beats them all. *RN* 1992;55(1):52–57.

Meyer C: Bedside computer charting: Inching toward tomorrow. *Am J Nurs.* 1992;92(4):38–44.

Mikuleky MP and Ledford C: *Computers in Nursing: Hospital and Clinical Applications.* Menlo Park, CA: Addison-Wesley, 1987.

Springhouse: *Nursing '92 Drug Handbook.* Springhouse, PA: 1991.

Saba V and McCormick K: *Essentials of Computers for Nurses.* Philadelphia: Lippincott, 1986.

Saba V et al., eds.: *Nursing and Computers: An Anthology.* New York: Springer-Verlag, 1989.

Saxton DF et al., eds.: *Mosby's Comprehensive Review of Nursing.* 13th ed. St. Louis: Mosby, 1989.

Tobias S: *Overcoming Math Anxiety.* Boston: Norton, 1980.

U.S. Pharmacopeial Convention: *United States Pharmacopeia, 22 rev. National Formulary.* 17th ed. Rockville, MD: U.S. Pharmacopeial Convention, 1989.

U.S. Pharmacopeial Convention: *United States Pharmacopeia Dispensing Information.* 12th ed. Rockville, MD: U.S. Pharmacopeial Convention, 1992.

Weinstein, S: Math calculations for intravenous nurses. JIN 1990;13(4):231–236.

INDEX

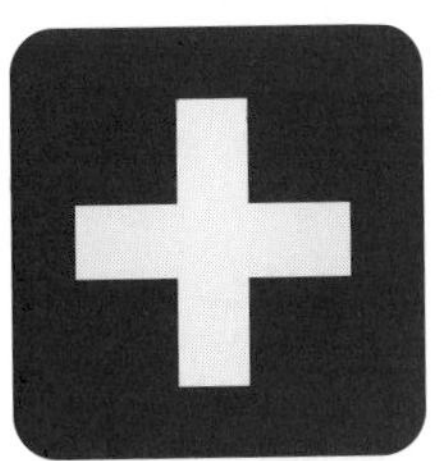

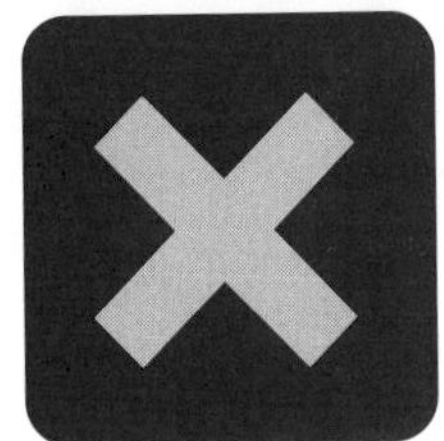
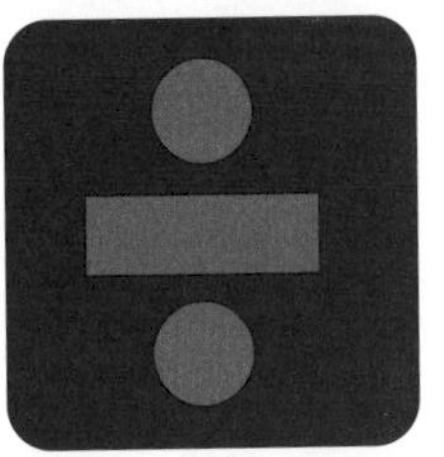

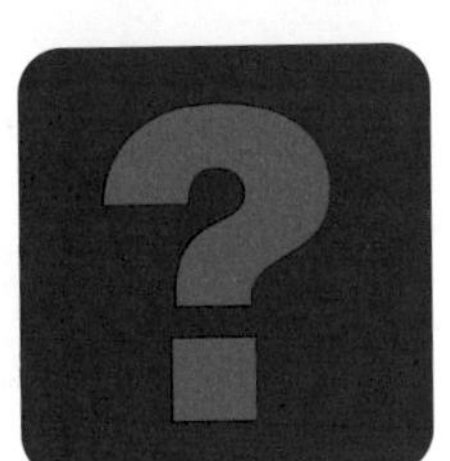

Note: Page numbers in *italics* refer to illustrations.

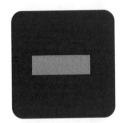

E

F

G

H

I

K

L

M